T0271905

Statistical Methods in Health Disparity Research

A health disparity refers to a higher burden of illness, injury, disability, or mortality experienced by one group relative to others attributable to multiple factors including socioeconomic status, environmental factors, insufficient access to health care, individual risk factors, and behaviors and inequalities in education. These disparities may be due to many factors including age, income, and race. ***Statistical Methods in Health Disparity Research*** will focus on their estimation, ranging from classical approaches including the quantification of a disparity, to more formal modeling, to modern approaches involving more flexible computational approaches.

Features:

- Presents an overview of methods and applications of health disparity estimation
- First book to synthesize research in this field in a unified statistical framework
- Covers classical approaches, and builds to more modern computational techniques
- Includes many worked examples and case studies using real data
- Discusses available software for estimation

The book is designed primarily for researchers and graduate students in biostatistics, data science, and computer science. It will also be useful to many quantitative modelers in genetics, biology, sociology, and epidemiology.

J. Sunil Rao, Ph.D. is Professor of Biostatistics in the School of Public Health at the University of Minnesota, Twin Cities and Founding Director Emeritus in the Division of Biostatistics at the Miller School of Medicine, University of Miami.

He has published widely about methods for complex data modeling including high dimensional model selection, mixed model prediction, small area estimation, and bump hunting machine learning, as well as statistical methods for applied cancer biostatistics.

He is a Fellow of the American Statistical Association and an elected member of the International Statistical Institute.

Chapman & Hall/CRC Biostatistics Series

Recently Published Titles

Model-Assisted Bayesian Designs for Dose Finding and Optimization
Methods and Applications
Ying Yuan, Ruitao Lin and J. Jack Lee

Digital Therapeutics: Strategic, Scientific, Developmental, and Regulatory Aspects
Oleksandr Sverdlov, Joris van Dam

Quantitative Methods for Precision Medicine
Pharmacogenomics in Action
Rongling Wu

Drug Development for Rare Diseases
Edited by Bo Yang, Yang Song and Yijie Zhou

Case Studies in Bayesian Methods for Biopharmaceutical CMC
Edited by Paul Faya and Tony Pourmohamad

Statistical Analytics for Health Data Science with SAS and R
Jeffrey Wilson, Ding-Geng Chen and Karl E. Peace

Design and Analysis of Pragmatic Trials
Song Zhang, Chul Ahn and Hong Zhu

ROC Analysis for Classification and Prediction in Practice
Christos Nakas, Leonidas Bantis and Constantine Gatsonis

Controlled Epidemiological Studies
Marie Reilly

Statistical Methods in Health Disparity Research
J. Sunil Rao, Ph.D.

For more information about this series, please visit: https://www.routledge.com/Chapman--Hall-CRC-Biostatistics-Series/book-series/CHBIOSTATIS

Statistical Methods in Health Disparity Research

J. Sunil Rao, Ph.D.

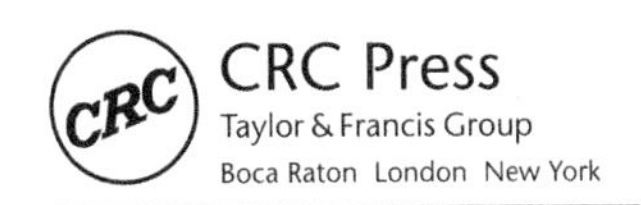

CRC Press is an imprint of the
Taylor & Francis Group, an **informa** business
A CHAPMAN & HALL BOOK

Designed cover image by Sau Ping Choi

First edition published 2023
by CRC Press
6000 Broken Sound Parkway NW, Suite 300, Boca Raton, FL 33487-2742

and by CRC Press
4 Park Square, Milton Park, Abingdon, Oxon, OX14 4RN

CRC Press is an imprint of Taylor & Francis Group, LLC

Library of Congress Cataloging-in-Publication Data

Names: Rao, J. Sunil, author.
Title: Statistical methods in health disparity research / J. Sunil Rao.
Description: First edition. | Boca Raton : CRC Press, 2023. | Series: Chapman & Hall/CRC biostatistics series | Includes bibliographical references and index.
Identifiers: LCCN 2022061985 (print) | LCCN 2022061986 (ebook) | ISBN 9780367635121 (hardback) | ISBN 9780367635169 (paperback) | ISBN 9781003119449 (ebook)
Subjects: LCSH: Health status indicators. | Health services accessibility--Research--Statistical methods. | Health surveys--Methodology.
Classification: LCC RA408.5 .R36 2023 (print) | LCC RA408.5 (ebook) | DDC 362.1072/3--dc23/eng/20230407
LC record available at https://lccn.loc.gov/2022061985
LC ebook record available at https://lccn.loc.gov/2022061986

ISBN: 978-0-367-63512-1 (hbk)
ISBN: 978-0-367-63516-9 (pbk)
ISBN: 978-1-003-11944-9 (ebk)

DOI: 10.1201/9781003119449

Typeset in LM Roman
by KnowledgeWorks Global Ltd.

Publisher's note: This book has been prepared from camera-ready copy provided by the authors.

To my wife, Darlene, and my children, Nalini and Dev

Contents

Foreword

Twenty years after the Institute of Medicine's landmark report, Unequal Treatment, was published, striking health disparities continue to be pervasive. The intractability of health disparities was on full display early in the COVID pandemic when marginalized and minoritized groups across the world experienced a greater burden of disease and excess deaths. Although these inequities was acute, they reflect long-standing disparities in health that many communities, clinicians, public health practitioners, and researchers have striven to address, often with too few resources, incomplete or inaccurate data, and lack of rigorous, tailored methods.

The spotlight on health inequities during the pandemic and the concurrent heightened awareness of structural racism and broader racial injustices have provided unique opportunities to make progress towards reducing and eliminating health disparities. Leveraging these opportunities will require innovative approaches to collecting, managing, and analyzing data using an equity lens. For example, the importance of key demographic data and social and structural determinants of health data to understanding health disparities cannot be overstated. Unfortunately, early in the pandemic, race and ethnicity were missing in data reported by the CDC in nearly half of COVID cases and a quarter of deaths. Without accurate sociodemographic information, data cannot be disaggregated to precisely identify disparities or implement more precise strategies to mitigate disparities. At Vanderbilt University Medical Center, we have prioritized the creation of dashboards that can be filtered by race, ethnicity, preferred language, and ZIP Code, which can be linked to community-level socioeconomic data and social vulnerability indices. This strategy has been vital to our population health and precision medicine efforts and enables innovative strategies to address health inequities.

Progress towards more impactful health disparities research has been hampered by disciplinary siloes and methods that cannot be applied broadly. Ideally, disparities research teams are transdisciplinary with researchers working collaboratively to decipher and eliminate health disparities through a deeper mechanistic understanding and broader incorporation of multifaceted scientific approaches and data analysis. Health disparities research requires a cadre of researchers from different backgrounds who can apply rigorous research methods with an equity lens across different disciplines. To enable transformative approaches to health disparities research, we must identify and disseminate tools and methods that transcend any single disease area or population.

This book, written by J. Sunil Rao, represents the first comprehensive reference on the statistical methods and theory for health disparity estimation and, as such, fills a vital gap as part of a roadmap to guide health disparities research. Fundamental health disparity concepts are presented including social and structural determinants of health and structural racism, which are often missing or insufficiently covered in reference books on general statistical methods. The emphasis on more precise and data-driven methodology integral to health disparities research will increasingly rely on complex data structures including clinical, social, environmental, and genomics data. The book brings together types of analyses (e.g., multilevel or survey-based or causal inference), which are often used in disciplinary or disease-specific silos. This book will be a valuable resource for faculty, students, and trainees to learn specific statistical methods in health disparities research and is a timely contribution.

Dr. Rao's book brings attention to a neglected area of health disparities research and will enhance measurement and improve investigative methods. I applaud Dr. Rao for this important service to the field and his stalwart commitment to eliminating health disparities and diversifying the scientific workforce.

Consuelo H. Wilkins, MD, MSCI
Senior Associate Dean and Senior Vice President, Health Equity
Professor of Medicine
Vanderbilt University School of Medicine

Preface

Healthy People 2020 defines a health disparity as a particular type of health difference that is closely linked with social, economic, and/or environmental disadvantage. Health disparities adversely affect groups of people who have systematically experienced greater obstacles to health based on their: racial or ethnic group; religion; socioeconomic status; gender; age; mental health; cognitive, sensory, or physical disability; sexual orientation or gender identity; geographic location; or other characteristics historically linked to discrimination or exclusion.

Over the years, efforts to eliminate disparities and achieve health equity have focused primarily on diseases or illnesses and on health care services. However, the absence of disease does not automatically equate to good health.

Powerful, complex relationships exist between health and biology, genetics, and individual behavior, and between health and health services, socioeconomic status, the physical environment, discrimination, racism, literacy levels, and legislative policies. These factors, which influence an individual's or population's health, are known as determinants of health.

Health disparities matter because they indicate a type of social injustice in society and thus fuse with basic human rights. They are useful for assessing the health status of groups of individuals and thus their estimation is of direct interest. However, while disparities may be apparently isolated to certain members of society, they ultimately affect everyone. For instance, reducing the rate of health disparities in one region of a city is a public good that will benefit individuals everywhere because it can limit overall gains in things like quality of care and health for the broader population.

Knowing why and how some populations suffer disproportionate health disparities and what role the environment, safe housing, race, ethnicity, education, socioeconomic status, and access play in that suffering can prepare us to begin to alleviate such hardships. Here is where the ever-growing tsunami of data that society is generating can be mined. Understanding evolving patterns of disparity can serve as red flags of ongoing inequities but data can also be used to focus on evidence-based interventions meant to reduce disparities in a population. Thus there is a strong need for a research resource that brings together statistical methods for health disparity research. Surprisingly, such a resource does not yet exist. This book aims to fill this troubling gap.

The main aim of this book is to provide a comprehensive account of the statistical methods and theory for health disparity estimation. A unique feature of the discussion is the focus on data and measurement ranging from experimental to observational to complex surveys. The distinction between these has to do with sampling designs employed, and the usage of appropriate methods must originate from here.

Chapter 1 introduces some basic terminology related to health disparities and presents some important applications as motivating examples. Chapter 2 focuses on the overall estimation of health disparities using non-model based indices, model-based approaches including linear, generalized linear, and survival models as well as multi-level modeling, generalized estimating equations, and fully Bayesian approaches. Chapter 3 re-orients the reader's attention to domain-specific disparity estimates where a domain can be a subpopulation defined by geography, socio-economic status, or other variables. Interest in reliable estimates of disparity from smaller and smaller domains has continued to increase as these can have important implications for the allocation of government funds and in regional planning. In Chapter 3, the bulk of the discussion revolves around traditional and robust small area estimation (Rao and Molina 2015; Jiang and Rao 2021). Chapter 4 discusses moderation and mediation – two concepts in causal inference which have particular relevance in health disparity estimation. Given a growing appreciation for the roles of multilevel determinants of disease including biological, social, and environmental determinants of health, understanding how these determine the mechanisms that underly disparities is of importance because then potential avenues for disparity mitigation and prevention can be implemented.

Chapter 5 switches gears quite dramatically and the focus turns to machine learning approaches to health disparity estimation, driven primarily by the tremendous growth of methods developed in the last two decades, accompanied by the ever-increasing size of datasets and improved computational power. Machine learning methods can allow for the relaxation of traditional modeling assumptions and bring forward an avalanche of new flexible or algorithmic-based approaches which are seeing broader and broader utilization in the health disparities research community. Chapter 5 spends time fleshing out some of these methods including their underlying theoretical motivation and optimality where appropriate, from tree-based methods and random forests to shrinkage methods to deep learning, and then illustrates their usage through a number of real-world applications.

Chapter 6 continues to drill down into the modern side of health disparities research, discussing the role of precision medicine-based thinking and how this might improve or enhance health disparity estimation. This paradigm may or may not employ machine learning approaches but can be thought of more as precision public health to reinforce the focus on health disparity being more "local" populations. Topics of interest are tree-based moderation methods, disparity subtyping, and classified mixed model prediction (CMMP)

Chapter 7 ends off with some miscellaneous topics which cannot easily be lumped into other chapters. These include prevalence estimation from biased samples, geocoding, disparity estimation with differentially privatized datasets, and a short discussion around health disparity estimation software.

Throughout the text, I discuss the advantages and limitations of the different methods and also emphasize the need for proper validation of findings including the use of cross-validation, sample splitting, and comparisons of estimates derived from a model with reliable external sources. Mathematical theorems and proofs are given as necessary, but lengthy details are omitted, and the reader is referred to relevant papers instead. This text does, however, provide some detailed discussion of direct estimation (Chapter 2), linear mixed models (Chapter 2), Bayesian estimation (Chapter 2), robust small area estimation (Chapter 3), and the more popular machine learning approaches (Chapter 5). However, complete treatment of these topics often results in each chapter being expanded significantly. Readers are referred to specific references for broader accounts of these topics. The focus here is to introduce these ideas and show how they are being used in health disparity research. Some prior exposure to standard courses in linear models and mathematical statistics would be helpful, as would a basic course in survey sampling, but it is not essential.

This book is intended to be first and foremost a research monograph, but it could also serve as a suitable text for a graduate course on health disparity estimation methods. In fact, if split carefully, the book could be used as a resource for students from (bio)statistics, epidemiology, and the social sciences. The first four chapters, say, could be an entirely appropriate introduction to statistical methods in health disparity research for students with less advanced quantitative backgrounds, and the inclusion of the remaining chapters would appeal to graduate students with more statistics and computing in their backgrounds. Practitioners interested in statistical methods for health disparity research may also find portions of the text useful, particularly Chapters 2, 3, 4, and 5, as well as the applications used throughout the book.

I would like to recognize Dean Henri Ford, who graciously approved a six month sabbatical so that I could begin work on this book, and my colleagues in the Division of Biostatistics and the Department of Public Health Sciences at the University of Miami, who have been a constant source of support and inspiration. I have important external collaborators that I would like to thank including Melinda Aldrich, Consuelo Wilkins, Ana Palacio, Nancy Cox, and Lea Davis for engaging in very enlightening conversations around a number of topics connected to health disparities. Much of my material was honed by our collective interactions as part of the NIH Center of Excellence on Precision Medicine and Health Disparities between 2015 and 2020. I would like to also extend my gratitude to Ping Choi for her artistic creativity in connecting together many underlying ideas in the design of the book cover image that truly brings the title to life. As any faculty advisor would agree, I'm extremely thankful for having a wonderful group of Ph.D. students over the years who may not fully appreciate how much I have learned from them as they matured into independent researchers of their own. I'm also grateful to Jiming Jiang and Hemant Ishwaran for our many years of close collaboration on various problems related to mixed models, small area estimation and high dimensional shrinkage estimation – some of which are included here.

I consider myself very lucky to have other strong professional influences in my father, J.N.K. Rao, and my advisor, Rob Tibshirani, both of whom are widely regarded as leading experts in their areas of statistics and machine learning. Their various books served as inspiration for me in that they also wrote the early major texts in growing areas of important research. I have also had tremendous support from my mother (Neela Rao), my in-laws (Pamela and Dennis Rebello), brothers (Elton Rebello and Sohail Robert) and sisters (Supriya Rao and Serena Rebello-Robert), and niece (Shalini Robert) and nephews (Elijah Robert and Xavier Robert). I thank them for always being there for me and the family. I have also been blessed with my wonderful children, Nalini and Dev (and Grassi), who have brought me never-ending joy and happiness. I could not be more proud of you. Finally, I am forever grateful to my incredible wife, Darlene. She has been there from the very start when I was a Ph.D. student in Toronto. I thank her for her unwavering love and encouragement, and belief in what I have done all throughout my career. I am truly her biggest fan.

J. Sunil Rao

Miami, Florida
December, 2022

1

Basic Concepts

1.1 What is a health disparity?

Health disparities are simply defined as population differences in health status outcomes or health care access, utilization, or quality. While historically many of these focused on comparisons between racial groups, these have been criticized over time as being imprecise and more of a human-made construct than something truly objectively measurable, comparisons may also involve geography (urban vs rural), gender, socioeconomic status, or age among other factors of interest. Health disparity determinants have historically been focused on social and environmental factors (see next sections), but today, with the advances made in genomics and other omic sciences, there is also growing attention to the role of biology in determining health disparities. Specifically, precision medicine is touted as a paradigm that might provide deeper insights into important biological determinants. For example, [124] found 20 unique somatic mutations which preferentially are detected in Black as compared to White colorectal cancer patients. The findings suggest differences in colon cancer development that, when combined with other important determinants of health, may be associated with differences in incidence and outcomes.

1.2 A brief historical perspective

Will Farr, the statistical superintendent who presided over Britain's censuses and vital registration system from 1840 onward, began doing life table comparisons (which then became the gold standard) with the goal of disseminating urban health problems that were arising as a result of the industrial revolution (Reference).

Around the same time, French epidemiologists Parent-Duchâtelet and Villermé were documenting mortality differences in various districts in Paris whilst relating them to the wealth of individuals and to sanitary facilities. Their work showed that for privileged individuals, health improved due to urbanization but that this effect was not felt by all socioeconomic groups in the city.

DOI: 10.1201/9781003119449-1

As the demand for government interventions grew through louder political voices, public infrastructure projects related to better water, sewer, food sanitization, safer housing, better work environments, and safer transportation began. Additionally, better educational opportunities for women slowly began to emerge. So the importance of social factors was clearly seen as vital to improving health outcomes for all, and this predated advances in germ theory or the discovery of antibiotics.

Other early evidence for the presence of health disparities includes a hypothesized association between environmental risk factors and breast cancer incidence in Catholic nuns which was noted by Ramazzini ([97]). In 1775, British surgeon Sir Percival Pott detected a cluster of testicular cancers among chimney sweeps ([41]). In 1840, British statistician Edwin Chadwick demonstrated mortality differences between social classes in Liverpool and concluded that these were likely due to poverty and lifestyle factors of being poor ([51]).

Throughout the 20th century national mortality trends were estimated using decennial census data in Britain. This led to sorting infant mortality rates by occupational social class which correlated inversely with infant mortality. Titmuss and Logan examined class-based mortality trends and found disparities in rates between upper- and lower-class children through 1950. Research in Europe continued to measure and document disparities, culminating historically in the so-called Black report which was authored by the Research Working Group on Inequalities in Health chaired by Sir Douglas Black. This was the British government's systematic study to try and explain health inequalities ([31, 333, 120]).

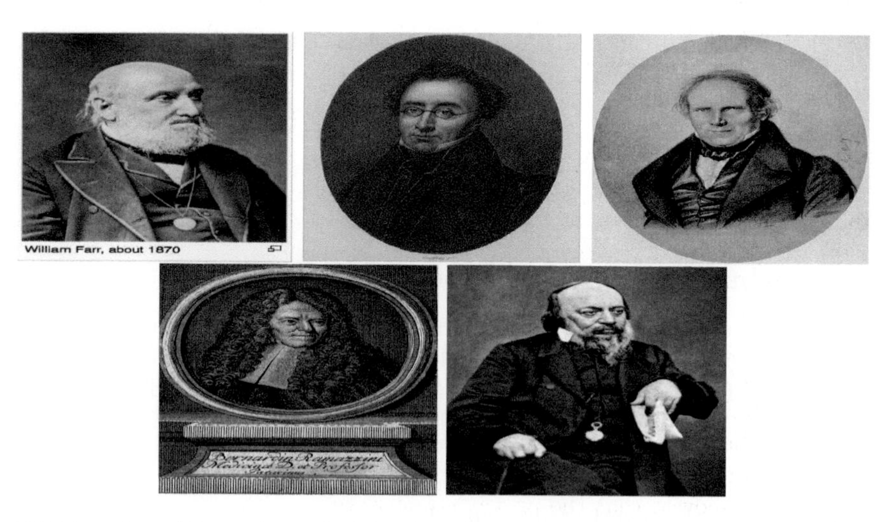

FIGURE 1.1: (Taken from Wikipedia, August 30, 2022): William Farr (top row left); Alexandre-Jean-Baptiste Parent-Duchâtelet (top row middle) Louis-René Villermé (top row right); Bernardino Ramazzini (second row left); Edwin Chadwick (second row right).

In the U.S., research was also moving forward in studying health outcomes in defined populations. This research pointed to gain the importance of the environment and social conditions as determinants of health outcomes. Methods being employed at this time included geographical information systems and small area methods ([245, 300]). In 1984, The U.S. Department of Health released the "Health, United States, 1983" report ([96]). This showed that significant disparities in illness and death rates were experienced by Blacks and other minority Americans as compared to the overall population. In 1985, the "Report of the Secretary's Task Force on Black and Minority Health" was released in an attempt to raise the public's awareness of the health disparities that were being measured. A number of large epidemiological studies have been conducted since 1980 which have demonstrated time and again disparities of one kind or another focusing attention on poor and/or minority populations.

Interestingly, other studies showed health disparities even amongst individuals in higher socioeconomic groups. These were later attributed to stress, early life experiences, social capital, and income inequality (see for example, [334, 13]).

1.3 Some examples

Adler and Rehkopf (2008)[7] provide a nice review of the causes and mechanisms of health disparities in the U.S. As they note, most of the early research has focused on health disparities due to race/ethnicity or social class/socioeconomic status. Other empirical work on gender and geography health disparities has also been done, but much has focused on how these moderate racial/ethnic or social health disparities.

Kitigawa and Hauser (1973)[200] examined all-cause mortality rates for Whites and non-Whites using data from 1960 matched records of persons aged 25 and over. They demonstrated that age-adjusted all-cause mortality rates were 34% higher in non-White females as compared to White females and 20% higher for non-White males as compared to White males. These estimates were adjusted for census-undercounting. Further comparisons by income, location, and education were also done and marked disparities in all-cause mortality were observed. For example, White men, mortality was 64% higher for the least educated versus the most educated groups. Similar trends were seen for White women. Pappas *et al.* (1986)[275] updated this analysis in 1986 and showed that the previously observed health disparities had only worsened and that higher income, more educated individuals were systematically having better outcomes overall and within racial/ethnic groups over time.

Deeper explorations were made into cause-specific mortality and whether systematic differences between racial/ethnic and social groups could be observed. Analyses from the National Longitudinal Mortality Study (NLMS) ([335]) of 1.3 million persons showed racial/ethnic mortality differences in many diseases. For instance, Black men had markedly higher standardized mortality ratios (SMR) than did Whites for esophageal cancer, heart disease, and homicide but lower SMRs for suicide, leukemia, and chronic obstructive pulmonary disease (COPD). Black women, on the other hand, showed higher SMRs for homicide, heart disease, nephritis, and stomach cancer (among others), and lower SMRs for suicide, COPD, and leukemia. Further study of this data by [150] demonstrated that much of these differences could be accounted for by differences in socioeconomic status between the groups. Wong *et al.* (2002)[370] showed the importance of education to racial/ethnic cause-specific mortality differences. They showed that differential mortality rates in cancer and lung disease were associated with differences in education status.

Geographic variation in mortality rates across the U.S. has been noted, but less work has gone into intersecting these differences with racial/ethnic and social factors. The NLMS validates this showing that locations with the lowest mortality rates for Whites and Blacks were similar even though overall rates were higher for Blacks ([310]). This study hints at the importance of area-level context and that racial/ethnic and social health disparities were not static across the U.S.

Time is another axis whose influence on disparities has been explored. Ward *et al.* (2004)[363] studied differences in cancer mortality by race/ethnicity during the time period of 1975–2000. From 2000 onward, they noted Black women had higher breast cancer mortality than White women and Black men had higher colorectal cancer mortality than did White men. Marked differences in prostate cancer mortality were observed throughout the time period studied. This might be linked to differences in access to healthcare and improved screening for these cancers but could also be due to differences in risk factors whose effects too have changed over time differentially between these groups. Figure 1.2 taken from Ward *et al.* (2004) shows these results clearly.

1.4 Determinants of health

"In rich white Streeterville, Chicagoans can expect to live to 90. In poor black Englewood, it's just 60 – the most divergent of any U.S. city" (The Guardian, June 23, 2019). Yet these two communities are only 8 miles apart in physical distance. Streeterville is a bustling, affluent community with easy access to fresh produce, low crime, open green spaces, high rates of post-secondary education and graduation rates, and low unemployment. Englewood is the polar opposite with boarded-up shops, a sparsity of grocery stores, weak

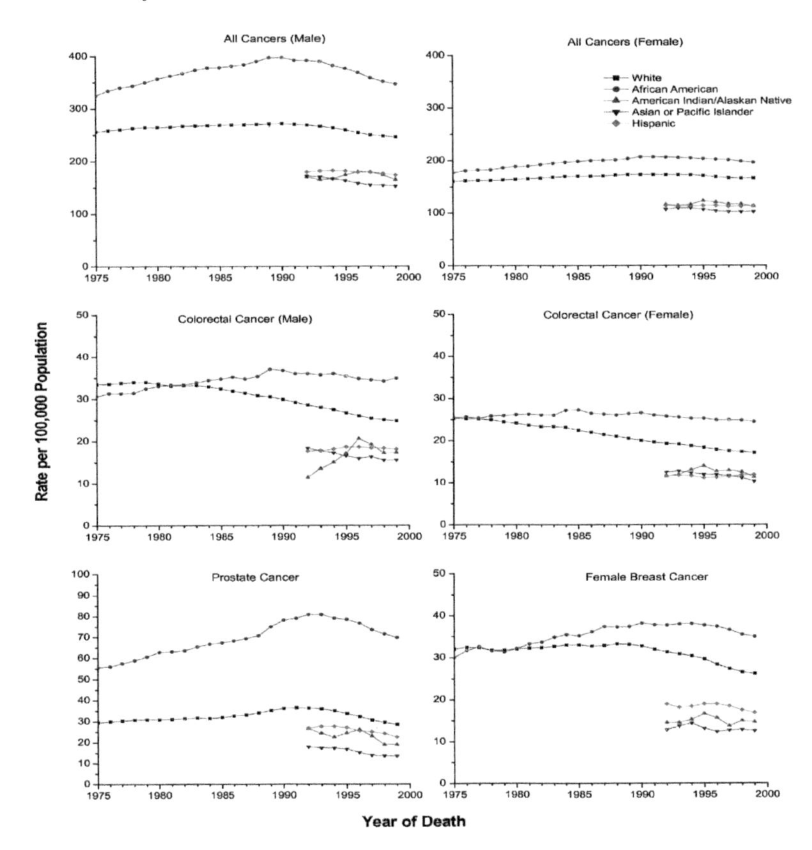

FIGURE 1.2: (Taken from Ward et al. (2004)[363]): Trends in cancer mortality by race/ethnicity between 1975 and 2000. Data is from the Surveillance, Epidemiology, and End Results (SEER) program.

educational outcomes, high unemployment, and high crime. Thus the fact that one community is predominantly White and the other predominantly Black only details a very small amount of the differences between the two communities. There is an increasing understanding that one's zip code (postal code) can contribute as much to health as one's genetic code. These complex determinants of health interplay in complex ways to help shape health outcomes and hence health disparities.

1.4.1 Biology and genetics

These factors are the ones that most easily come to mind when thinking about determinants of health. Some biological and genetic factors affect certain populations more than others. Older individuals are more prone to physical and cognitive decline as compared to adolescents. Sickle cell anemia, a condition in which both parents carry the gene for sickle cell, is more common in people with ancestry from West Africa, the Mediterranean countries, South and Central America, the Caribbean islands, India, and Saudi Arabia. HIV-positive patients are much more vulnerable to opportunistic infections. Individuals carrying the BRCA1 or BRCA2 gene have a markedly increased risk for breast and ovarian cancer. Individuals with strong family histories of heart disease are themselves more vulnerable.

1.4.2 Individual behavior

Behavior modification programs have long been associated with improved health outcomes. This can include things like smoking cessation programs which can improve a host of health outcomes, from heart disease to cancer. Interventions focused on changing individual behavior around substance abuse, diet, and physical activity have all been associated with improved outcomes. It's the disparity in risky behaviors that can contribute to health disparities. Another interesting example is handwashing. This simple behavior is known to reduce risk for a number of communicable diseases. Yet during the COVID-19 pandemic of 2020–2021, it was observed that certain populations simply did not have access to clean water or sanitizer which left them at a higher risk of contracting the disease (see for example, [33, 284]).

1.4.3 Health services

Access and quality of health services can impact health outcomes. Barriers include availability, cost, lack of insurance, and language access. This translates into increased unmet health needs, delays in receiving care, reduced preventive services, and increased hospitalizations. The Finding Answers program ([57]) provided healthcare organization interventions by designing a variety of quality improvement initiatives that led to better delivery of care and ultimately better health care for minority populations ([57]). Cultural competency programs for providers and empowerment programs that encourage more patient advocacy are other examples of useful interventions.

1.4.4 Social determinants of health

Social determinants of health refer to factors that involve social and physical conditions of the environment in which people are born, live, learn, play, work, and age (see, for example, [34, 271, 236]). These include living wages, healthy foods, social attitudes, exposure to crime and violence and social disorder, social interactions, poverty, quality education, transportation access, residential segregation, the natural environment, including green spaces and built environment, climate change and weather, housing and neighborhoods, exposure to toxic substances or other physical hazards.

There are many examples where intervention on social determinants of health has led to a reduction in health disparities (see, for example, [367, 15, 351]). Improving access to better quality education like structured early childhood education and parental support programs have positive impacts on the health of children and parents but also can reduce economic and health disparities ([367, 144]) by strengthening families, enhancing educational achievement, improving economic outcomes and preventing neurodevelopmental issues that arise as consequences of being disadvantaged. For example, the Perry Preschool Project is a two-year program for Black children aged 3 and 4 from a disadvantaged community in Michigan. These children were randomized to an intervention or control group where the intervention was designed to improve educational outcomes. This resulted in higher rates of safety belt use and less engagement in risky health behaviors such as smoking and drug use as an adult ([364]). Urban planning and community development can also yield significant reductions in health disparities. The community development project in East Los Angeles where over 90% of residents are Mexican-American, involved transforming corner neighborhood stores into healthy stores ([273]). Project U-Turn in Michigan increased cycling in a target region and included the creation of safe routes to school. This resulted in a 63% increase in active transportation across the region. Here the groups being compared would be those of varying levels of physical activity. Other important examples of social determinant interventions involve improving housing quality, income supplements, and improving employment access ([349]).

1.4.5 (Health) policies

Health disparities exist and persist through complex interactions between the various levels of determinants. In order to accelerate disparity reduction, interventions are needed that act upon the so-called structural determinants of health often determined by health policymaking ([40]). Structural interventions attempt to change determinants that may shape or constrain health behaviors. They target factors like economic instability, access to quality education and employment, systemic racism, lack of resources to healthy food, clean water, physical activity spaces, transportation, and healthcare.

The Moving to Opportunity Study ([218]) is a randomized housing mobility trial that offered housing vouchers to low income families who resided in public housing in high poverty communities in the hope to encourage families to move to lower poverty areas. After 15 years of follow-up, the intervention group had measurable and statistically significant improvements in physical and mental health including outcomes of obesity, diabetes, stress, and depression. Another example is the Earned Income Tax Credit which aims to increase wealth among low income families. This has had important effects including higher rates of prenatal care among pregnant women, reductions in low birth weight rates among African American mothers, and improved

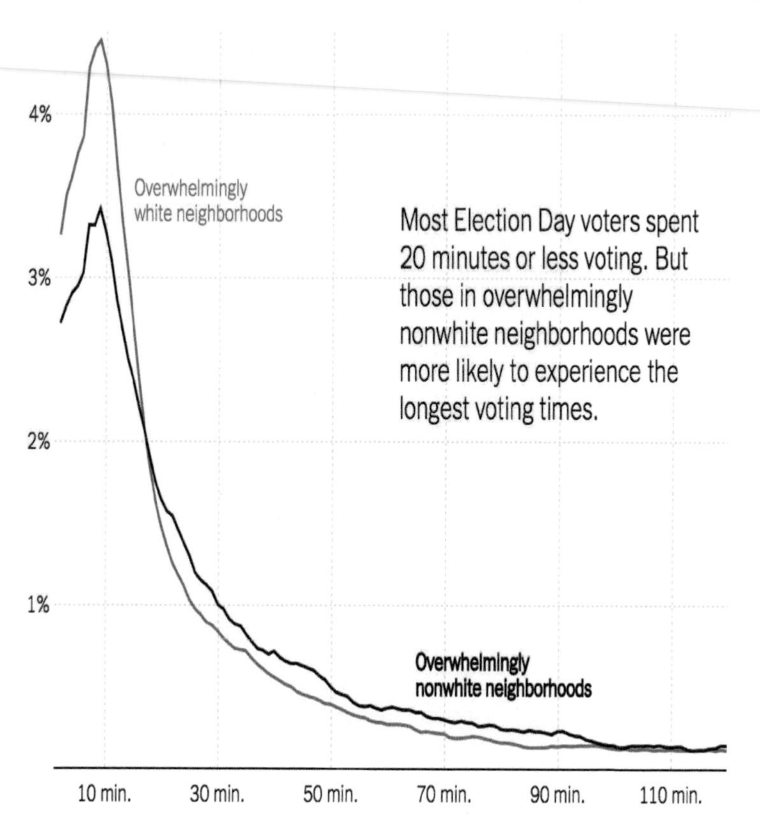

FIGURE 1.3: (Taken from New York Times, Jan 4, 2021): Distribution of vote times in White and non-White neighborhoods

child nutrition ([151, 127, 235]). These are two examples that focus on education and fiscal policy that has resulted in long-term improvements in minority health outcomes and reductions in health disparities.

More indirectly consider the following much more upstream example. Figure 1.3 shows a New York Times analysis of voting times in the 2020 federal U.S. election. Clearly largely non-White neighborhoods have a larger propensity for longer wait times. Small variations in voting time are likely not that important. But at the extremes, they may lead to people leaving the line and not voting and this appears to be more probable for non-White neighborhoods.

1.5 The challenging issue of race

Race has never had a precise meaning. This is largely because the concept of race, which is closely linked to social inheritance, was developed as a method for implementation of discriminatory policies ([241, 158]). Genetic ancestry, on the other hand, is rooted in the idea of genetic inheritance. It refers to the population differentiated genetic markers that are transmitted from parent to child over the course of many generations. Genetic ancestry generally reflects the correlation between allele frequencies and geographic clines, not social identities and can be affected by factors like genetic drift and selection pressures which influence allele frequencies. It has been observed that these frequencies are often correlated with geographical locations along which ancestral populations lived. This results in some genetic variants that can be found in high frequencies among some populations and low in other populations.

Collectively, these types of variants are referred to as Ancestry Informative Markers (AIMs) ([241]). When a particular variant of an AIM is observed, it can be interpreted as coming from a region of the world where said AIM is in high frequency among populations. AIMs and other genetic variants are useful for inferring genetic ancestry (17,18), which is now thought of as a mosaic that includes information from different regions of the world.

Still, genetic ancestry does not always correlate to how an individual socially identifies their race. Despite the lack of a direct relationship, race and biology intertwine at the level of effect. Consequently, race is often used as an (imperfect) proxy for both biological and social factors that are correlated with human health ([330, 329]). Thus, race (more precisely racism) can become a major confounder in human genetic studies of complex traits, even among analyses restricted to African-descent populations as all African-descent individuals do not share the same racial identity or experience of discrimination ([314]). A schematic of this relationship and how it relates to health disparities is presented in Figure 1.4.

Actkins *et. al.* (2022) performed an interesting analysis to see if self-identified race could be disentangled from genetic ancestry using a residual-based analysis, and then if the associated residuals could be related to different disease phenotypes in a phenome-wide association study (PheWAS). They used data from a de-identified version of the electronic health record (EHR) database at Vanderbilt University known as the Synthetic Derivative (SD) which includes patient records on more than 2.8 million individuals. Demographic variables and EHR-reported (self-reported and third-party reported) race were extracted on nearly 40,000 patients comprising a training sample and over 82,000 patients that made up a validation sample. These individuals also had genetic data available in a linked biobank. Blacks and Whites comprised approximately 11% and 89% of the discovery sample and 20% and 80% of the replication sample.

A principal component analysis (PCA) was then performed on over 9500 so-called ancestral genetic markers (AIMs) in the training sample and 250,000 AIMs in the validation sample. PCA is a technique used as a dimension reduction tool to reduce variation across many thousands of genetic variants into orthogonal vectors that explain maximal variance within a genotyped sample. It is well-known that the first principal component (PC1) represents

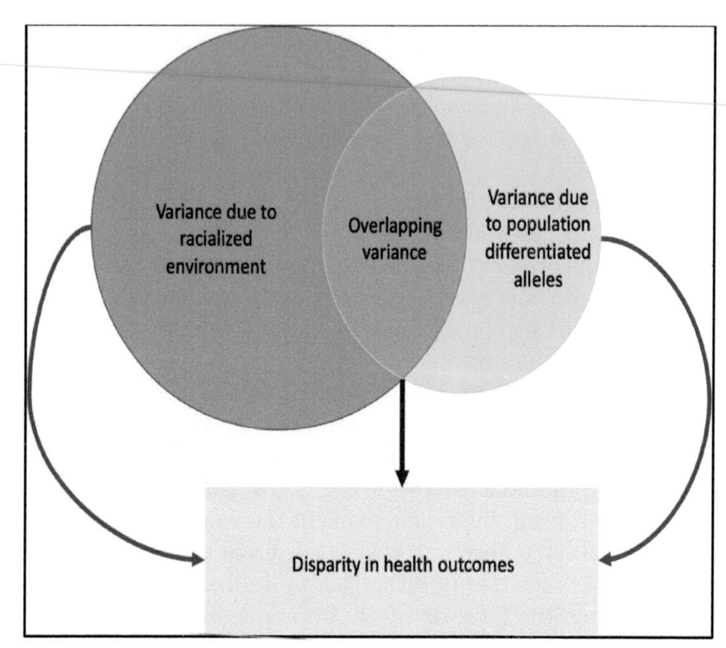

FIGURE 1.4: (Taken from Actkins *et al.* (2022)[6]) : Conceptual framework for the relationship of genetics ancestry and race in determining health disparities.

the geographical cline from Northernmost Europe to Southernmost Africa. Actkins *et al.* (2022)[6] then calculated regression residuals for EHR-reported race and PC1 after adjusting for the variance of the other variable. What this means is that the residuals of PC1 represent variance due to the remaining biological construct of genetic ancestry after adjusting for the variance due to EHR-reported race and the residuals of EHR-reported race represent the variance due to the remaining social construct of race after adjusting for the variance explained by PC1.

They then performed a PheWAS study using phenotype data extracted from billing codes in the medical records using the PC1 residuals as the predictor. They also conducted a PheWAS using the EHR-reported race residuals as the predictor and then asked the question if associations to disease were different between the two. What they found was that from each testing sample PheWAS, there was significant overlap in phenotypic associations but that EHR-reported race (thought of as a social construct) had larger effect sizes. The implication of their study was that "racialized environments" ([6]) may confound genetic analyses.

1.5.1 Racial segregation as a social determinant of health

Racial segregation or dissimilarity within communities ([154]) has been shown to impact health outcomes ([104]) and is more frequently being considered an important factor for predicting individual and community health outcomes

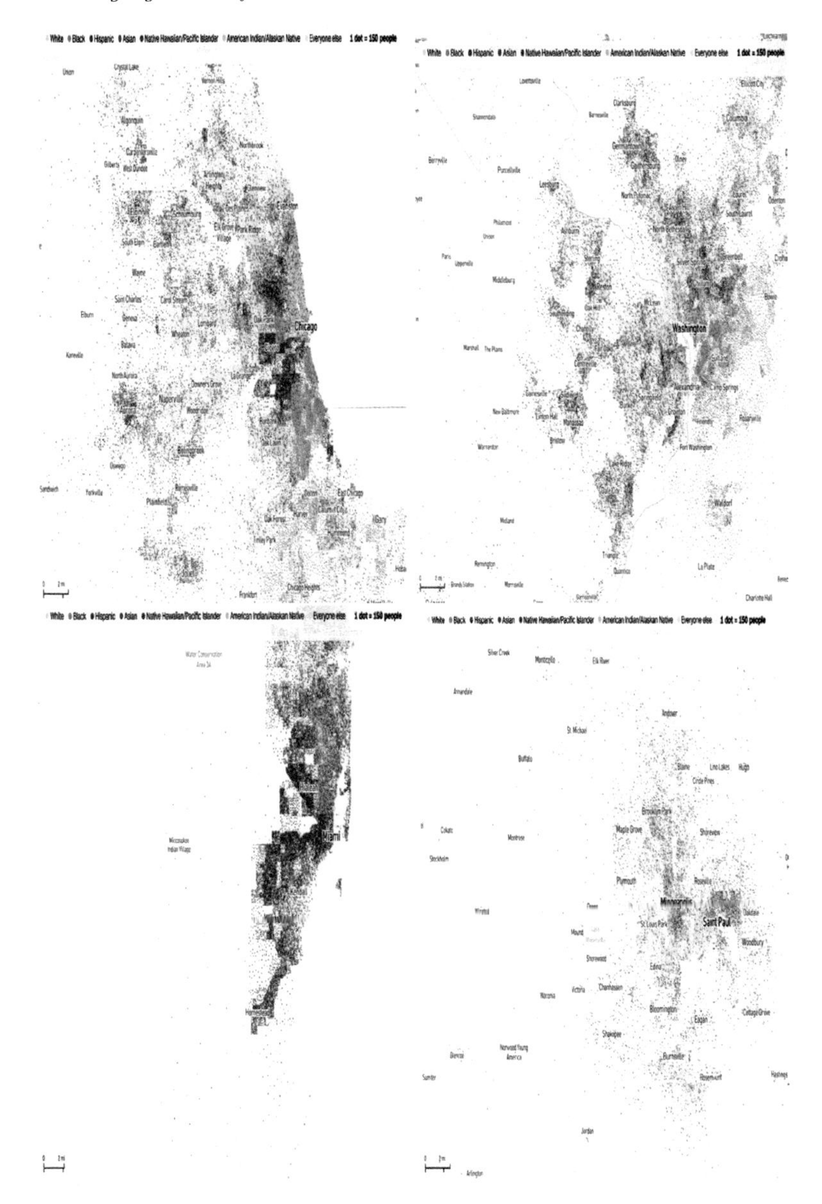

FIGURE 1.5: (Source: U.S. Census Bureau): Racial segregation for four different communities in the U.S. Each dot corresponds to 150 people and each color a different racial/ethnic category.

([306, 155]). Figure 1.5 shows racial segregation for four different communities from the 2020 U.S. Census data. The four cities are Chicago, Washington DC, Miami, and Minneapolis-St.Paul. Each dot on the plot represents 150 people and each color, a different racial/ethnic category. Segregation is evident by sharp boundaries between clusters of (mostly) homogeneous colored dots as is seen in Miami, Chicago and DC but less so in Minneapolis-St. Paul. In the *Color of Law*, Richard Rothstein discusses how from Reconstruction to the present day, local, state, and federal policies and laws have been used to segregate the American population along racial lines resulting in persistent inequalities in social, economic, and educational opportunities. Minorities tend to live in poorer neighborhoods, attend lower-quality schools and receive health care at lower-quality hospitals ([64]).

Indeed most of the research around racial segregation and health outcomes has been focused in urban areas. One notable exception is the work by [246] who empirically evaluated county-level data in Georgia to test the relationship between racial segregation and other social determinants of health using dissimilarity indices in order to predict measures of health status and quality of life. Racial segregation was found to have a significant and negative relationship with quality of life measures but had no effect on measures of health status. This suggests that more segregated counties have fewer percentage reporting aspects of poor health.

1.5.2 Racism, segregation, and inequality

Racism, segregation, and inequality contribute to disparities in health outcomes across the life course. Beck *et al.* (2020)[25] explored three causal pathways that adversely affect outcomes for newborn infants and their families. These are increased risk, lower quality care, and persistent socioeconomic disadvantage.

Structural racism refers to mutually enforcing forms of discrimination ([14]) including neighborhood deprivation, economic inequalities, educational disparities, and differences in access to health care leading to nutritional deficiencies and unhealthy environmental exposures. So clearly, structural racism is potentially causally linked to levels of social determinants of health that might adversely affect health outcomes. But as [25] discussed, exposure to a social determinant of health in itself is insufficient to increase the risk of preterm birth. Additional stressors and exposures are needed including exposures during the perinatal period such as maternal stress and depression increase preterm birth and infant mortality risk. They also make the point that genetics must be taken into account by that genetics alone likely plays a small role in differential risk but rather, gene-environment interactions may explain some differences ([342, 44]). Additionally, there appears to be some suggestive evidence that epigenetics may play a role in preterm birth in that immigrant African women are less likely to give birth preterm than native-born Black women ([43]).

1.6 Role of data visualization in health disparities research

Data visualization or the process of communicating the analytical results of large amounts of data in a visual context is a very effective strategy to help simplify and justify decision making. Data visualization strategies can help understand underlying patterns, trends and correlations in datasets and such information may not be apparent in a spreadsheet of data itself. These strategies are typically linked to the analysis of so-called big or massive datasets but they need to be limited to those applications. Indeed the advocacy for the use of effective graphics can be traced to the foundational work of Edward Tufte (see, for example, Tufte's classic *The Visual Display of Quantitative Information*). Tufte's famous six principles of effective data visualization include:

1. Show a comparison: when creating graphics, plot comparison groups in the same plot, thus giving readers the sense of effect sizes
2. Show causality and explanation: provide an explanation that shows a causal framework for thinking about the question you are trying to answer
3. Show multivariate data: since the real world is complex, relationships between variables are not always linear; thus show as much data as you can in your plots
4. Don't let the tools drive the analysis: have the ability to expand from one form of visual expression to multiple modes of presentation
5. Document graphics with appropriate labels and scales and data sources
6. Content above all else: before reporting a result, make sure it's something interesting and important.

Since health disparities research is a heavily quantitative science, it's not surprising that there is increasing attention on designing interesting data visualization tools to understand disparities. Here is one recent example:

Example 1.1 Why COVID-19 death rates are rising in some groups – source: New York Times, December 28, 2021

As of April 2021 when vaccines became more widely available, COVID-19 death rates declined in the U.S. But from April to December 2021, nearly 250,000 people in the U.S. died from the virus and a NY Times article presented a useful set of data visualizations to understand emerging pattern changes – namely that a higher share of deaths from all causes was now affecting younger Americans and White Americans than it was prior to vaccine distribution. Without going into all of the nuances of the emergence of new virus variants, Figure 1.6 effectively shows these changes in patterns. Clearly, the disparity patterns have altered since the widespread distribution of the vaccines.

Share of each age group that is fully vaccinated

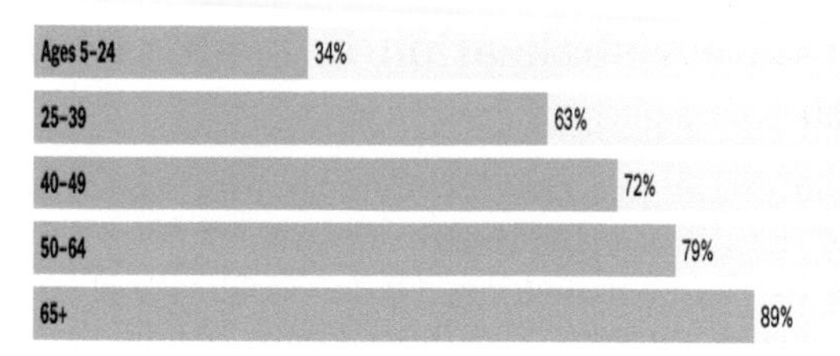

Sources: Centers for Disease Control and Prevention, Census Bureau • Note: Vaccination rates are as of Dec. 22. Fully vaccinated include those who have received Johnson & Johnson's single-dose vaccine or the two-dose series made by Pfizer-BioNTech and Moderna.

Covid-19 deaths before and after universal adult vaccine eligibility

Covid-19 deaths increased as a share of deaths from all causes

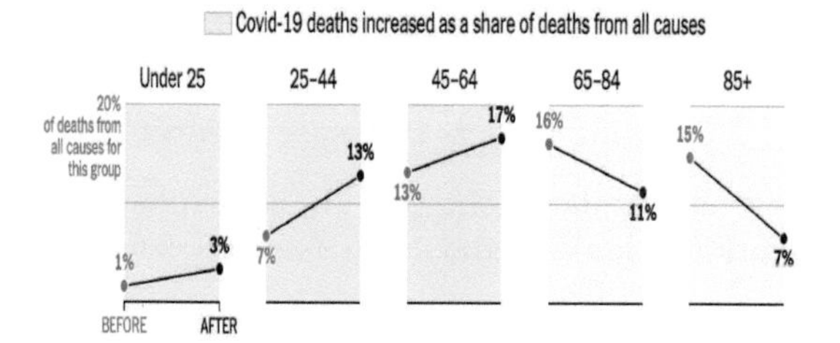

Source: Provisional weekly death data from the C.D.C. through Nov. 27. • Note: Universal vaccine eligibility was April 19, the date when all adults in the United States were eligible for vaccination.

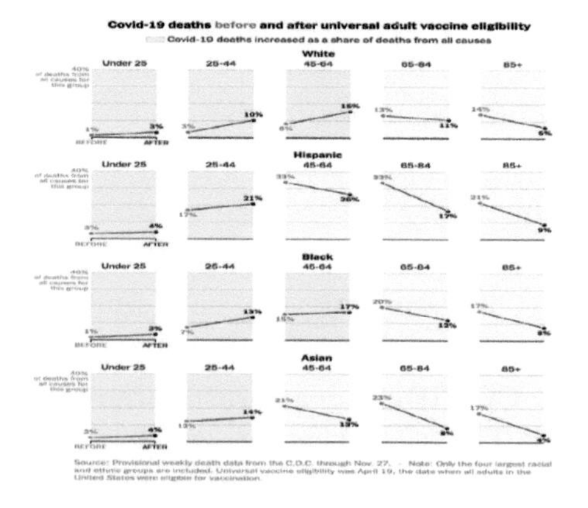

FIGURE 1.6: (Source: NY Times, December 28, 2021): COVID-19 deaths before and after adult vaccine eligibility by age group (middle figure) and further broken out by racial group (bottom figure).

1.7 A note on notation adopted in this book

In probability and mathematical statistics, it has been the norm to use capital letters, such as X_i or Y_i, to indicate a random variable, whereas lowercase letters like y_i and x_i, to indicate an observed value for the random variables Y_i and X_i, respectively (i.e., the actual data). However, this distinction is not widely adopted in many areas of applied statistics where in fact, lowercase letters refer to both a random variable and a realized value of that random variable. For instance, this has been the convention for small area estimation models, linear and generalized linear mixed models, and many other areas of applied statistics, although admittedly, this is not the convention in areas like causal inference. In this book, we will use lowercase letters throughout and clearly state assumptions as required to avoid confusion.

2

Overall Estimation of Health Disparities

2.1 Data and measurement

Major sources of data for health disparity estimation can be experimental, observational, or from complex surveys (refer to examples from Chapter 1). The distinction between these has mostly to do with the sampling designs employed. While complex surveys are especially seen as a separate topic from mainstream statistical analyses, it's most useful to try and unify notation across these designs. This will aid in the presentation of health disparity estimation methods which will at times require specialized treatment to deal with differences in sampling designs. Skinner and Wakefield (2017)[331] provide a very nice introduction to the analysis of complex survey data but in their article, they also provide a unified notational framework for these different sampling designs. We will adopt their notation here.

Let $y_i, i = 1, \ldots, N$ represent values of a survey variable of interest on all N units of a well-defined finite population. It's typical to also use $i \in U$ to index this collection. A sample of these units $S \subset U$ is drawn based upon a probability mechanism $p(s)$ which is the probability of selecting $S = s$ such that $\sum_s p(s) = 1$. The only observed values are then y_i for $i \in S$. The probability of unit i being selected can be denoted $\pi_i = \sum_{i:i \in s} p(s)$ (This is sometimes noted $\varpi(s)$). The inverse of these are termed *design weights* $d_i = \pi_i^{-1}$. Examples of sampling designs include simple random sampling (srs), cluster sampling, stratified sampling, etc. It is the inclusion of the latter complications that distinguishes complex surveys from other designs. These complications drastically alter the probability mechanism and for estimation and inference to be done correctly, these must be taken into account. In *design-based* inference, the population values (e.g., means, totals, ratios) are of interest and considered fixed constants with the collection of units in S considered random ([61, 113, 114, 115]).

The contrast to design-based inference is *model-based* inference. What distinguishes these is the source of randomness, the former being the randomization associated with the probability mechanism, the latter from a model assumed to generate the population values y_i. In model-based inference, the y_i are considered realized values of random variables $Y_i, i = 1, \ldots, N$ which follow some underlying model. This paradigm views the population as drawn from

DOI: 10.1201/9781003119449-2

a hypothetical infinite superpopulation. Inference amounts to characterizing variation across repeated realizations from the model. Thus, it's typical to use the $Y_i, i = 1, \ldots, n$ notation to reflect a sample drawn from the population under the model. The change of notation reflects the fact that the set of units S selected from N is no longer relevant. What's more, as a matter of convention, we will resort to writing all random quantities in lowercase notation unless they are random matrices. In model based inference, it's typical to ignore the sampling design features and assume the sampled individuals are independent observations. Interest here focuses on model parameters ([316, 317]). This is more in line with the paradigm of traditional statistical modeling.

There is a third approach called *model-assisted* inference. Here again, interest lies on finite population parameters as in the design-based approach and inference is with respect to the probability sampling design. But here, inference and associated estimators are motivated through an assumed model. So then, the model-assisted paradigm is really design-based but is known to gain efficiency when the finite population is well described by the underlying model ([48]). Sources of randomization include then the probability sampling design for the finite population and the assumed model for a superpopulation. These can be considered jointly ([48]). Thus the finite population is regarded as a random sample from the superpopulation model and the survey sample is viewed as second phase sampling from the superpopulation. In this book, when discussing health disparity estimation from complex survey data, we will employ design-based or model-assisted approaches as appropriate.

2.2 Disparity indices

Much of the work in health disparity estimation has stemmed from producing summary measures or indices aggregated from data from sample surveys or registries. These indices provide a birds-eye view that can be used for disease surveillance ([130, 56]). If the focus is on a single population, then one can measure total disparity which provides a summary index of health differences across a population. While sometimes informative, these measures do not inform about systemic variation in health among population subgroups. However, total disparity measures are often used by large agencies like WHO for assessing the performance of health systems in different countries. These are also popular measures of population health for health economists.

2.2.1 Total disparity indices

Examples of total disparity indices include the individual-mean difference (IMD) measures and the inter-individual difference (IID) measures. The IMD is based on calculations of the difference between the health of every individual in a population and the population average. This family of measures can be defined by

$$IMD(a,b) = \frac{\sum_{i=1}^{N} |y_i - \mu|^a}{N\mu^{b|}},$$

where N is the total population size, and a and b are parameters that specify the significance attached to health differences in the tails of the population distribution. For example, $a = 2, b = 0$ gives the (finite) population variance, $a = 2, b = 1$ is the coefficient of variation. Note that IMD is dimensionless (without units) since it is always relative to the population mean.

IID measures can be generally represented as,

$$IID(a,b) = \frac{\sum_{i=1}^{N} \sum_{j=1}^{N} |y_i - y_j|^a}{2N^2\mu^b}.$$

Here, when $a = 2, b = 1$, the IID becomes the Gini coefficient ([130]). Other weights have been used. For instance, [101] compared total disparity in child survival across 50 countries and used $a = 3, b = 1$. A value of $a = 3$ indicates that the measure gives more weight to larger than smaller pairwise deviations between individuals.

2.2.2 Disparity indices measuring differences between groups

Disparity estimation is not just concerned with total disparity measures. In fact, it's often of interest to compare groups within a population to better understand the structural components in the population that could be responsible for the disparity as well as to measure the progress towards reducing disparities between groups. For simplicity, we will detail pairwise comparisons but these naturally extend to more than two groups. Such disparity indices are generally classified as absolute or relative measures ([130]). Absolute measures typically use simple (mean) differences and relative measures are calculated as differences relative to a particular reference group. Absolute disparity can generically be represented as $AD = r_1 - r_2$, where r_1 and r_2, are indicators of health status in two groups and where r_2 can be thought of as a reference group. AD is thus expressed in the same units as r_1 and r_2. Relative disparity can be generically written as $RD = r_1/r_2$ where r_2 is the reference group. Sometimes this rate ratio is converted to percentages for convenience of interpretation. Figure 2.1 shows the absolute and relative Black-White disparity for prostate and stomach cancer incidence from 1992 to 1999 ([130]). The AD for prostate cancer is much larger than for stomach cancer because the rates for both groups is high as compared to stomach cancer. On the other hand, RD is higher for stomach cancer than prostate cancer by a little amount. This reflects the difference between using a difference versus a ratio estimator.

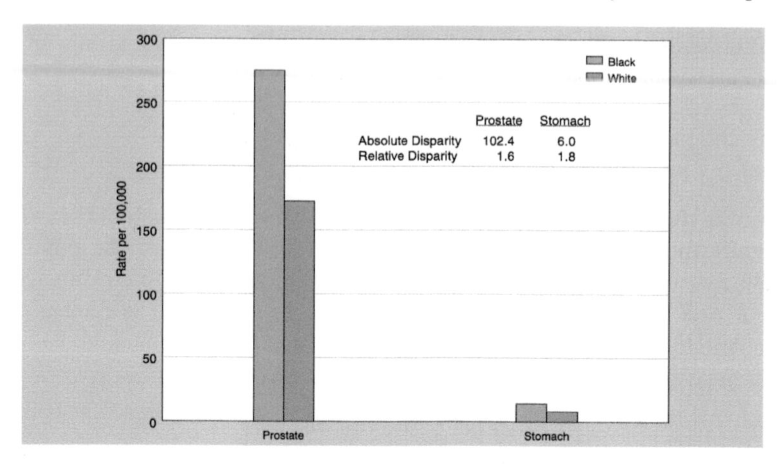

FIGURE 2.1: (Taken from Harper and Lynch (2010)[131]): Absolute and relative disparity estimates between Blacks and Whites in prostate cancer and stomach cancer incidence 1992–1999 in the U.S.

Further absolute measures include the absolute concentration index and the slope index of inequality. Concentration indices are built off of the bivariate distribution of health and group ranking and derived from a concentration curve. To do so, the population is ordered first by group status and then the cumulative percentage of the population is plotted against the group's share of total (ill) health. The absolute concentration index (ACI) is arrived at by plotting the cumulative share of the population against the cumulative amount of ill health. The slope index of inequality is derived by ordering the groups from lowest to highest. The population of each group category is given a score based on the midpoint of its range in the cumulative distribution of the population. Health status is then plotted against this midpoint variable and an ordinary regression line is fitted. The slope of this line is the slope index of inequality (SII). By weighting the groups by their population share, the SII is able to incorporate changes in the groupwise distribution that can affect health disparities.

Additional relative measures include the relative concentration index (RCI), index of disparity (IDisp), mean log deviation, Theil index, relative index of inequality, and the Kunst-Mackenbach index (KMI). How these measures differ amount to which reference group is used, whether a measure considers all socioeconomic groups, and whether the difference in health is weighted by population shares in each social group, whether a measure considers the ordinality of a social determinant, and whether the measure allows social value judgment.

The RCI is similarly derived to the ACI except that the y-axis is the share of ill health. The general formula for RCI for grouped data is

$$RCI = \frac{2}{\mu}(\sum_{j=1}^{J} p_j \mu_j R_j) - 1,$$

where p_j is the jth group's population share, μ_j is the group's mean health and R_j is the relative rank of the jth group defined as $R_j = \sum_{j=1}^{J} p_\gamma - 1/2p_j$ where p_γ is the cumulative share of the population up to and including group j. R_j reflects the cumulative share of the population up to the midpoint of each group interval. ACI and RCI can be related by the formula,

$$ACI = \mu RCI,$$

where μ is the mean level of health in the population as a whole. The index of disparity (IDisp) looks at the total (i.e., sum) difference in group rates relative to a reference rate and expresses this as a percentage of the reference rate. Originally introduced by [277], it can be formulated as,

$$IDisp = (\sum_{j=j}^{J-1} |r_j - r_{ref}|)/r_{ref} \times 100,$$

where r_{ref} represents the reference group rate and this group is one of the J groups under consideration. Gastwirth (2007)[103] modified IDisp to allow weighting of each group's deviation from the reference rate by its population size giving the disparity index U,

$$U = \sum_{j=j}^{J-1} (r_j - r_{ref}).$$

U can also be expressed relative to the health status of the total population.

Theil's index (1967)[350] was developed by economist Henri Theil and is a measure of general entropy. It is derived from Shannon's measure of information entropy which is a measure of randomness in a given set of information. This general form of entropy is,

$$S = k \sum_{i=}^{N} (p_i log_a(1/p_i)),$$

where i is an individual item from the set, p_i is the probability of finding i from a random sample from the set, k is a constant, and $log_a(x)$ is the logarithm to base a. For grouped data, Theil's index of disparity is the sum of two parts: the between-group disparity and a weighted average of within-group disparity,

$$T = \sum_{j=1}^{J} p_j r_j ln(r_j) + \sum_{j=1}^{J} p_j r_j T_j,$$

where $T_j = \sum_{i=1}^{N_j} p_i r_i ln(r_i)$ where p_i is an individual's population share (typically $1/N_j$) and r_i is the ratio of the individual's health status to the population average for group j. The decomposition also makes it clear that between-group disparity can be estimated without having information at the individual level.

The relative index of inequality (RII) is derived from the SII (an absolute disparity measure) as,

$$RII = SII/\mu,$$

where μ is the mean population health. Its interpretation differs from SII in that it measures the proportionate rather than absolute increase or decrease in health between the highest and lowest groups. Kunst and Mackenbach (1994)[208] modified this as,

$$KMI = \beta_0/(\beta_0 + SII),$$

where β_0 is the intercept of the line which is used to estimate SII. Thus KMI compares the health of the extremes of the groupwise distribution but is estimated using all groups and is weighted to account for group sizes.

Li, Yu and Zhang (2018)[220] provide a summary of a wide range of health disparity indices focusing on the so-called HD*Calc measures put forward by the National Cancer Institute. HD*Calc was intended to provide multiple summary measures of health disparity which users can then apply to analyze data from population-based surveillance systems like SEER or the National Vital Statistics System. HD*Calc provides an expanded range of both absolute and relative measures.

Point estimates and variance estimates assuming i.i.d. observations have been proposed for each of the measures (for example, see [220]).

2.2.3 Disparity indices from complex surveys

Lin, Yu and Zhang (2018)[220] show how to estimate HD*Calc disparity indices from complex survey data as well as how to estimate variances using Taylor linearization methods. In a stratified complex survey say, let p_j be the population share of the jth socioeconomic group ($j = 1, \ldots, J$) and μ_j as the mean "health" for the jth group. With H strata and t_h primary sampling units in stratum h, let n_{ha} be the number of sampled units from the ath primary sampling units in the hth stratum. Then [220] showed that all disparity indices can be written as functions of μ_j and p_j. For example,

$$RCI = \frac{2}{\mu} \times [\sum_{j=1}^{J} p_j \mu_j R_j] - 1,$$

with $\mu = \sum_{j=1}^{J} p_j \mu_j$ and $R_j = \sum_{r=1}^{j-1} p_r + 0.5 p_j$.

Generically they write all of these indices as $g(\mu_j, p_j); j = 1, \ldots, J$ where g is a differentiable function of μ_j and p_j corresponding to a particular disparity index. Plug-in estimation is then done producing a complex survey estimate of each index – namely $g(\hat{\mu}_j, \hat{p}_j)$. These are combined across all socioeconomic groups to produce a population estimate of disparity.

Plug-in estimation uses the following,

$$\hat{\mu}_j = \frac{\sum_{i=1}^{n} I(hai \in j) w_{hai} y_{hai}}{\sum_{i=1}^{n} I(hai \in j) w_{hai}},$$

and

$$\hat{p}_j = \frac{\sum_{i=1}^{n} I(hai \in j) w_{hai}}{\sum_{i=1}^{n} w_{hai}},$$

where $y_{hai} \in (0, 1)$ is the binary health status for individual i in cluster a in stratum h and w_{hai} the sampling weight for that same individual.

For variance estimation, Taylor linearization (sometimes called the delta method) is used which is a common technique employed in the analysis of complex survey data. These are known to provide design-consistent estimates of variance. This approach tries to account for the variability due to differential sampling weights, stratification, and clustering effects induced by the complex survey design. Lin, Yu and Zhang (2018)[220] provide derivations for each of 11 HD*Calc disparity indices.

To describe in general terms what they do, consider a first order Taylor series approximation for $g(\hat{\mu}_j, \hat{p}_j)$ about the point (μ_j, p_j) is

$$g(\hat{\mu}_j, \hat{p}_j) = g(\mu_j, p_j) + g'_{\mu_j}(\mu_j)(\hat{\mu}_j - \mu_j) + g'_{p_j}(\hat{p}_j - p_j) + R$$

where R is a remainder term. Therefore, $E(g(\hat{\mu}_j, \hat{p}_j)) = g(\mu_j, p_j)$. By definition of variance of $g(\hat{\mu}_j, \hat{p}_j)$

$$Var(g(\hat{\mu}_j, \hat{p}_j)) = E[g(\hat{\mu}_j, \hat{p}_j) - E(g(\hat{\mu}_j, \hat{p}_j)]^2$$

which then implies,

$$Var(g(\hat{\mu}_j, \hat{p}_j)) \approx E[g'_{\mu_j}(\mu_j)(\hat{\mu}_j - \mu_j) + g'_{p_j}(\hat{p}_j - p_j)]^2.$$

These are then aggregated across strata and socioeconomic groups. Specifically, they define

$$Var(g(\hat{\mu}_j, \hat{p}_j)) = \sum_{h=1}^{H} \frac{t_h}{t_h - 1} \sum_{a=1}^{t_h} (Z_{ha} - \bar{Z}_h)(Z_{ha} - \bar{Z}_h)',$$

where $Z_{ha} = \sum_{i=1}^{n_{ha}} w_{hai} z_{hai}$ and $\bar{Z}_h = 1/t_h \sum_{a=1}^{t_h} Z_{ha}$. Here z_{hai} are the Taylor deviates of $g(\hat{\mu}_j, \hat{p}_j)$ for unit hai.

Example 2.1 Estimating disparity in child and adolescent obesity among SES groups from NHANES: Lin, Yu and Zhang (2018)[220]

SES Group	Sample-Weighted Results		Unweighted Results	
	Obesity Prevalence (Proportion)	Population Share	Obesity Prevalence (Proportion)	Population Share
Low SES	0.206	0.250	0.203	0.348
SES group 2	0.203	0.242	0.207	0.271
SES group 3	0.169	0.275	0.176	0.222
High SES	0.110	0.233	0.100	0.159

Abbreviation: SES, socioeconomic status.

FIGURE 2.2: (Taken from Lin, Yu and Zhang (2018)[220]): Obesity prevalence estimates by SES group.

analyzed data from the National Health and Nutritional Examination Survey (NHANES) survey from 2011 to 2016 of 9016 individuals to estimate disparities in obesity rates between socioeconomic (SES) groups. They defined SES as family poverty ratio and created 4 SES groups ($0-100\%$ of federal poverty level, 101–200% of federal poverty level, 201–400% of federal poverty level and >400% of federal poverty level). Obesity was defined as a body mass index (BMI) greater than or equal to the 95th percentile adjusted for age and sex based on the 2000 CDC growth charts (NCHS, 2018).

NHANES uses a stratified multistage cluster design with oversampling of some socioeconomic groups. Figure 2.2 from Lin, Yu and Zhang (2018) shows the weighted versus unweighted estimates of obesity prevalence by SES group. Weighted and unweighted estimates are similar across SES groups but population shares are not. Groups with lower SES tend to be oversampled. Also note that Low SES and SES group 2 appear to have similar prevalence estimates (0.206 and 0.203, respectively). Figure 2.3 shows 11 indices that provide point estimates of disparity across the 4 SES groups and 95% CIs. For comparison, [220] also includes estimates and CIs for simple random sampling which fails to incorporate sampling weights. This results in biased point estimates. In addition, by assuming i.i.d. sampling and constant population shares, the standard errors are consistently smaller which leads to shorter 95% CIs.

2.3 Randomized experiments: an idealized estimate of disparity

Here we discuss an idealized estimate of disparity which often is not realizable in practice. The goal is to estimate a causal effect between levels of a focus variable f. This effect represents precisely the disparity that we are interested in. Here we describe this effect and an idealized estimate based on randomization. For details beyond our exposition, [319] provides a very nice summary discussion of these ideas.

HD*Calc Measure	NHANES Design		Simple Random Sampling Design	
	Estimate (SE)	95% CI	Estimate (SE)	95% CI
Absolute measures				
RD	0.003 (0.016)	−0.029, 0.034	0.004 (0.011)	−0.019, 0.024
BGV	0.001 (0.000)	0.001, 0.002	0.001 (0.000)	0.001, 0.002
ACI	−0.019 (0.003)	−0.025, −0.014	−0.017 (0.002)	−0.024, −0.015
SII	−0.125 (0.019)	−0.163, −0.087	−0.107 (0.014)	−0.152, −0.098
Relative measures				
RR	1.013 (0.080)	0.856, 1.171	0.979 (0.052)	0.911, 1.115
IDisp	21.836 (5.012)	12.012, 31.660	21.977 (2.374)	17.182, 26.489
MLD	0.028 (0.010)	0.007, 0.048	0.028 (0.006)	0.016, 0.040
Theil index	0.025 (0.009)	0.008, 0.043	0.024 (0.005)	0.016, 0.035
RCI	−0.113 (0.019)	−0.150, −0.076	−0.091 (0.012)	−0.136, −0.090
RII	−0.722 (0.121)	−0.960, −0.484	−0.591 (0.075)	−0.870, −0.575
KMI	2.131 (0.298)	1.547, 2.714	1.839 (0.152)	1.833, 2.429

Abbreviations: ACI, absolute concentration index; BGV, between-group variance; CI, confidence interval; HD*Calc, Health Disparities Calculator; IDisp, index of disparity; KMI, Kunst-Mackenbach index; MLD, mean log deviation; NHANES, National Health and Nutrition Examination Survey; RCI, relative concentration index; RD, rate difference; RII, relative index of inequality; RR, rate ratio; SE, standard error; SII, slope index of inequality.

FIGURE 2.3: (Taken from Lin, Yu and Zhang (2018)[220]): Various disparity index point estimates and 95% CIs. Left-hand side is based on the NHANES sampling design; right hand side assumes simple random sampling only.

Notationally, let's assume our focus variable f has two levels $f = 0, 1$, and our goal is to estimate the causal effect between the two "exposures". This is the average difference between an outcome y at each level of f. If this difference is not 0, then it represents a disparity. Following [319], let's begin with a situation where one sampling unit is exposed to $f = 0$ and another to $f = 1$. The disparity would be

$$\delta = 1/2[y_1(f = 1) - y_1(f = 0) + y_2(f = 1) - y_2(f = 0)],$$

which cannot be directly realized since each unit was exposed to either $f = 0$ or $f = 1$. Hence, an estimate of the disparity could be $y_1(f = 1) - y_2(f = 0)$ or $y_2(f = 1) - y_1(f = 0)$ depending on which unit was assigned to $f = 0$. Neither of these is actually close to the disparity for either unit. However, if the units were randomly assigned to exposure levels, then it's equally likely to observe either estimate. Thus the average effect is

$$\hat{\delta}_r = 1/2[y_1(f = 1) - y_2(f = 0)] + 1/2[y_2(f = 1) - y_1(f = 0)],$$

which precisely is the disparity. Thus randomization produces an unbiased disparity estimate. This logic extends naturally when n units are randomly exposed to each of $f = 0$ and $f = 1$ (call it $\hat{\delta}_{rn}$). When additional potential confounding variables may exist $x_j; j = 1, \ldots, p$, then randomization still produces an unbiased estimate of disparity. Why? Due to randomization, it's equally to see x_j in half of the equally likely unit allocations as it is to see $-x_j$. Thus averaged over all allocated units, the x_j has no effect on the disparity estimate. Specifically,

$$\hat{\delta}_{rn}(x_j) = 1/n \sum_{i \in f=1} [y_i(f=1) - x_{ij}] - 1/n \sum_{i \in f=0} [y_i(f=0) - x_{ij}] = \hat{\delta}_{rn},$$

remains an unbiased estimate of disparity over the randomization set.

2.4 Model-based estimation: adjusting for confounders

When data are observational in that either randomization did not occur or was not possible, then statistical adjustments for potential confounding must be used. Randomization not taking place is common but what about randomization not being possible? In disparity studies, it's not uncommon to be interested in disparities between levels of the exposure f for which randomization cannot happen. Examples include race, ethnicity, age, etc.

In this section, we assume that data are captured at the individual level only and our goal is to estimate group differences whilst adjusting for other covariates which may differ across the groups. Two primary approaches are considered – the regression approach and the Peters-Belson approach ([119]). There are subtle differences between the two in setup and in interpretation.

2.4.1 Regression approach

Notationally, let y_i be the outcome measured on the ith individual with accompanying grouping (or focus) variable f_i and individual level covariate $p-$vector x_i. For now we assume simple that the focus variable has only two levels. For the regression approach, we assume fit the linear model

$$y_i = x_i'\alpha + f_i\delta + e_i,$$

where α and δ are the unknown regression parameters and e_i the random errors. Normality assumptions on the errors are allowed but not necessary. Independence of the errors is usually assumed for these models. Constancy of variance for the errors can easily be relaxed via heteroscedastic regression techniques. Given a sample of n independent such observations, least squares or maximum likelihood estimation is used to estimate the regression parameters and error variance. Specifically, re-write the parameter vector as $\beta = (\alpha, \delta)$

and $\tilde{x}_i = (x_i, f_i)$ as the concatenated covariate vector containing both individual level and group indicator variables and $\tilde{X}$ to indicate the $n \times (p+1)$ full design matrix. Then $y_i = \tilde{x}_i'\beta + e_i$. Parameter estimation yields,

$$\hat{\beta} = (\tilde{X}'\tilde{X})^{-1}\tilde{X}'y.$$

Thus $\hat{\delta} = \hat{\beta}_{p+1}$ gives the estimate of disparity in outcome between the focus variable levels conditional on the other covariates x. When the focus variable has more than two levels, this can be accommodated by specifying a baseline or reference level (group) and using dummy variables for each of the other levels. Corresponding parameter estimates would be interpreted as disparity estimates between a focus variable level and the reference level. Furthermore, statistical contrasts could be estimated which allow for model-based estimation of disparities between other combinations of levels.

Confounding between x and f can be made more explicit by considering the following two linked equations:

$$logit(P(f_i = 1|x_i)) = x_i'\eta,$$

where η is the linear predictor unknown parameter vector and

$$y_i = x_i'\alpha + f_i\delta + e_i.$$

The first equation indicates that the probability of being level $f = 1$ is a function of covariates x and the second equation is the response function above. The fact that x appears in both indicates that there is clear confounding between x and f in terms of predicting y.

2.4.1.1 Model-assisted survey regression

For complex surveys, the regression model is taken to be a working model used to motivate estimators of finite population totals and is not assumed to hold. The covariates are considered ancillary data and one way to use these is to compute model-assisted estimators of finite population totals by specifying a working model for the mean of y given the covariates x and then use this model to predict y values (reference). These linear working models can lead to classical survey post-stratification, ratio, and regression estimators. These are all considered special cases of generalized regression estimation (GREG). Solutions for regression parameter estimation take into account the complex sampling design namely,

$$\hat{\beta}_s = argmin_{\beta}(y_s - \tilde{X}_s\beta)'\varpi_s^{-1}(y_s - \tilde{X}_s\beta) = (\tilde{X}_s'\varpi_s^{-1}\tilde{X}_s)^{-1}\tilde{X}_s'\varpi_s^{-1}y_s,$$

where $\tilde{X}_s = [\tilde{x}_i']_{i\in s}$, $y_s = [y_i]_{i\in s}$ and $\varpi_s = diag(\pi_i)_{i\in s}$ is a diagonal matrix of inclusion probabilities.

2.4.2 Peters-Belson approach

A second approach is the Peters-Belson method ([63]). Rather than use a model-based estimate of disparity directly, it uses the observed difference between focus variable levels. Since some of this observed difference is likely due to differences in individual-level variables between focus variable levels, the difference is then partitioned into what is explained by the individual level variables and what is left unexplained.

To estimate these portions, we again fit a regression model as above but now only to members of the so-called assumed advantaged level. This model incorporates individual-level covariates. We then take this fitted model and apply it to the observations in other focus variable levels *at the same covariate values* (regression prediction). These predicted outcomes are compared to the observed outcomes from the advantaged group.

Specifically, we'll write the linear model more generally as $s(x, f)$ to indicate dependence on x and f. Let $\hat{y}(f = 0) = \hat{s}(x, f = 0)$ indicate the vector of fitted values of the model fit to the data of the assumed advantaged group only. Then $\hat{y}(f = 1) = \hat{s}(x, f = 1)$ is the vector model predicted values for the $f = 1$ level. Hence $\hat{\delta} = mean(y(f = 1) - \hat{y}(f = 1))$ gives a point estimate of disparity explained by the individual level covariates. A formal statistical test can be conducted to draw conclusions about whether this disparity is statistically significant or not (more below). The Peters-Belson approach imposes certain restrictions by design: i) the choice of the model for the advantaged group is assumed to be appropriate for all other groups including the functional forms of the predictors and ii) there are no measured predictors that were excluded from the model for the advantaged group but which are important for predicting outcomes in the other groups.

Each of the regression method or the Peters-Belson method brings with it advantages and disadvantages. For the Peters-Belson approach, partitioning disparity into an explained and unexplained portion is more intuitive and generalizations to other types of outcomes and multiple levels is intuitively straightforward. However it requires multiple fits of the model on separate portions of the data. When sample sizes are small for the assumed advantaged level, this can lead to inefficient and unreliable predictions. For the regression approach, the interpretation of the disparity estimate is conditional on the other covariates in the model. There is an implicit assumption in both approaches the underlying model is correctly specified for all levels of the focus variable. In order to confirm this, various diagnostic methods can be run ([63]).

2.4.2.1 Peters-Belson approach for complex survey data

Li, Graubard, Huang and Gastwirth (2015)[219] applied the Peters-Belson approach to estimate disparities across multiple groups using complex survey data. In their case, they focused on binary outcomes and logistic regression (see later). To adjust for the complex survey design, they used (sample) weighted estimates of observed and predicted probabilities (proportions) for each group for of an outcome of interest. They fit appropriate binomial, multinomial or proportional odds logistic regression models to accommodate the multiple groups being compared. Model coefficients were estimated by maximizing a sample weighted pseudo-likelihood. For variance estimation of disparity estimates, they used Taylor linearization or leave-one-out jackknifing and then conducted Wald-type hypothesis tests against a composite null of no disparities across groups being compared.

2.4.2.2 Peters-Belson approach for clustered data

When clustering is present in the data, one can account for this using stratification, adding additional cluster-specific fixed effects, and the use of random effects. Stratification requires sufficient sample sizes within each stratum ([88]). The addition of random effects can complicate matters with regard to predicting responses for the disadvantaged groups since it's unclear how best to handle the random effects when generating predictions for new observations. However, as we will see in Chapter 6, some new methods on classified mixed model prediction (CMMP) ([178]) may provide a path forward.

2.4.3 Disparity drivers

The Peters-Belson approach does not reveal which covariates are contributing most to the estimated disparity. The approach can be exploited further to elucidate this. It relies on the fact that $\hat{\delta} = \hat{y}(f = 1) - \hat{y}(f = 0)$ and be written as $\hat{\delta} = x_i'(\hat{\beta} + \hat{\gamma}) - x_i'\hat{\beta}$ where $\hat{\gamma}$ is the estimated covariate effect *shift* due to being in the disadvantaged group.

So now, we can make use of the data enriched regression method of [54] or the extended version of this known as the data shared lasso of [123] to directly provide estimates of γ. Some additional notation is needed.

Assume our sample of data consists of (x_i, y_i, f_i) where $f \in 0, 1$ indicates focus group level membership. We assume the following model structure,

$$y_i = x_i'\beta + e_i; i \in f = 0,$$

and

$$y_i = x_i'(\beta + \gamma) + e_i; i \in f = 1,$$

where $var(e_i|f = 0) = \sigma_0^2$ and $var(e_i|f = 1) = \sigma_1^2$. To keep exposition consistent, let's assume that the error variances in the two groups are equal ($\sigma_0^2 = \sigma_1^2 = \sigma_2$). Then we estimate β and γ by minimizing

$$\sum_{i \in f=0} (y_i - x_i'\beta)^2 + \sum_{i \in f=1} (y_i - x_i'(\beta + \gamma))^2 + \lambda P(\gamma).$$

The first part of the above objective function is the pooled sum of squares of error from the above two models. The second part is a penalty applied to the γ only. The penalization tuning parameter is λ. It is assumed that $\lambda \in [0, \infty]$ and $P(\gamma) \geq 0$. A most interesting choice for $P(\gamma)$ is $||\gamma||_1$ which is the $L1$ norm penalty. The solution for γ would then yield what are termed lasso ([352]) estimates of γ. The lasso penalty imposes a size constraint on γ and also provides the opportunity for the γ_j solutions to be shrunken to zero.

The penalty tuning parameter λ is interesting in its own right. Setting $\lambda = 0$ leads to separate fits $\hat{\beta}$ and $\hat{\beta} + \hat{\gamma}$ in the two groups. Taking $\lambda = \infty$ constrains $\hat{\gamma} = 0$ and is the same as pooling the groups. Chen *et al.* (2015)[54] have a much more detailed discussion of this framework from the perspective of borrowing strength for prediction across two datasets – one of which may be larger or more expensive to collect than the other.

Gross and Tibshirani (2016)[123] describe the data shared lasso which generalizes data enriched regression to allow more than two groups. It also assumes a slightly different formulation. For the case above with only two groups, the following underlying models is assumed

$$y_i = x_i'(\beta + \gamma_0) + e_i; i \in f = 0,$$

and

$$y_i = x_i'(\beta + \gamma_1) + e_i; i \in f = 1,$$

where $var(e_i|f = 0) = \sigma_0^2$ and $var(e_i|f = 1) = \sigma_1^2$. Again, for simplicity, assume these are equal. Now each group's covariate effects are assumed shifted from some pooled overall value β. They solve the following optimization problem:

$$(\hat{\beta}, \hat{\gamma}_0, \hat{\gamma}_1) = argmin \frac{1}{2} \sum_i (y_i - x_i'(\beta + \gamma_{f_i}))^2 + \lambda(||\beta||_1 + \sum_{f=0}^{1} r_f ||\gamma_f||_1).$$

Unequal error variances can be incorporated as weights in the first part of the penalized least squares objective function. Here the parameters r_0 and r_1 control the degree of sharing between data at the two levels (a type of fusion penalty). That is, the can work to move the γ values closer together – at the extreme making them the same and hence pooling the data entirely across levels and hence identifying no disparity drivers. Gross and Tibshirani (2016)[123] detail a data augmentation approach for fitting. Define,

$$Z = \begin{pmatrix} X_0 & r_0 X_0 & 0 \\ X_1 & 0 & r_1 X_1 \end{pmatrix}.$$

Let $\tilde{y} = (y_0, y_1)'$ and $\tilde{\beta} = (\beta', \frac{1}{r_0}\gamma_0', \frac{1}{r_1}\gamma_1')'$. A lasso fit of $\tilde{y}$ on Z yields a potential solution. Beyond the model formulation difference to data enriched regression, the data shared lasso penalizes both β and γ_f. Now that everything has be mapped to a standard lasso framework, efficient estimation algorithms ([99]) can be used. These are readily available for instance in the **glmnet** package in R. Note that not all parameters are penalized by default. The intercept for instance is not and glmnet uses mean centering to estimate it outside of the penalized optimization step ([99]). The interesting part of this type of an analysis is that not only can disparity drivers be identified amongst the covariates, but focusing on matching covariate patterns between the two groups is not necessary since the same regression relationship is assumed across the range of x.

Example 2.2 Racial disparity in age of smoking onset based on National Longitudinal Mortality study: We will use the tobacco-use data from the National Longitudinal Mortality Study (NLMS), which has a maximum follow-up time of 5 years and consists of data centered around the year 2000. There are 493,282 records from the tobacco use file. For illustration purposes, we only focus on completed cases with no missing value, which results in 718 cases. There are 653 White population, 48 Black population, 1 American Indian or Alaskan Native, 9 Asian or Pacific Islander, and 7 other non-Whites. We use a log transformation of their smoking age as our response variable (i.e., the age at which they began smoking). The transformation makes the response variable approximately normal. The output below shows the covariates we used as the fixed effects in the model. Figure 2.4 shows boxplots for smoking age by racial group. We can see that when Blacks (race=2) have higher median smoking age than Whites (race=1). The following R output shows the linear model fit on the Black subpopulation only:

```
Coefficients:
              Estimate Std. Error t value Pr(>|t|)
(Intercept)  3.068e+00  1.972e-01  15.560   <2e-16 ***
age          5.205e-05  2.596e-03   0.020   0.9841
wt          -1.147e-04  1.469e-04  -0.781   0.4301
hhnum       -3.407e-02  1.846e-02  -1.845   0.0719 .
follow      -2.092e-05  5.435e-05  -0.385   0.7022
---
Signif. codes:  0 ?***? 0.001 ?**? 0.01 ?*? 0.05 ?.? 0.1 ? ? 1

Residual standard error: 0.234 on 43 degrees of freedom
Multiple R-squared:  0.08749,   Adjusted R-squared:  0.002611
F-statistic: 1.031 on 4 and 43 DF,  p-value: 0.4024
```

A naive examination of this would indicate that the hhnum variable is marginally significant but that none of the other covariates are. But this conclusion says little about disparity drivers since this determination is not based on disparity (i.e., it does not use the $y(f = 1)$ values).

A Peters-Belson analysis reveals the disparity estimate between Blacks and Whites using the individual level covariates listed in Table 2.1 is -0.108 years meaning Whites age of smoking onset is estimated to be lower than Blacks based on a Peters-Belson analysis. Note that no exact matches between Black and White individuals was found and hence a nearest neighbor propensity score matching (see next section) was used. Figure 2.5 shows boxplots of the

TABLE 2.1: NLMS tobacco use covariates

Number	Variable	Description
1	age	age at time of survey
2	wt	adjusted weight using age-sex-race group totals by state
3	hhnum	number of persons residing in household at time of interview
4	follow up	length of follow up period in days

four covariates after matching indicating that the covariate distributions are reasonably well balanced. A histogram of the differences between observed and predicted values for the matched samples is shown in Figure 2.6. The disparity estimate is indicated by the red vertical line.

Suppose now we want to identify disparity drivers using the data sharing lasso. Figure 2.7 reveals a trace plot from the lasso fit (see Friedman, Hastie and Tibshirani date for more on traceplots). Each line corresponds to a particular $\hat{\beta}_j$ (labeled 1-4), $\hat{\gamma}_{0j}$ (labeled 5-8) or $\hat{\gamma}_{1,j}$ (labeled 9-12) estimated value as a function of the amount of shrinkage applied. Typically what is done is to draw a vertical line at a given amount of appropriate shrinkage (i.e., a given value for the L1 norm). This can be done using cross-validation for instance. So if a cutoff of L1norm $= 0.04$ is used say, then variable numbers 1, 9, 4, 3 and 6 would be the only ones estimated as non-zero. Of these, variable 6 is $\hat{\gamma}_{03}$ and variable 9 is $\hat{\gamma}_{11}$. These correspond to a unique effect for Whites on wt

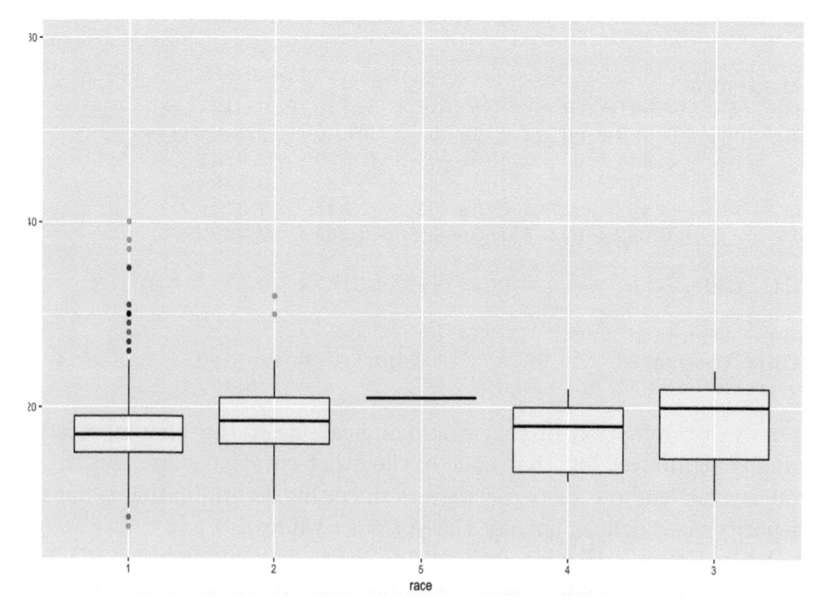

FIGURE 2.4: Boxplots of raw smoking age response by race.

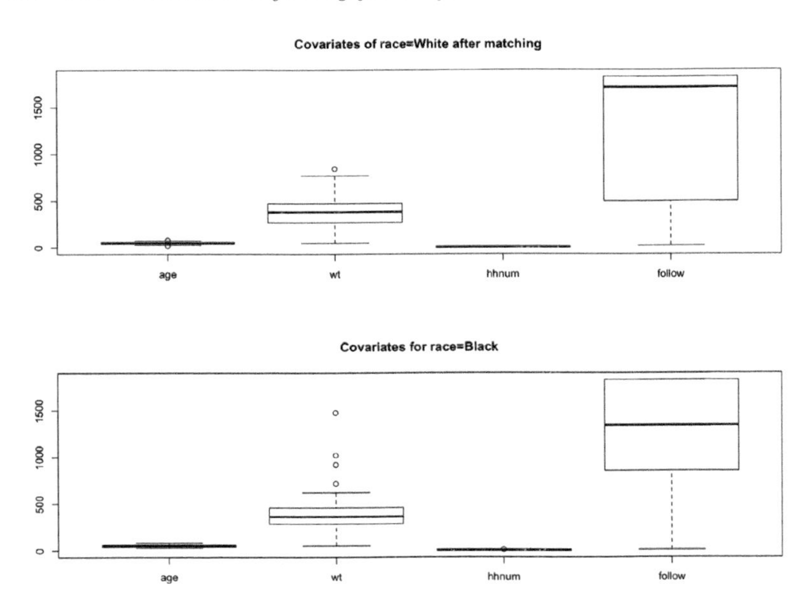

FIGURE 2.5: Histogram of Black-White differences in age of smoking based on Peters-Belson analysis.

and a unique effect for Blacks on age (above and beyond the overall estimated effects $\hat{\beta}$). Thus smoking age increases with increasing age in Blacks, whereas smoking age decreases with increasing weight in Whites. Taken together, this would indicate that weight and age could be candidate disparity drivers.

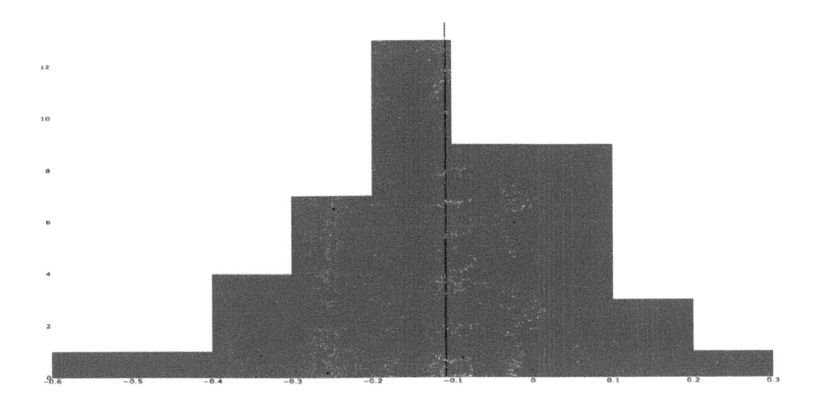

FIGURE 2.6: Histogram of Black-White differences in age of smoking based on Peters-Belson analysis.

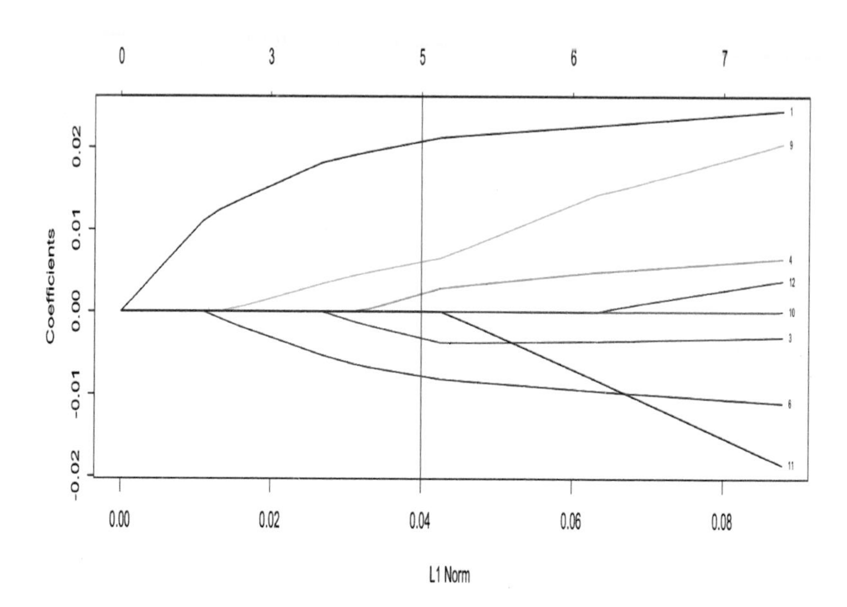

FIGURE 2.7: Disparity driver traceplots for NLMS data.

2.4.3.1 Disparity drivers for complex survey data

For complex survey data, one can make use of the survey regression estimation with lasso as described in McConville *et al.* (2017). To do so, we simply define $\tilde{y}^* = \varpi_s^{-1/2}\tilde{y}_s$ and $\tilde{Z}_s^* = \varpi_s^{-1/2}Z_s$ where $\tilde{y}_s$ and $\tilde{Z}_s$ incorporate the square root of the design weights $d_i = \pi^{-1}$. Then standard lasso fitting algorithms like that found in glmnet in R can be used to estimate the survey regression parameters.

2.5 Matching and propensity scoring

Let's return to the ideal causal effect of disparity and the case where we have two units one being exposed to $f = 0$ and the other to $f = 1$. Recall that we could naively estimate disparity as $y_1(f = 1) - y_2(f = 0)$ or $y_2(f = 1) - y_1(f = 0)$ (i.e., no randomization). Suppose now that the two units respond very similarly. In other words, there is some significant correlation in the way their outcome values. Then we say that the two units are closely matched with respect to the effects of the two exposures. Then both individual naive estimates of disparity are approximately equal and thus their average is approximately equal to δ. Taken to the limit, if the two units respond identically, then this approximation is exact. Thus matching has a beneficial effect irrespective of randomization. It should be clear then that the Peters-Belson method utilizes a form of matching.

In general, matching produces greater balance between covariate distributions for the levels of f. One caveat of matching is that it may become challenging when many potential confounders are present. Propensity scores ([313, 171]) can facilitate matching (and other methods of analysis). Propensity scores are defined as the probability that a unit will be in $f = 1$ given its set of covariates x_i. This naturally relies on a suitable model typically fit as a logistic regression, but should such a plausible model exist, then matching can be reduced from examining p covariates to examining a univariate propensity score. An illustration of this can be found in [372]. They examined a combined dataset from the U.S. National Alcohol Survey (NAS) which were two comparable probability samples of U.S. adults generated using computer-assisted telephone interviews based on random dialing. The data of interest was on so-called *at risk* drinkers defined in terms of their alcohol consumption and relationship to ethnicity which was self-identified. Demographics and SES covariates were collected and considered confounders. Effect modifiers included gender, age, education, annual household income and health insurance coverage. The outcome of interest was whether a subject had one or more primary care visits in the prior year.

Propensity score stratification was done by first estimating propensity scores via a logistic regression model using gender, age, education, annual household income and health insurance coverage as covariates. Here propensity scores were defined as the probability of being Hispanic versus White. Estimated scores were then stratified into quintiles depending on what was considered the *reference sample*. Table 2.2 shows the results when the combined Whites/Hispanics were treated as the reference sample. Here the pooled sample is divided into 5 equal-sized strata based on the sorted score

TABLE 2.2: (Adapted from Ye et al. (2012)[372]): Illustration of propensity score matching. The table shows the odds ratio estimates by propensity score strata when the combined Whites/Hispanics are used as a reference sample.

PS Stratum (ordered by propensity for being Hispanic)	Group	N	Odds ratio
1	White	751	1.56
	Hispanic	43	
2	White	571	1.04
	Hispanic	58	
3	White	581	1.38
	Hispanic	97	
4	White	553	1.83
	Hispanic	141	
5	White	342	3.39
	Hispanic	345	
Overall	White	2798	1.57 (1.23, 2.00)
	Hispanic	684	

distribution. The table shows the effect estimates both overall and within each stratum. Larger odds ratio (Whites vs Hispanic) (i.e., disparity estimates) were observed for strata with higher score estimates.

The usual cautionary note for all statistical adjustments is that their effectiveness relies on the assumption of no unobserved confounders and correct model specifications (including functional form). More details on the underlying methodology of particular matching strategies will be discussed in Chapter 4.

2.6 Discrete outcomes

For binary, count and other discrete outcomes, the regression approach can be extended by using generalized linear models (GLMs) ([242]). Disparity estimates then become more explicitly differences in model-predicted outcomes between focus variable levels ([87]).

A GLM contains a three-layered specification: i) the random component, ii) a systematic component and, iii) a link function between the two. The random component describes the variability in y. For the normal linear model, this is a location-scale model and does not depend on the mean. For non-normal outcomes, the GLM employs unification under the exponential family of distributions which contain the normal, Poisson, binomial, gamma, inverse gaussian, etc as members and has form,

$$f(y;\theta,\psi) = exp\{(y\theta - b(\theta))/a(\psi) + c(y,\psi)\},$$

for known functions $a(\cdot), b(\cdot)$, and $c(\cdot)$. For known ψ, this represents an exponential-family model with canonical parameter θ. Let $l(\theta,\psi;y)$ be the log-likelihood function which is defined for given y. Following [242], the mean and variance of the response can be derived as $E(Y) = \mu = b'(\theta)$ and $var(Y) = b''(\theta)a(\psi)$.

A link function g connects the linear predictor $\eta = \tilde{x}'\beta$ to the expected value μ. Canonical links are situations where $\theta = \eta$. Iteratively re-weighted least squares (IRLS) (equivalently maximum likelihood) techniques ([242]) can be used for estimating regression parameters. Predicted focus variable level differences are estimated by taking the g^{-1} transformation at a particular set of individual level covariates $\tilde{x}$ (which recall contains the focus variable f). Thus the interpretation of disparity between levels is once again conditional on the particular values of x. Inference on the focus variable (comparison between levels) is based on either a likelihood ratio tests (LRT), a score test or a Wald-like test ([242]). Goodness of fit using deviance functions or Pearson's χ^2 statistics are usually readily derivable.

2.6.1 Binary outcomes

Let's consider the case of a binary outcome with $\mu = E(y|x) = P(y = 1|x) = p(x)$. Then the model being fit can be a logistic regression model (amongst others) in which the mean of the responses μ is modeled as,

$$g(\mu) = \tilde{x}'\beta,$$

where g is the link function that links the mean μ to the linear predictor $x'\beta$. For ease of discussion, let's assume we only have a single covariate in x. To ensure that $p(x)$ is restricted to be in $[0, 1]$, we can model it using a cumulative distribution function,

$$p(x) = \int_{-\infty}^{x} f(s)ds,$$

where $f(s) \geq 0$ and $int_{-\infty}^{\infty} f(s)ds = 1$. The probability distribution $f(s)$ is called the tolerance distribution. Well-known models for binary outcomes arise by different specifications of this tolerance distribution. For example, if $f(s)$ is a $N(\mu, \sigma^2)$, the $p(x) = \phi(\frac{x-\mu}{\sigma})$ where ϕ is the cumulative probability function for a $N(0, 1)$ distribution. Therefore,

$$\phi^{-1}(p(x)) = \beta_0 + \beta_1 x,$$

where $\beta_0 = -\mu/\sigma$ and $\beta_1 = 1/\sigma$. This is called the probit regression model. However, if

$$f(s) = \frac{\beta_1 exp(\beta_0 + \beta_1 s)}{[1 + exp(\beta_0 + \beta_1 s)]^2},$$

this gives,

$$p(x) = \int_{-\infty}^{x} f(s)ds = \frac{exp(\beta_0 + \beta_1 x)}{1 + exp(\beta_0 + \beta_1 x)}.$$

This gives the logit link function $g(\mu) = logit(p(x)) = log(p(x)/(1-p(x))$ with $p(x) = \frac{exp(x'\beta)}{1+exp(x'\beta)}$ and is the basis of logistic regression. Here the regression parameter estimates are interpreted as log odds-ratios on the logit scale.

Other popular tolerance distributions exist. For instance, if $f(s)$ is the extreme value distribution,

$$f(s) = \beta_1 exp[(\beta_0 + \beta_1 s) - exp(\beta_0 + \beta_1 s)],$$

then $p(x) = 1 - exp[-exp(\beta_0 + \beta_1 x)]$ so thus $log[-log(1 - p(x))] = \beta_0 + \beta_1 x$.

This is called the complementary log-log link function and behaves similarly to the logistic and probit models for values of $p(x)$ near 0.5 but differs from them for values near 0 or 1. The extension to multiple covariates in x is then straightforward.

2.6.2 Nominal and ordinal outcomes

Consider now the situation where the response y has J unordered categories. This is called a nominal random variable. Let $p_1, \ldots, p_J$ denote the probabilities for each in the population with $\sum_{j=1}^{J} p_j = 1$. Thus for n independent observations in sample, y_1 outcomes in category 1, y_2 in category 2 up until y_J in category J. The joint probability distribution is then a multinomial distribution for which the Binomial distribution is a special case when $J = 2$. The nominal logistic regression model is used when there is no natural ordering to the categories and one category is chosen as the reference category. Let's say that $j = 1$ is the reference. Then logits for the other categories can be defined as,

$$logit(p_j(x)) = log(p_j/p_1) = x'_j\beta_j; j = 2, \ldots, J.$$

All $(J-1)$ logits are used to estimate the β_j parameters. Once these have been estimated, then one can calculate,

$$\hat{p}_j = \hat{p}_1 exp(x'_j\hat{\beta}_j), j = 2, \ldots, J.$$

Since $\sum_{j=1}^{J} \hat{p}_j = 1$, this allows back calculation for $\hat{p}_1$.

When y has J ordered categories, ordinal logistic regression can be used. This can take the form of a cumulative logit model, proportional odds model or continuation ratio logit model ([78]). The cumulative logit model assumes,

$$log\frac{p_1 + \ldots + p_j}{p_{j+1} + \ldots + p_J} = x'_j\beta_j.$$

The proportional odds model assumes,

$$log\frac{p_1 + \ldots + p_j}{p_{j+1} + \ldots + p_J} = \beta_{0j} + \beta_1 x_1 + \ldots + \beta_{p-1}x_{p-1},$$

which assumes that only the intercept β_{0j} depends on j. It's based on the assumption that the covariate effects are the same for all categories on the logarithmic scale.

2.6.3 Poisson regression and log-linear models

If y is the number of occurrences, the probability distribution function can be written as,

$$f(y) = \frac{\mu^y e^{-\mu}}{y!}, y = 0, 1, 2, \ldots.$$

Here, μ is the average number of occurrences, and $E(y) = Var(y) = \mu$. Often μ is described as a rate. For example, the number of cancers in a given time period, or the number of violent crimes per unit area. Generally speaking, the rate is specified in terms of units of exposure. Another example includes person-years at risk. The effect of the covariates on y is modeled through μ.

Two situations are described here – i) events relate to varying amounts of exposure which need to be taken into account and ii) exposure is constant and therefore not relevant to the model. The second scenario typically involves covariates that are categorial and hence the response is distributed across a cross-classified contingency table. Poisson regression is used for the first scenario and log linear models for the second.

For Poisson regression, we assume $E(y_i) = \mu_i = n_i\theta_i$. Here n_i is the exposure and i represents a particular covariate pattern. The dependence of θ_i on x is modeled by,

$$\theta_i = exp(x_i'\beta).$$

The natural link function is then,

$$log(\mu_i) = log(n_i) + x_i'\beta.$$

Here the $log(n_i)$ term is referred to as an offset (known constant) which gets incorporated into the estimation procedure for the regression parameters. For binary focus variables say $f = 0$ or $f = 1$ (embedded as part of the vector x), the corresponding regression coefficient represents the log relative risk of one level of f to the other.

The form of particular log-linear models derives the underlying contingency tables which describe the response variable as well as the constraints (or lack thereof) imposed on the table by experimental design. For instance, when there are no constraints on the values the y can take for any cell in a contingency table, then the joint pdf of the table can be represented by as the product of independent Poisson random variables with mean parameters μ_i. If the only constraint is that the sum of the y_i's is n, then a multinomial distribution can be used as the joint pdf. If there are more fixed marginals than just the overall total n, the product multinomial distributions are used to model the data.

However, all of the probability models are at their root, based on the Poisson distribution and in all cases μ_i can be transformed to be a function of the linear predictor via the log link function.

2.7 Survival analysis

Consider outcomes defined as the time from a well-defined starting point until some event (or failure) occurs. These duration times are known as survival times. A random variable describing such outcomes possesses some unique features – i) the times are non-negative and usually have skewed distributions with long tails and ii) not all individuals may have observable survival times and are described as censored. Various forms of censoring are possible including loss to follow-up or having another event type that prevents an individual from having the event of interest. Loss to follow-up can be due to reasons inherent in the study design (e.g., study window closed) or could be due to reasons completely outside of the study design.

If the survival time commenced before the study began, then the recorded survival time is denoted as left censored. Otherwise, losses to follow-up are typically considered right censored. It's also typical to assume that a random censoring mechanism is present and that the survival times for censored observations are independent from those of uncensored observations.

2.7.1 Survivor and hazard functions

If we let a random response y denote the survival time and $f(y)$ its pdf, then some important functions pertinent to survival analysis can be derived. Note that in many instances, it's typical to use t as the random variable indexing survival times. However, we choose to stick with y to stay consistent with previous notation as much as possible. We can first define the cumulative distribution function,

$$F(y) = \int_0^y f(t)dt.$$

The survivor function is the complement of this and quantifies the probability of survival beyond time y. This is given by,

$$S(y) = 1 - F(y).$$

The hazard function is the instantaneous risk of having an event which can also be expressed as the probability of having an event in an interval $[y, y + \delta]$ as $\delta \to 0$. This can be expressed mathematically as,

$$lim_{\delta \to 0} \frac{F(y + \delta) - F(y)}{\delta} \times \frac{1}{S(y)}.$$

The first part of the above equation is just $f(y)$. This then means that the hazard $h(y)$ can be also written as,

$$h(y) = \frac{f(y)}{S(y)},$$

or equivalently,

$$h(y) = -\frac{d}{dy}[log(S(y))].$$

Furthermore,

$$S(y) = exp(-\int_0^y h(t)dt).$$

The term inside the exponentiation is called the cumulative hazard function and is denoted $H(y)$.

The analysis of survival data has many nuances and procedures but we will focus on the most commonly used ones. These include parametric models where fully parametric assumptions are attached to y or the Cox proportional hazards model ([66]) which is a semi-parametric model that does not pre-specify a particular probability distribution for y. Advantages of the fully parametric specifications typically include more exact inference as well as a wider range of models to describe the data. Note that the also widely used accelerated failure time (AFT) model is classified as a parametric model.

2.7.2 Common parametric models

Commonly used parametric models include the exponential model, the Weibull model, and the AFT model. For the exponential model, y follows the exponential distribution,

$$f(y;\theta) = \theta e^{-\theta y},$$

where $\theta > 0$ is the parameter of the distribution and also $y \geq 0$. The cumulative distribution function is,

$$F(y;\theta) = \int_0^y \theta e^{-\theta y} = 1 - e^{-\theta y}.$$

Therefore,

$$S(y;\theta) = e^{-\theta y},$$

and

$$h(y;\theta) = \theta.$$

Thus the cumulative hazard $H(y;\theta) = \theta y$. Notice that the hazard function does not depend on y which means that the instantaneous risk is not related to how long someone has already survived. This is known as the memoryless property of the exponential distribution.

Covariates x are introduced into this model through the mean, namely $E(y) = 1/\theta$ through the relationship $\theta = e^{x'\beta}$ which ensures that $E(y)$ remains positive. Then the hazard function has multiplicative form $h(y;\beta) = \theta = e^{x'\beta}$. If considering a binary-valued focus variable f (contained as part of the vector x) which takes values 0 or 1, then the hazard ratio,

$$\frac{h_1(y;\beta)}{h_0(y;\beta)} = e^{\beta_f},$$

provided that the contribution from the other covariates is constant. Thus, $h_1(y;\beta) = h_0(y;\beta)e^{\beta_f}$. Models of this form are known as proportional hazards models and $h_0(y;\beta)$ is known as the baseline hazard function. Similarly the cumulative hazard functions are related by $logH_1(y;\beta) = logH_0(y;\beta) + \beta_f$.

Another widely used parametric model for survival outcomes is the Weibull model. Here, the pdf of y can be written as,

$$f(y;\lambda,\theta) = \frac{\lambda y^{\lambda-1}}{\theta^\lambda} exp(-(y/\theta)^\lambda), y \geq 0, \lambda > 0, \theta > 0.$$

The parameter λ is known as the shape parameter and θ the scale parameter. Note that when $\lambda = 1$, the Weibull distribution reduces back down to the exponential distribution. The survivor function is,

$$S(y;\lambda,\theta) = \int_0^y f(t)dt = exp(-\phi y^\lambda),$$

where $\phi = \theta^{-\lambda}$. Hence, $h(y;\lambda,\theta) = \lambda\phi y^{\lambda-1}$ and $H(y;\lambda,\theta) = \phi y^\lambda$. Thus the hazard function can be influenced by λ and can increase or decrease with y. This thus leads to the AFT model which is understood from the relation $logH(y;\lambda,\theta) = log\phi + \lambda logy$.

To introduce covariates x, we note that $E(y) = \phi^{-1}\Gamma(1 + 1/\lambda)$ where the gamma function is given by $\Gamma(u) = \int_0^\infty s^{u-1}e^{-s}ds$. This suggests that introducing x via ϕ in a multiplicative fashion is correct. Specifically if

$$\phi = \alpha e^{x'\beta},$$

then the hazard function is $h(y; \lambda, \theta) = \lambda \alpha y^{\lambda-1} e^{x'\beta}$. Once again a proportional hazards interpretation can be achieved for a binary valued focus variable f if the contribution of all other variables is constant between levels of the focus variable. Interestingly, the Weibull model is the only one that has features of the proportional hazards model and the AFT model.

2.7.3 Estimation

Data consists of the following: for the ith individual, we have the survival time y_i, a censoring indicator δ_i which takes the value 0 if individual i is censored and 1 otherwise, and a vector of covariates x_i which contains the focus variable f_i. In total, we assume we have a sample of n individuals with such data. We start by dividing the dataset into the$y_1, \ldots, y_r$ uncensored individuals and the $y_{r+1}, \ldots, y_n$ censored ones. Assuming all observations are independent, the likelihood function for the uncensored observations is,

$$\prod_{i=1}^{r} f(y_i).$$

For the censored individuals, we know that we know that the survival times are at least $y_i, i = r+1, \ldots, n$ and thus adding their contributions to the likelihood gives the full likelihood,

$$L = \prod_{i=1}^{n} f(y_i)^{\delta_i} S(y_i)^{1-\delta_i}.$$

The likelihood function (and the log likelihood function) depend on the covariates x through the linear predictor $x'\beta$ as described above. Thus maximum likelihood estimates of relevant parameters can be found typically using iterative numerical optimization methods like Newton-Raphson.
Remark:. Note that another approach to estimation exists based upon using Poisson regression. Take for example, exponential model. The full likelihood function is,

$$L(\theta; y) = \prod_{i=1}^{n} (\theta_i e^{-\theta_i y_i})^{\delta_i} (e^{-\theta_i y_i})^{1-\delta_i}.$$

The log likelihood function is then,

$$l(\theta; y) = \sum_{i=1}^{n} (\delta_i log\theta_i - \theta_i y_i).$$

If we consider the censoring indicators δ_i as random variables, then the expression on the right-hand side of the log likelihood function is proportional to the log likelihood function of n independent Poisson random variables with rate parameter $\theta_i y_i$. Thus as shown in Aitkin and Clayton (1980), since $E(\delta_i) = \mu_i = \theta_i y_i$, then $log(\mu_i) = log\theta_i + log y_i$. Thus the survival times are included as an offset in this Poisson regression model. A similar derivation is available for the Weibull model ([8]).

2.7.4 Inference

The estimation procedure used to get the maximum likelihood estimates also yields the information matrix which can be inverted to give the approximate variance-covariance matrix for the vector of estimated parameters. Thus inferential procedures can be based on Wald-type tests which take the ratio of $\hat{\beta}_f$ (where f reflects the focus variable) and the hypothesized value of β_f and the standard error of $\hat{\beta}_f$ (from the square root of the fth diagonal element of the inverted information matrix). This test statistic has an approximate $N(0, 1)$ sampling distribution which can be used to derive p-values or confidence intervals. Alternative forms of inference include likelihood ratio tests or score tests.

2.7.5 Non-parametric estimation of $S(y)$

While survivor functions can be derived based on fully parametric assumptions as above, it's often useful to relax those assumptions and estimate $S(y)$ non-parametrically. The most common estimator is the Kaplan-Meier estimate ([196]) (also called the product limit estimate). To do so, we first arrange the unique survival times from smallest to largest $y_{(1)}, \ldots, y_{(K)}$. Then let n_k be the number of subjects still at risk before time y_k and let d_k the number of events that occur at $y_{(k)}$. Thus the estimated probability of survival past $y_{(k)}$ is $(n_k - d_k)/n_k$. If the ordered survival times are independent, the Kaplan-Meier estimate of $S(y)$ is,

$$\hat{S}(y) = \prod_{k=1}^{K} \frac{(n_k - d_k)}{n_k}.$$

Kaplan-Meier survivor functions for each level of the focus variable f can also be estimated and then tested for equality using the log-rank or generalized Wilcoxon test. We will describe the log-rank test here for comparing 2 levels of the focus variable f. First order the K unique survival times from smallest to largest $y_{(1)}, \ldots, y_{(K)}$. Define $n_f(y_{(k)})$ as the number of individuals at risk for each level $f = 1, 2$. Also define the total number at risk at $y_{(k)}$ as $n(y_{(k)})$ and let d_{fk} be the number in level f who have the event at $y_{(k)}$ and d_k be the total number of events in all levels of f at $y_{(k)}$.

Define the expected value and variance of d_{1k} as,

$$E_k = \frac{n_1(y_{(k)})}{n(y_{(k)})} d_k,$$

$$V_k = \frac{n_0(y_{(k)})n_1(y_{(k)})d_k(n(y_{(k)}) - d_k)}{n(y_{(k)})^2(n(y_{(k)}) - 1)}.$$

Now let $O_{1k} = d_{1k}$ be the observed number of events at ordered time k. Then define the log-rank statistic,

$Z = \frac{O-E}{\sqrt{V}}$ where O, E and V are summed across all K time points. So we are combining 2×2 tables across all of the ordered time points into a Fishers'-style test which tests the null hypothesis of equality of empirical survival curves. The sampling distribution for this test statistic is typically approximated as a $N(0, 1)$ from which p-values can be derived. The generalized Wilcoxon test is simply a weighted log rank test that emphasizes certain times (late, early) more than others and enters these weights into both the numerator and denominator of the log rank statistic. Once again, a normal approximation to the sampling distribution is used for testing purposes. When more than 2 levels of f are under consideration, then the 2×2 tables generalize to $2 \times F$ tables aggregated over the K distinct ordered event times where F represents the total number of levels in f.

2.7.6 Cox proportional hazards model

To introduce additional covariates (continuous or otherwise), the log rank and related tests do not generalize. However, there may be a desire to steer away from fully parametric survival models as described earlier. So [66] developed the ingenious version of his proportional hazards model which is described as semi-parametric. Define the hazard function as,

$$h(y|x) = h_0(y)exp(x'\beta).$$

Here the covariates (which can include the focus variable f) are explicitly modeled in a multiplicative fashion through $x'\beta$ and do not depend on time. A so-called baseline hazard function $h_0(y)$ is added but remains unspecified and hence the model is termed semi-parametric. No constant term is added because it is absorbed into the baseline hazard function. Note that for two different individuals with different set of covariates x_1 and x_2, the ratio of the hazard functions is $exp(x_1'\beta)/exp(x_2'\beta)$ which does not depend on time. Hence this model is also a proportional hazards model. In fact, the model formulation is based on such an assumption.

For estimation, [66, 67] proposed a partial likelihood for β that does not involve $h_0(y)$. Suppose for individual i we observe the triple (y_i, δ_i, x_i). Now suppose there are K distinct event times that are ordered as above. To simplify the discussion, let's assume there are no ties for now. Now define the risk set $R(t) = \{i : y_i \geq t\}$. These are the set of individuals who are at risk to have an event at time t. From this concept, we can construct the partial likelihood as the product over the observed event times of conditional probabilities of seeing the observed event given the risk set at that time given that only one event is to happen. At each event time y_i, the contribution to the likelihood is,

$$\begin{aligned} L_i(\beta) &= P(\text{individual i has event}|\text{one event from } R(y_i)) \\ &= h(y_i|x_i)/\sum_{l \in R(y_i)} h(y_l|x_l). \end{aligned}$$

Accumulations from all distinct event times fills out the partial likelihood. Now invoking the proportional hazards assumption for incorporation of covariates $h(y|x) = h_0(y)exp(x'\beta)$, this can be plugged into the partial likelihood and numerical methods used to solve for $\hat{\beta}$. Inferential procedures include score tests and Wald tests among others ([195]).

Many adjustments for tied event times have been proposed. These include those of [66] which is termed the discrete method that assumes that tied even times truly happened at the same time. The exact method of [195] is based on the assumption that if there are ties, that is due to measurement error and that there must be some true ordering. All possible orderings of tied event times are calculated and probabilities of each are summed. Breslow and Peto's method ([39, 280]) approximated the discrete partial likelihood by modifying the denominator of the partial likelihood by raising the terms to a power corresponding to the number of events at $y_{(k)}$. Efron (1977)[89] suggested an even closer approximate to the discrete partial likelihood that like Breslow and Peto, will yield estimates of β that will be biased toward 0 when there are many ties, however, Efron's approximation is faster and yields less biased estimates.

Finally, once estimates of β are produced, then the baseline hazard can be estimated (or a function of it). One example is the baseline cumulative hazard function which reduces to the Nelson-Aalen ([3, 265]) estimator when there are no covariates.

2.8 Multi-level modeling

Multi-level modeling describes an analytical approach that models individual-level outcomes on group/area/context level covariates and individual level covariates at the same time. As [76] notes in an excellent review, this can be contrasted to traditional epidemiological studies which only use individual-level covariates and ecological studies which typically use only group level outcomes and group level covariates. The first of these assumes independence of observations and if this is violated, then incorrect inferences can result. The second of these focuses on between-group variation and eliminates the non-independence issue but ignores how individual-level covariates. Introducing group-level indicator variables into the first approach is similar to fitting separate regressions for each group and does not facilitate the elucidation of group characteristics that may explain the outcome. Multi-level analysis addresses many of these issues.

The analysis is described in terms of levels. In the first level, an individual level analysis is conducted:

$$y_{ij} = \beta_{0j} + x_{ij}\beta_{1j} + e_{ij}, \tag{2.1}$$

where $e_{ij} \sim N(0, \sigma^2)$. Here x_{ij} is an individual level variable for individual j in group i. The second level analysis focuses on group-specific covariates w_i in that,

$$\beta_{0i} = \gamma_{00} + \gamma_{01}w_i + \alpha_{0i}, \tag{2.2}$$

and,

$$\beta_{1i} = \gamma_{10} + \gamma_{11}w_i + \alpha_{1i}, \tag{2.3}$$

where $\alpha_{0i} \sim N(0, g_0)$ and $\alpha_{1i} \sim N(0, g_1)$. Hence the group-specific intercept and slopes are assumed to be random effects. We also allow $cov(\alpha_{0i}, \alpha_{1i}) = g_{01}$ which introduces a correlation between the random effects. The α_{0i} and α_{1i} are sometimes called macro errors. So in other words, we are saying that the group-specific intercept and slope randomly vary around some overall values as a function of group-specific covariates w_i.

We can combine these equations together giving,

$$y_{ij} = \gamma_{00} + \gamma_{01}w_i + \gamma_{10}x_{ij} + \gamma_{11}w_i x_{ij} + \alpha_{0i} + \alpha_{1i}x_{ij} + e_{ij}. \tag{2.4}$$

This is what is termed a mixed effects model which in addition to the random effects, includes fixed effects group-level variables, individual-level variables, and their interaction. Observations within groups are correlated because they share common random effects. Additionally, the variance of the responses y_{ij} is not constant because it depends on the variance of the random effects and x_{ij}. So the interpretation of the model can be had through the final combined equation or equivalently through examination of the component equations. Notice how the estimation of g_{01} and g_1 and how they change as individual-level or group-level covariates are introduced, allowing examination of between-group variability and the extent to which it's explained by individual and group level covariates. The multilevel model separates the effect of context and individuals.

2.8.1 Estimation and inference

Parameters to be estimated include the fixed effects regression coefficients and the variance components associated with the random effects and errors. Following distributional assumptions of the model, maximum likelihood estimation (ML) can be used. Let's first write the mixed effects model out more generally:

$$y_i = X_i\beta + z_i\alpha_i + e_i; i = 1, \ldots, m. \tag{2.5}$$

with $\alpha_i \sim N(0, G)$ and $e_i \sim N(0, R)$. We will for now assume that $R = \sigma^2 I_{n_i}$ and that the errors and random effects are independent. G and R are the covariance matrices of multivariate normal distributions and m is the total number of groups. The random effects help distinguish the group-specific mean and the marginal (population average) mean:

$$E(y_i|\alpha_i) = X_i\beta + z_i\alpha_i$$

versus

$$E(y_i) = X_i\beta.$$

The group-specific covariance is $cov(y_i|\alpha_i) = R$ and population average covariance is $cov(y_i) = V_i = z_i G z_i' + R$. Thus for each group we have

$$y_i \sim N(X_i\beta, V_i).$$

This permits full maximum likelihood estimation for the unknown parameters assuming independent groups (i.e., the full likelihood is the product of the group-specific components). Typically, V_i is parameterized by parameter vector ψ such that we can write $V_i = V_i(\psi)$.

Maximum likelihood estimates of the variance parameters ψ are known to be biased downwards due to the lack of acknowledgment of using up degrees of freedom when estimating the fixed effects parameters. This can sometimes provide negative estimates of variance components (reference). To avoid this, restricted (or residual) maximum likelihood (REML) can be used.

REML can be intuitively explained through a simple illustration. Let's consider estimation for the mean μ and variance σ^2 of a random sample from a normal distribution. Consider the following decomposition:

$$\sum_{i=1}^{n}(y_i - \mu)^2 = \sum_{i=1}^{n}[(y_i - \bar{y}) + (\bar{y} - \mu)]^2 = \sum_{i=1}^{n}(y_i - \bar{y})^2 + n(\bar{y} - \mu)^2.$$

Thus the log likelihood is,

$$logL = -\frac{n}{2}ln(2\pi) - \frac{n}{2}ln(\sigma^2) - \sum_{i=1}^{n}\frac{(y_i - \bar{y})^2}{2\sigma^2} - \frac{n(\bar{y} - \mu)^2}{2\sigma^2}.$$

This can be rewritten as

$$[-\frac{1}{2}ln(2\pi) - \frac{1}{2}ln(\sigma^2) - \frac{n(\bar{y} - \mu)^2}{2\sigma^2}] - [\frac{(n-1)}{2}ln(2\pi) + \frac{(n-1)}{2}ln(\sigma^2) + \sum_{i=1}^{n}\frac{(y_i - \bar{y})^2}{2\sigma^2}].$$

The first part is almost the log likelihood of the sample mean $\bar{y}$ and the second part does not depend on μ. This second part is known as the restricted or residual log likelihood. So to carry out maximization, the second part is maximized first with respect to σ^2, and then this value is plugged into the first part which is subsequently maximized with respect to μ. More generally, one has formed a set of linear contrasts of y that do not depend on the mean parameters but only the variance components.

For the linear mixed model, these are sometimes called error contrasts. More specifically, if vector a is orthogonal to all columns of X such that $a'X = 0$, then $E(a'y) = 0$. We can find $n - p$ such vectors that are linearly independent. So if we defined $A = (a_1, a_2, \ldots, a_{n-p})$, then $A'X = 0$ and $E(A'y) = 0$. A candidate for A is $S = I - X(X'X)^{-1}X'$. Additionally, here $AA' = S$ and $A'A = I$. Stacking all of the m groups observations together, we write out the linear mixed model as the general linear model,

$$y = X\beta + e,$$

where $var(e) = V(\psi)$. Then we note the error contrast vector

$$w = A'y = A'(X\beta + e) = A'e,$$

which is distributed as $N(0, A'V(\psi)A)$ and is free of β. Patterson and Thompson (1971) show that no information is lost about ψ when inference is based on w rather than on y. Thus, REML estimates for ψ can be found by maximizing the restricted log likelihood of w with respect to ψ. These can be plugged back into the generalized least squares solution for β namely, $\hat{\beta} = (X'V(\hat{\psi})X)^{-1}X'V(\hat{\psi})y$. Efficient methods for computing these estimates are based on numerical methods including the Newton-Raphson method or "scoring" algorithms (see [223, 283]).

Example 2.3 Multilevel analysis of variations in excess mortality among Black populations in Massachusetts:

Subramanian *et al.* (2005)[345] performed a multilevel analysis of all-cause mortality data in Massachusetts for the time period 1989–1991 where they explored racial disparities while adjusting for individual-level covariates (level 1) as well as the hierarchical effects of census tract (level 3) and block level

TABLE 2.3: (Adapted from Subramanian *et al.* (2005)[345]): Summary of the estimated variance components from Models 1, 2, and 3.

		Estimate (SE)	
Term	Model 1	Model 2	Model 3
		Between Census Tract Variation	
Constant/constant (σ^2_{v0})	0.095 (0.005)	0.085 (0.005)	0.066 (0.004)
Constant/Black (σ^2_{v0v1})		0.050 (0.015)	−0.017 (0.012)
Black/Black (σ^2_{v1})		0.337 (0.053)	0.158 (0.034)
Constant/other (σ^2_{v0v2})		0.054 (0.016)	−0.034 (0.013)
Black/other (σ^2_{v1v2})		0.136 (0.047)	0.028 (0.030)
Other/other (σ^2_{v2})		0.325 (0.064)	0.120 (0.040)
		Between Block Level Variation	
Constant/constant (σ^2_{u0})	0.111 (0.004)	0.111 (0.004)	0.108 (0.004)

(level 2) nested within census tract. Individual level covariates included age (as quintiles), race/ethnicity, and gender. Census tracts were characterized by the percentage of the population living below the poverty line (as quintiles). The response was defined as the number of deaths as a proportion of the total population in each cell. Cells were defined as cross-tabluations of age by gender by racial/ethnic categories. The focus of the analysis was on White-Black racial comparisons.

Three-level binomial logit mixed models were fit with over-dispersion being allowed in level 1. Three different models were entertained. Model 1 fit all three levels with fixed effects for age, gender and race/ethnicity as well as all second-order interactions. The random part included random intercepts for the census tract and block level within the census tract. This model allows for an examination of overall racial differences in mortality as well as the magnitude of variation in mortality across block levels and census tracts. Model 2 had the same fixed effects and random effects as Model 1, but also included an additional random slope for race at the census tract level. This model can further test the hypothesis of whether census tract level variation in mortality is different across racial groups. Model 3 extended Model 2 to include a fixed cross-level interaction between census tract poverty level and race/ethnicity. Thus Model 3 could assess the relationship between census tract poverty, race and mortality as well as the extent to which census tract level poverty accounted for census tract racial variation in mortality.

Their findings included the following depicted in Table 2.3:

1. Between census tract variation in mortality was nearly six times greater for Blacks than for Whites.

2. Census tract poverty contributed heavily to area variations in Black excess mortality. Specifically, they found that the mortality odds ratio for Blacks

compared to Whites (i.e., disparity) ranged from 0.31 to 5.36 (the average disparity being 1.30).

2.9 Generalized estimating equations

For non-normal responses that may be clustered, one popular option of estimating model-based disparity estimates is through the machinery of generalized estimating equations (GEE) ([221]). We assume that we have responses $y_{ij}, i = 1, \ldots, m, j = 1, \ldots, n_i$ which consist of m clusters each of n_j observations. Observations within a cluster may be correlated. In addition, the responses y_{ij} may be non-normal and hence GEE extends the framework of generalized linear models (GLMs) to allow marginal inference on model parameters (i.e., covariate effects). GEE models can be characterized by the following three components:

1. The conditional mean response $\mu_{ij} = E(y_{ij}|x_{ij})$ is related to the linear predictor $\eta_{ij} = x'_{ij}\beta$ through a monotone link function g such that $\mu_{ij} = g^{-1}(\eta_{ij}) = g^{-1}(x'_{ij}\beta)$.

2. The conditional variance of y_{ij} given x_{ij} is $Var(y_{ij}|x_{ij}) = \phi v(\mu_{ij})$ where v is the variance function with known form and $\phi > 0$ is the dispersion parameter.

3. The conditional covariance matrix of y_i is given by $V_i = Cov(y_i|x_i) = A_i^{-1/2} R_i(\nu) A_i^{-1/2}$, where $A_i = diag(\phi v(\mu_{i1}), \ldots, \phi v(\mu_{in_i}))$. $R_i(\nu)$ is a working correlation matrix with a specified structure involving parameter ν.

4. The response vectors in different clusters given their covariate vectors are assumed to be independent.

Regression coefficients are estimated as solutions to the so-called quasi score equations which derive from the quasi-likelihood (QL) which is in place since the GEE specification relies only on the first two moments of the distribution of y_{ij} (MN, 1993). Specifically,

$$\sum_{i=1}^{m} \frac{\partial \mu_i'}{\partial \beta} V_i^{-1}(y_i - \mu_i) = 0.$$

Iterative algorithms like quasi-scoring are used to find the solutions. Importantly, these solutions are robust against misspecifications of the working correlation matrix in the sense that point estimates for the regression parameters are still consistent. Robust variance estimates for regression parameters can be found using so-called sandwich estimators (Huber, date). These are also consistent under misspecification of the working correlation matrix. The price paid for misspecification however is a loss of efficiency in finite samples (References). Hypothesis testing can proceed using robust score tests or robust Wald tests ([221]).

2.9.1 Pseudo GEE for complex survey data

Carillo, Chen and Wu (2010)[48] extended GEE to the case of the analysis of non-normal complex longitudinal survey data. That is, a model-assisted framework under the so-called joint randomization framework. Their set up was as follows: a well defined finite population of N subjects with response and covariate values $(y_{ij}, x_{ij1}, \ldots, x_{ijp})'$ for the ith subject at the time of the jth cycle of the survey with $j = 1, \ldots, T_i$. This can be simplified if $T_i = T$ for all subjects. Then let s be the set of n units selected from the finite population under a complex sampling design and let d_i be the design weights. Thus the full data from the longitudinal survey is $(y_{ij}, x_{ij1}, \ldots, x_{ijp}); j = 1, \ldots, T_i, i \in s$. They then took the usual GEE estimating equation over the full N subjects and treated this as the finite population total which is to be estimated by the survey sample s. This led to the sample-based pseudo-GEE estimator for β which was defined as the solution to the set of estimating equations,

$$\sum_{i \in s} d_i \frac{\partial \mu_i'}{\partial \beta} V_i^{-1}(y_i - \mu_i) = 0.$$

Once again, the solutions are found using iterative techniques (Newton-Raphson) and consistency under the joint randomization of the model was established. Variance estimation for the estimated regression parameters was done by a form of Taylor linearization resulting in a survey-adjusted version of the sandwich variance estimator from usual GEE.

2.10 Bayesian methods

2.10.1 Intuitive motivation and practical advantages to Bayesian analyses

Consider the example studied in [369] who wanted to study if sexual minority populations (SM) in New Zealand reported more stress relative to heterosexuals. Their main data source was the New Zealand Household Survey (NZHS) using pooled data from 2016 and 2017. This is a nationally representative survey of about 10,000 individuals each year to investigate increased risk of hazardous drinking among SMs. However, they only were able to identify 626 people as SM (i.e., homosexual or bisexual) from a total multiyear pooled survey of 26,218 individuals (exact details of how this number was arrived at are described in [369]. Stress was measured using a version of Kessler Psychological Distress Scale which asks 10 questions about feelings of distress in the last month. A score of 11 (max is 54) is considered a high level of stress. A logistic regression model was fit with stress as the binary outcome and age, homosexual, bisexual, heterosexual orientation, gender, the New Zealand deprivation index (derived from socioeconomic variables from the New Zealand Census which is used as a measure of socioeconomic status of a household (Atkinson, 2014), and various interactions as covariates.

The authors recognized that they needed reliable measures on SMs due to their over-representation in measures of poor health, but due to the small sample size in their survey, this would prove difficult. So they proceeded to also carry out an informed Bayesian analysis which might help produce more accurate effect estimates in groups with small sample sizes. In order to do this, they incorporated external information by using pooled data from the 2016 and 2017 National Survey of Drug Use and Health (NSDUH) from the U.S. which contained information on 83.661 individuals who completed the stress questions, of which 44,424 self-identified as female. They fit a similar logistic regression model but used household income as a proxy for the New Zealand Deprivation Index in the other survey. Stress was measured using a shorter version of the Kessler scale with a score over 12 (max of 24) being considered a high level of stress. A prior range of plausible effect estimates for homosexuals and bisexuals was derived from the NSDUH model. This was used to inform (or constrain) the plausible range of NZHS model effect estimates through the posterior distribution (discussed below). This distribution summarizes the state of knowledge about an unknown quantity conditional on the prior and the current data. For instance, the (posterior mean) effect estimate for homosexuals went from an odds ratio of 1.58 under the unconstrained model to 2.22 in the constrained model. Figure 2.8 shows how the prior and posterior distributions for the effect estimates differ from one another.

However, even though the ease and flexibility with which this type of informed analysis can be done can be a major advantage of the Bayesian approach, it's the development of efficient computational algorithms and marked improvements in computing speed that have greatly facilitated the adoption of this approach to analysis. In addition, the posterior distributions can provide intuitively appealing interpretations for the end user. For instance, while $100(1-\alpha)$ percent confidence intervals represent the range of values containing the true parameter $100(1-\alpha)$ percent of the time in repeated sampling, a so-called credible interval based on the posterior distribution can be interpreted as the interval containing the true parameter with some probability given the data that has been observed (Dunson 2001). In addition, posterior probabilities can serve as alternatives to usual p-values and are sometimes advocated as being more intuitive to understand ([84]).

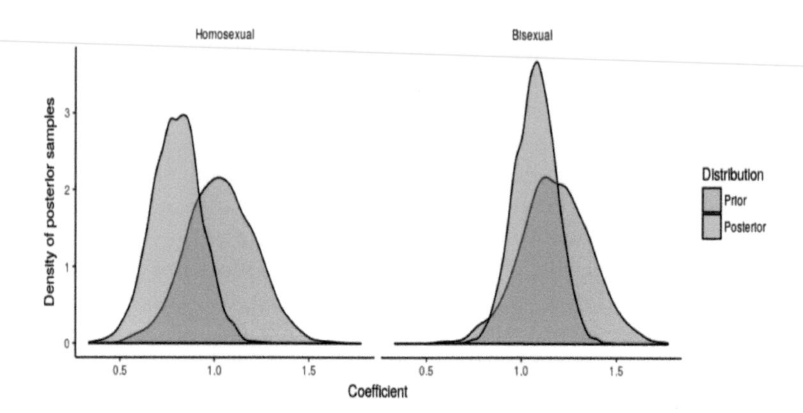

FIGURE 2.8: (Taken from Winter *et al.* (2020)[369]): Prior distributions derived from NSDUH and posterior distributions for NZHS which are constrained by the priors.

2.10.2 An overview of Bayesian inference

In addition to describing random variables, Bayesian inference assumes (model) parameters are not fixed population quantities and thus the knowledge about them can be summarized via their own probability distributions. This framework's backbone rests on conditional probabilities and Bayes theorem. In its simplest form, consider two events A and B. The conditional probability $P(A|B)$ can be written as,

$$\begin{aligned} P(A|B) &= \frac{P(AB)}{P(B)} \\ &= P(B|A)\frac{P(A)}{P(B)} \\ &= \frac{P(B|A)P(A)}{P(B|A)P(A) + P(B|A^c)P(A^c)}. \end{aligned}$$

Bayes theorem can also be generalized to random variables and their probability densities. Specifically,

$$f(x|y) = f(y|x)\frac{f(x)}{f(y)},$$

or in other words, $f(x|y) \propto f(y|x)f(x)$. Bayesian inference goes beyond just using Bayes theorem. As stated above, inference around model parameters incorporates the belief that these parameters do not hold fixed population values and thus bring with them additional uncertainty as captured through probabilistic arguments.

Before formally defining the paradigm, it's useful to recall what frequentist based inference inherently involves – the notion of repeated sampling from the population. Take for instance the construction of a traditional 95% confidence interval for a parameter of interest θ. This confidence interval implies that for 100 samples drawn of the same size from the population, that 95/100 of the constructed 95% confidence intervals would contain the population θ.

Bayesian inference on the other hand acknowledges that only one dataset is at hand. Uncertainty in θ is captured by a prior distribution $\pi(\theta)$. The data itself is characterized through a likelihood $f(y|\theta)$. Bayes theorem is applied which updates the prior distribution to a posterior distribution,

$$g(\theta|y) \propto f(y|\theta)\pi(\theta).$$

No repeated sampling is involved, and given modeling assumptions and the prior, generation of the posterior distribution is "automatic". As one keeps adding data and updating knowledge, the posterior will concentrate around the (so-called) true θ. Rather, more precisely, more plausible values of θ given the data. Point estimation and inference are done via the posterior distribution. Examples of this include maximum posterior (MAP) estimation (posterior mode), the posterior mean $E(\theta|y)$, or credible interval construction using quantiles of the posterior. The latter is useful for say hypothesis testing where one may be interested in whether $\theta \leq \theta_0$ for some hypothesized value θ_0. In this case, a reasonable posterior measure would be the posterior probability $P(\theta \leq \theta_0|y)$. Large values would indicate evidence that there was not enough information in the data to reject the (null) hypothesis.

Similarly, credible intervals can be constructed as a means to communicate findings from a Bayesian analysis (see, for example, [142, 86]). A $(1 - \alpha)$ credible interval for θ is defined as $[-c(\alpha), c(\alpha)]$ where $c(\alpha)$ satisifes,

$$P(-c \leq \theta \leq c|y) = \int_{-c}^{c} f(\theta|y)d\theta = 1 - \alpha.$$

Priors can be elicited from knowledge external to the current study or subject matter experts. Clearly the prior can have a marked influence on posterior inference. But they can also be made less subjective and assign more equalized prior weight across possible values of θ. A limiting version of this is the flat prior. Flat priors do not actually represent prior ignorance because most of their support is given for more extreme parameter values. Priors can be conjugate if the family of densities they lie in is the same as the posterior distribution. Conjugacy is useful for elicitation and computational purposes. The influence of different priors can be studied through so-called sensitivity analysis but as more and more data is collected and added, most priors are dominated by the likelihood and give very similar posteriors.

Bayesian inferential arguments are often seen in multilevel models. In the Bayesian world, these are often called hierarchical models. Here, priors can depend on other parameters with their own prior distributions. As such, uncertainty is propagated through the hierarchical model by Bayes theorem and generation of the posterior. For instance,

$$Y|\theta \sim f(\cdot|\theta)$$
$$\theta|\nu \sim g(\cdot|\nu)$$
$$\nu \sim h(\cdot)$$

2.10.3 Markov Chain Monte Carlo (MCMC)

The increased use of Bayesian methods in recent years can partly be attributed to advancements in Bayesian computing algorithms and specifically Markov Chain Monte Carlo (MCMC) algorithms. These algorithms iteratively generate samples of the parameters in a statistical model ([84]). Upon convergence, these samples reflect correlated draws from the joint posterior distribution of the model parameters. Marginalizing the joint posterior allows estimation of the posterior distribution of any parameters or function of parameters in the model. These algorithms enjoy a great deal of flexibility allowing one to fit very realistic models to complex datasets. Wiecki (2015)[365] provides a very nice intuitive summary of MCMC. Taking another look at the posterior distribution $f(\theta|y)$, we note that,

$$f(\theta|y) = \frac{f(y|\theta)g(\theta)}{f(y)}.$$

The numerator is generally easy to solve but looking at the denominator, we can write

$$f(y) = \int f(y,\theta)d\theta,$$

which amounts to integrating the joint probability of y and θ over all possible parameter values. For even slightly non-trivial models, it's difficult to compute the posterior in a closed-form way.

One strategy then to approximate the posterior is to draw samples from it using Monte Carlo approximation. Directly sampling however means we not only have to solve Bayes formula but also invert it. Markov chain Monte Carlo (MCMC) represent a general class of algorithms that construct a Markov chain to do the Monte Carlo approximation.

The intuitive steps of MCMC posterior generation under the simple model above are:

1. Specify an initial value of θ. This can be randomly chosen
2. Proposal to jump somewhere else. For example, take a sample from a normal distribution centered around the current θ value with a certain standard deviation.

3. Evaluate if the jump is good or not. If the resulting normal distribution with the proposed θ explains the data better than the old θ, then accept the proposal. Explaining the data better can be evaluated through the likelihood. So we end up moving in directions that increase the likelihood.

4. Eventually we'll get to the prior mean value of θ and no more moves are possible.

5. To avoid this, we'll also accept sometimes, moves in other directions. This is done by creating an acceptance probability which is the ratio of the proposal probability and the current probability. If the proposal probability is greater, then we will accept, otherwise, there is some chance to keep the current value.

6. Repeating this procedure gives us samples from the posterior of interest.

The reason this all works has to do with the acceptance ratio idea. Specifically,

$$\frac{\frac{f(y|\theta_p)g(\theta_p)}{f(y)}}{\frac{f(y|\theta_o)g(\theta_o)}{f(y)}} = \frac{f(y|\theta_p)g(\theta_p)}{f(y|\theta_o)g(\theta_o)},$$

where θ_p and θ_o represent the proposed and current (old) values of θ. Thus $f(y)$ cancels out and the challenging computational piece is removed. Intuitively, we are dividing the posterior at one position by the posterior at another position and visiting regions of high posterior probability relatively more often than regions of low posterior probability. There are many additional details about different samplers, guarantees of posterior representation and computational details which can be found in many good books on Bayesian modeling and MCMC. Examples include [105, 244] and [47] among others.

Example 2.4 Teenage conception rates across Scottish health boards between 1990-1992: In 1992, the Scottish government established the Clinical Outcomes Working Group under the Scottish Office. Their charge was to produce comparative clinical outcome indicators for the country. These indicators were first generated in 1993 covering a wide range of health and healthcare issues. An annual indicators report has been published ever since. The reason for these indicators is to provide local National Health Service (NHS) physicians with information they can use to improve patient care. Their main usage is to highlight variations which can then be further probed and strategies for mitigation taken. The indicators are developed at three levels: NHS Board, Operating Division or hospital thus facilitating comparisons between providers over time.

Goldstein and Spiegelhalter (1996)[117] examined statistical issues in comparisons of institutional performance based on league tables. In their paper, one of the illustrations they provided was using unadjusted outcomes from the Scottish outcomes study (Scottish Office, 1994) focusing on conception rates for girls between 13 and 15 years old during the time period of 1990-1992, focusing on comparisons across health boards. They noted that an established target for reduction by the year 2000 was set at 4.8 per 1000 (National Health Service Management Executive, 1992). They fit both an independent Poisson model within each board as well as Bayesian multilevel models assuming a normal population distribution with locally uniform priors on the population mean and log(variance). Their analysis is shown in Figure 2.9 with the boards along the y-axis and the conception rate on the x-axis. Drawn are fixed effect point estimates (solid circles) and their corresponding 95% confidence intervals. Also overlaid are the posterior mean estimates (open circles) and corresponding 95% credible intervals from the multilevel model. What is evident is that the random effects model shrinks the point estimates towards the overall mean (resulting in bias) but also narrows the width of the intervals (reduction in variance). In essence, the uncertainty in the point estimates has become more comparable across boards. However, they further advocated for the use of adjustment procedures for initial disease severity (Goldstein and Spiegelhalter 1996).

These kinds of analyses have been continuously expanded upon over time. For instance, in the COPSS-CMS White Paper Committee (2012), researchers examined 3100 dialysis centers around the U.S. using data from 1998 to 2001. Each center had at least 10 patients represented. The interest was in comparing centers with respect to standardized mortality ratios. Let Y_k be the observed death number; μ_k the expected death number and ρ_k the SMR. Their proposed hierarchical model was built as a more direct comparison to

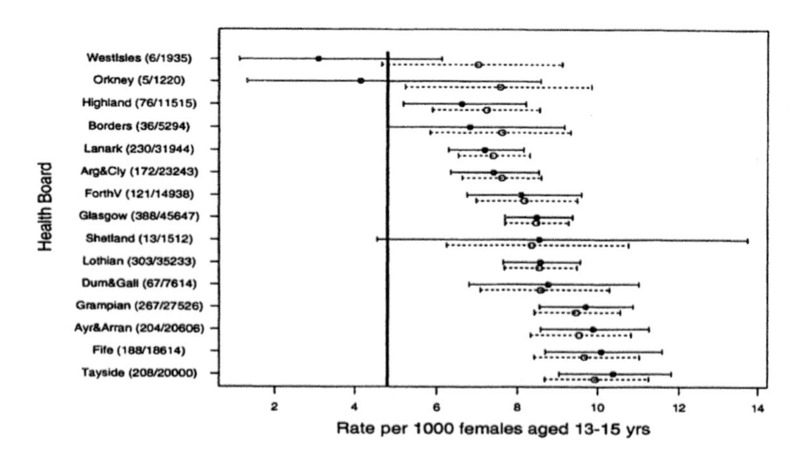

FIGURE 2.9: (Taken from Goldstein and Spiegelhalter (1996)[117]): Analysis of teenage conception rates across Scottish health boards between 1990 and 1992. Fixed point estimates (solid circles) and their corresponding 95% confidence intervals are shown and overlaid are the posterior mean estimates (open circles) and corresponding 95% credible intervals the multilevel model.

the Poisson fixed effects model,

$$\begin{aligned} Y_k|\mu_k, \rho_k &\sim Pois(\mu_k * \rho_k) \\ \rho_k &= exp(\theta_k) \\ \theta_k &\sim N(\psi, \lambda^{-1}) \\ \lambda &\sim Gamma(\alpha, \beta). \end{aligned}$$

Once again, they found that the standard maximum likelihood estimates and their confidence intervals (top plot) as compared to the posterior mean (PM) for the SMRs and their credible intervals were harder to interpret in terms of comparing centers due to the uneven variance estimates across centers. They also found that the posterior means were shrunken towards the prior mean as would be expected.

Example 2.5 Ethnic disparities in cancer incidence in Texas: Sparks (2015)[336] conducted a Bayesian analysis to explore disparities in cancer risk between different ethnic groups in Texas. He used cancer from the Texas Cancer Registry from 2000 to 2008 and built a Bayesian hierarchical model to incorporate various levels of uncertainty. As background, respiratory and digestive cancers have long been associated with behavior like smoking and poor diet and environmental influences like air pollutants. The Hispanic population in Texas is known to face socioeconomic disadvantages linked to these risk factors as compared to other ethnic groups. This includes higher poverty rates ([65]), and occupational risk which could expose them to environmental carcinogens.

Sparks (2015)[336] modeled the number of cancers y_{Cijk} using a Poisson distribution. Here, C is type of cancer, i is county, j is year, and k ethnicity. Thus,

$$y_{Cijk}|\theta_{Cijk} \sim Pois(e_{Cijk} * \theta_{Cijk}),$$

where e_{Cijk} is the expected number of cases calculated by assuming each county has the average incidence rate for the whole state for the period 2000-2008. The relative risk function in the model is θ_{Cijk}. Sparks (2015) looked at three different parameterizations. Focusing only on the first,

$$ln(\theta_{Cijk}) = \alpha_C + \delta_C * f_{Ci} + \sum_k \beta_{Ck} x_{ik} + u_{Ci} + \nu_{Ci} + t_{Cj} + \psi_{Cij}.$$

The variable f_{Ci} represents the focus variable ethnicity. The hierarchical model specification used was as follows:

$$
\begin{aligned}
\alpha_C &\sim U(-inf, inf) \\
\delta_C &\sim N(0, 0.0001) \\
\beta_{Ck} &\sim N(0, 0.0001) \\
\nu_{Ci}|\tau_{C\nu} &\sim N(0, \tau_{C\nu}) \\
u_{Ci}|\tau_{Cu} &\sim N(\frac{1}{n_j}\sum_{j\sim i} u_{Cj}, \tau_{Cu}/n_i) \\
t_{Cj}|\tau_{Ct} &\sim N(0, \tau_{Ct}) \\
\psi_{Cij}|\tau_{\psi C} &\sim N(0, \tau_{\psi C}).
\end{aligned}
$$

These represent an improper flat prior for α_C high variance normal priors for δ_C, β_C and ν_{Ci}, normal prior for t_j and vague Gamma priors for the other components. Note that as is custom in Bayesian model, normal distributions are specified in terms of their means and precision, with the latter being the inverse of the variance.

Table 2.4 gives a summary of the means of the (marginal) posterior distributions along with 95% credible intervals for all parameters. The results are adapted from Sparks (2015) showing results for respiratory and digestive cancers. The disparity parameter of interest δ is indicated as "Hispanic Disparity". For both diseases, elevated risks are seek for Hispanics versus non-Hispanics as estimated by e^{δ_C}.

TABLE 2.4: (Adapted from Sparks (2015)[336]): Posterior inference examining Hispanic versus non-Hispanic disparity in digestive and respiratory cancer incidence in Texas from 2000–2008.

Parameter	Posterior Mean (95% credible interval)	Posterior Mean (95% credible interval)
	Digestive	Respiratory
α	−0.81 (−0.119, −0.043)	−0.66 (−0.095, −0.037)
β's		
% in poverty	−0.016 (−0.052, −0.010)	−0.002 (−0.027,0.033)
hospitals per capita	−0.016 (−0.037, 0.004)	−0.007 (−0.032, 0.016)
% in construction work	−0.011 (−0.027, −0.005)	0.050 (0.028, 0.072)
metro county	0.023 (0.038, 0.66)	0.052 (0.007,0.095)
disparity (δ)	0.052 (0.038, 0.066)	0.107 (0.087,0.126)

3

Domain-Specific Estimates

3.1 What is a domain?

Domains are often thought of as representing specific subgroups, and can be defined by geographic areas, socio-economic groups, or other subgroups. Some common geographic domains include states, counties, municipalities, school districts, metropolitan areas, and health service areas ([300, 189, 110]). Socio-economic domains could refer to specific age, sex, race groups, or other areas of society.

3.2 Direct estimates

Domain estimates (discrepancies) can be direct if they are based only on domain-specific sample data. Direct estimation uses summary statistics based on a given domain or small region to estimate features of interest related to a small region. Typical features of interest are the small area mean, proportion, and total; the corresponding summary statistics are the sample mean, sample proportion, and the product of the sample mean and the domain size (i.e., the population size of the small area), assuming the latter is known of. See, for example, Chapter 2 of [300]).The direct estimates don't borrow strength in the sense that the estimate for a given domain doesn't use information from other domains, but they can also use information from a known auxiliary variable x related to the variable of interest y. A direct estimator is usually termed *design-based* because it is derived from designed sample surveys however they can also be motivated by and justified under certain models (see ch. 2 [300]). Direct estimators make use of survey weights and inferences use the probability distribution induced by the sampling design with population values held fixed.

Example 3.1 Disparities in the number of self-reported health older adults in the United States from 2000 to 2014: Davis *et al.* (2017)[73] examined the distribution of good health among older adults in the United States from 2000 to 2014. They wanted to understand whether improvements in health were equally distributed across various socioeconomic

DOI: 10.1201/9781003119449-3

groups including race/ethnicity, level of education and annual family income. Here the domains represent time periods and the focus groups for disparity estimation are the various socioeconomic groups.

They used data from the Medical Expenditure Panel Survey to identify older adults who reported their general health to be either excellent or very good twice in the same calendar year ([73]). They calculated rates of good health using survey estimation techniques described in Chapter 2 and adjusted for changes in age and sex composition over time using the direct adjustment method with the 2010 U.S. Census population as the reference distribution. They showed the rates differed significantly by race/ethnicity, level of education, and family income. For instance, older non-Hispanic White individuals reported being healthy at a rate of 442 per 1000 population in 2000 versus Hispanic individuals who at the same time period reported a rate of just over 300 per 1000 population. By 2014, the rate for non-Hispanic Whites increased to over 500 per 1000 population while the rate for Hispanics actually dropped to less than 300 per 1000 population. For education level, those older individuals with a graduate degree saw their rates increase from just under 600 per 1000 population to just over 600 per 1000 population whereas those with high school or less essentially saw no increase over time. A similar conclusion is reached when looking at high-family-income individuals versus poor or near-poor individuals.

3.3 Indirect estimates

On the other hand, indirect estimators can borrow strength from other domains or sources. Here we talk about indirect estimators without extensive use of statistical models, and leave the model-based methods to the next section. Methods of indirect estimation include synthetic estimation, composite estimation, and shrinkage estimation. See [300] (2015, ch. 3) for details. To illustrate with a simple example, suppose that the domain sizes under post-stratification (i.e., the strata in the population are formed after the samples are taken; e.g., Lohr 2010, sec. 4.4) are available, say, $N_{ig}, 1 \leq i \leq m, 1 \leq g \leq G$, where i represents the domain and g the post-stratum. Also suppose that an estimate of the post-stratum total, $\hat{Y}_{\cdot g}$, is available for $1 \leq g \leq G$. Let $N_{\cdot g} = \sum_{i=1}^{m} N_{ig}$ be the post-stratum size. Then, a synthetic estimator of the domain total is given by $\hat{Y}_i = \sum_{g=1}^{G}(N_{ig}/N_{\cdot g})\hat{Y}_{\cdot g}$. It is clear that $\hat{Y}_i$ is a weighted average of estimators of the post-stratum totals, where the weights depend on the domain. Furthermore, the same post-stratum total estimators are used in all of the domain total estimators, the only difference being the weights; this way, different domains can borrow strength from each other.

3.4 Small area model-based estimates

3.4.1 Small area estimation models

A domain is regarded as large if the domain-specific sample is large enough to produce sufficiently precise direct estimates. Conversely, a domain is considered *small* if the domain-specific sample cannot produce direct estimates with precision. Small domains are sometimes given other names that include "local area", "subdomain", "small subgroup" or "minor domain".

In recent years there has been substantial, and growing, interest in small area estimation (SAE) that is largely driven by practical demands. Here the term *small area* typically refers to a subpopulation or domain of interest for which a reliable direct estimate, based only on the domain-specific sample, cannot be produced due to small sample size in the domain. Examples of small areas include geographical regions (e.g., state, county, municipality), demographic groups (e.g., specific age × sex × race groups), demographic groups within geographic regions, etc. Such small areas are often of primary interest, for example, in policymaking regarding allocation of resources to subgroups, or determination of subgroups with specific characteristics (e.g., in health and medical studies) in a population. It is desirable that the decisions regarding such a policymaking be made based on reliable estimates. For such reasons, demands and interest in SAE research have increased rapidly in recent years. For example, SAE is nowadays routinely used for effective planning of health, social and other services, and for apportioning government funds in the United States, Canada and many European countries. Since 2013, there has been an Annual International Conference on SAE and related topics in various locations worldwide. Reviews on SAE and related topics can be found, for example, in [184], [72], [281], and [300]. Following these, [189] wrote a review on robust small area estimation methods.

According to [184], and [281], there are three "basic" SAE models in the sense that other models may be viewed as extensions, or variations, of these models. The first is the Fay-Herriot model ([95]), also known as area-level model; the second is the nested error regression (NER) model ([24]), also known as unit-level model; the third is the mixed logistic model ([182]), which is often used for binary outcomes, or binomial proportions.

A Fay-Herriot model may be expressed as $y_i = x_i'\beta + v_i + e_i$, $i = 1, \dots, m$, where m is the total number of small areas (for which data are available), y_i is a direct survey estimator for the ith small area, x_i is a vector of associated covariates, or predictors, β is a vector of unknown regression coefficients, v_i is an area-specific random effect that accounts for variation not explained by the predictors, and e_i is a sampling error. It is assumed that $v_i, e_i, i = 1, \dots, m$ are independent such that $v_i \sim N(0, A), e_i \sim N(0, D_i)$, where A is an unknown variance but D_i is assumed known, $1 \leq i \leq m$. In practice, D_i may not be exactly known but can be estimated with a high degree of accuracy. For example, typically D_i can be expressed as an unknown variance divided by the sample size for the ith area, and the unknown variance can be estimated using a (much) larger data set. See [300] (ch. 6) for further explanation. Thus, in the sequel we will use the notation D_i with the understanding that in most cases it is $\hat{D}_i$, an estimate of D_i.

An NER model can be expressed as $y_{ij} = x'_{ij}\beta + v_i + e_{ij}$, $i = 1, \dots, m$, $j = 1, \dots, n_i$, where m is the same as above, n_i is the number of units sampled from the ith small area, y_{ij} is the jth sampled outcome measure from the ith area, and x_{ij} is a corresponding vector of auxiliary variables. The meanings of β and v_i are the same as in the Fay-Herriot model, and e_{ij} is an additional error. It is assumed that the v_is and e_{ij}s are independent with $v_i \sim N(0, \sigma_v^2)$ and $e_{ij} \sim N(0, \sigma_e^2)$, where σ_v^2 and σ_e^2 are unknown variances.

As for the mixed logistic model, it is assumed that, given $v = (v_i)_{1 \le i \le m}$ with the v_i's having the same meaning as above, binary responses $y_{ij}, i = 1, \dots, m, j = 1, \dots, n_i$ are conditionally independent such that $\text{logit}(p_{ij}) = x'_{ij}\beta + v_i$, x_{ij}, β having the same meanings as in the NER model and $\text{logit}(p) = \log\{p/(1-p)\}$, and $p_{ij} = \text{P}(y_{ij} = 1|v)$. Note that the x_{ij}'s are considered non-random here, so the latter conditional probability is the same as $\text{P}(y_{ij} = 1|x'_{ij}\beta + v_i)$ due to the independence of the v_i's. Furthermore, it is assumed that v_i is distributed as $N(0, \sigma^2)$ with σ^2 unknown.

The assumptions underlying these models are considered strong in that they completely specify the underlying distribution of the data. Such assumptions would allow, for example, maximum likelihood (ML) or restricted maximum likelihood (REML) inference (e.g., [173]), but the latter may not be robust when the assumptions fail. For example, for computing the empirical best linear unbiased predictor (EBLUP; see below) one can use other types of consistent estimators of variance components than ML or REML estimators (e.g., [287]), but measures of uncertainty are more sensitive to the distributional assumptions. See below for more details.

3.4.2 Estimation

We refer to [300] for details of traditional methods of inference for small areas. A mainstream approach relies on using a statistical model in order to borrow strength. These models likely involve area-specific random effects, specification of the conditional mean and variance given the random effects, and normality assumption about the random effects and other additional errors that are involved in the model. The model-based approach can be non-Bayesian or Bayesian. These approaches lead to the EBLUP, empirical best predictor (EBP), empirical Bayes (EB) and hierarchical Bayes (HB) estimators, including their variations. The EB approach is different from the HB approach in the way that hyper-parameters at the bottom of the model hierarchy are estimated from the data in the former, while a prior will be assigned to the hyper-parameters in the latter. Note that there are also design-based approaches which do not use any model in deriving the estimators, such as the direct survey estimators are used.

Consider, for example, the Fay-Herriot model. The small area means can be expressed as $\theta_i = x_i'\beta + v_i, 1 \leq i \leq m$. The EBLUP of θ_i can be expressed as

$$\hat{\theta}_i = (1 - \hat{B}_i)y_i + \hat{B}_i x_i'\hat{\beta}, \tag{3.1}$$

where $\hat{B}_i = D_i/(\hat{A}+D_i)$, and $\hat{\beta}, \hat{A}$ are estimators of β, A, respectively. Expression (3.1) shows that the EBLUP is a weighted average of the direct estimator, y_i, and an indirect regression estimator, $x_i'\hat{\beta}$, with weights $(1 - \hat{B}_i)$ and $\hat{B}_i$, respectively. Alternatively, the EBLUP may be viewed as shrinking the direct estimator towards the regression estimator with the shrinkage factor $\hat{B}_i$. To understand the weights or shrinkage factor, note that if A is large compared to D_i, which means that the between area variation is large, there is not much strength that the direct estimator can borrow from other areas through the regression estimator; as a result, the shrinkage factor is expected to be close to zero, meaning little or no shrinkage. On the other hand, if A is small compared to D_i, the between-area variation is small, therefore, there is a lot of strength that the direct estimator can borrow from other areas; as a result, the shrinkage factor is close to one, meaning substantial shrinkage. The following example illustrates the *small area model-in-action.*

Example 3.2 Hospital kidney transplant graft failure rates:

Morris & Christiansen (1995)[260] presented a data set involving 23 hospitals (out of a total of 219 hospitals) that had at least 50 kidney transplants during a 27 month period. Specifically, the y_i's are graft failure rates for kidney transplant operations, that is, y_i = number of graft failures $/n_i$, where n_i is the number of kidney transplants at hospital i during the period of interest. The variance for graft failure rate, D_i, is approximated by $(0.2)(0.8)/n_i$, where 0.2 is the observed failure rate for all hospitals. Thus, the D_i's are treated as known. The severity index, x_i, is considered as a covariate. Ganesh (2009)[102] proposed a Fay-Herriot model as $y_i = \beta_0 + \beta_1 x_i + v_i + e_i$ to fit the data.

A graphic illustration of the model-in-action is shown in Figure 3.1. In the top figure, the direct estimate and EBLUP are plotted against $\sqrt{D_i}$; in the bottom figure, the absolute difference of the direct estimate and EBLUP is plotted against $\sqrt{D_i}$. A lowess smoother running through the bottom figure shows that this absolute difference increases as D_i increases or in other words, this is where the EBLUP estimator is most affected by underlying small area model. Also note that the estimators, $\hat{\beta}$, $\hat{A}$, are based on data from all of the areas; this is how the EBLUP for one area borrows strength from other areas. In fact, the weights in (3.1) are optimal when the $\hat{A}$ is replaced by A, the true variance of the random effects. Therefore, assuming that $\hat{A}$ is a consistent estimator of A, EBLUP borrows strength in a way that is nearly optimal. The standard estimators of β and A include REML, ML (e.g., [173]) or ANOVA (e.g., [287]) estimators. As noted earlier, typically D_i is also estimated.

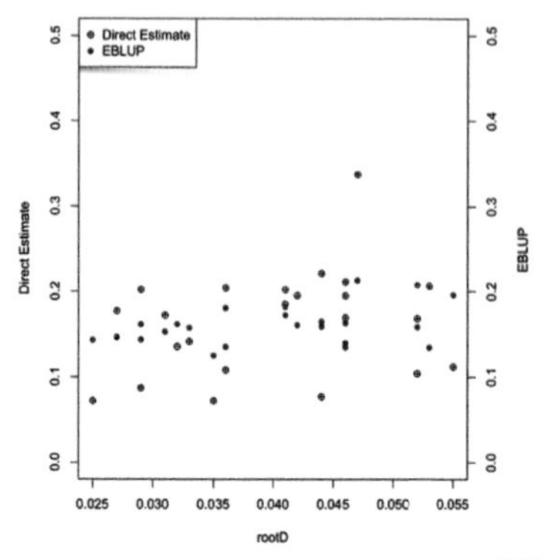

(a) Direct Estimate, EBLUP vs $\sqrt{D_i}$

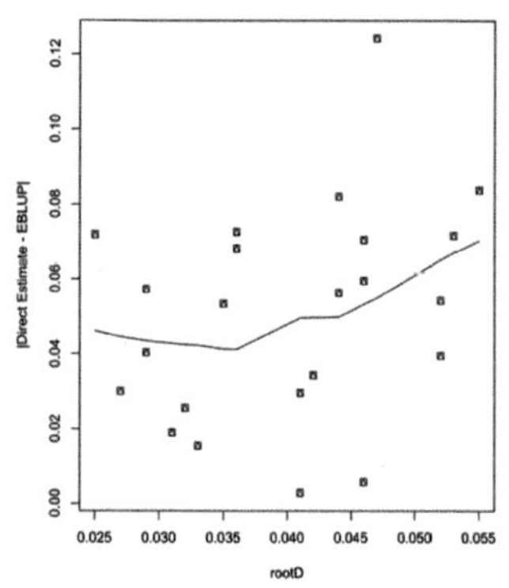

(b) Absolute Difference between Direct Estimate and EBLUP vs $\sqrt{D_i}$

FIGURE 3.1: (Taken from Jiang and Rao (2020)[189]): Illustration of a small area model-in-action.

Example 3.3 Characterizing the disparities in the dark figure of crime from the crime survey for England and Wales (CSEW): Buil-Gil (2020)[111] performed a small area analysis to understand disparities in local areas in the dark figure of crime using the crime survey for England and Wales. Crime surveys are used to address limitations of police statistics as crime data sources due to biases arising from uneven tendencies to report crime. So [111] focused on the crime survey to produce small area estimates of crimes unknown to the police at local authority districts (LADs) and middle layer super output areas (MSOAs) in order to understand the geographical disparities in the dark figure of crime. They discovered that this is larger in small cities that are deprived but also in wealthy areas. It's also larger in sub-urban, low-housing neighborhoods with higher concentrations of immigrants and non-Asian minorities.

They used data from CSEW from 2011 to 2017 with sample sizes varying from a low of 33,350 in 2013–2014 to a high of 46, 013 in 2011–2012. The CSEW is an annual victimization survey conducted since 1982 which is based on a multistage stratified random sampling design in which adults (defined as 16 and older) are randomly selected from within random selected households. Individuals are asked about whether they had been a victim of a crime in the last 12 months. The questionnaire is a mixture of face-to-face questions and online surveys (for more sensitive questions around alcohol, drug use and domestic abuse). Crimes are classified from misdemeanour-type offenses to major felonies. Each victim of crime is also asked if the crime was reported to the police from which information used to estimate dark crime numbers can be derived. Small area estimates are produced at both LADs and MSOAs. LADs reflect local governments with an average of 168,000 citizens and MSOAs are smaller areas designed to improve the reporting of statistical information. They average 7200 individuals in size. There are 7201 MSOAs and 348 LADs in England and Wales.

Buil-Gil (2020)[111] compared the following small area estimates: 1) direct estimates based on the Horvitz-Thompson estimator[149]; 2) regression synthetic estimates using direct estimates as a dependent variable and relevant area-level auxiliary information as covariates; 3) EBLUP estimates in each area from a Fay-Herriot model; 4) the Rao-Yu model [302] which extends the area-level EBLUP to allow for temporally autocorrelated random effects to allow borrowing of information across time; 5) the spatial EBLUP that allows spatially correlated random effects thus borrowing information from neighboring areas ([289]); and 6) spatio-temporal EBLUP estimates from a model proposed by [234]. Bootstrap estimates of relative root mean squared errors (RRMSEs) for the model-based estimates were generated (Maruhuenda *et al.* 2020) to allow for assessment of which methods produced reliable estimates. Any areas with RRMSE less than 25% were regarded as reliable and those with RRMSE greater than 50% as unreliable.

Auxiliary variables were derived from literature and preliminary data analyses. Only variables with information available from 2011 to 2017 were used. These variables were extracted from the Office of National Statistics (ONS) and the Consumer Data Research Centre (CDRC). Variable selection using a forward stepwise selection approach was used to select a smaller subset of variables although alternative approaches specifically designed for SAE problems can be used ([179]) as described later in this Chapter. Figure 3.2 shows the different small area model-based estimates and direct estimates by LAD (ordered by sample size) versus their respective estimated RRMSE values. The Rao-Yu and spatio-temporal model-based estimates have the lowest percentage of estimates with RRMSE greater than 50% (1.5% and 1.4%, respectively). Table 3.1 shoes that the strongest covariate is the measure of small urban areas as opposed to conurbations and rural areas. Dark figure crime is significantly larger in small urban districts. Also, LADs whose income is far above the average income have a larger percentage of crimes unknown. Finally, mean house

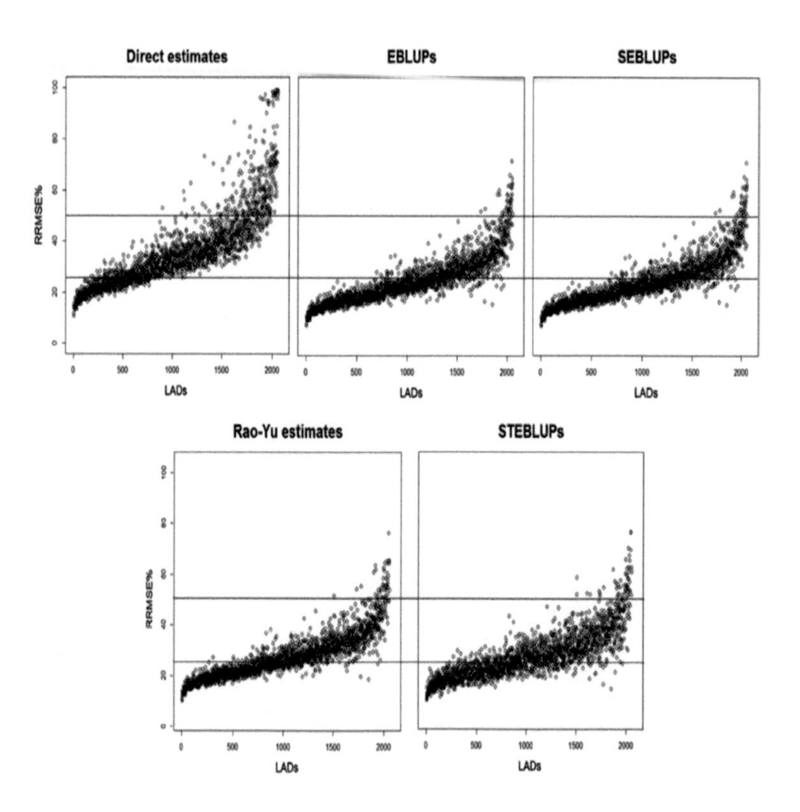

FIGURE 3.2: (Taken from Buil-Gil (2020)[111]): Various small area estimates for dark crime at the LAD level (ordered by sample size) versus their RRMSE values.

price indicates that dark crime is slightly lower in LADs with more expensive homes.

3.4.3 Inference

In addition to producing point estimates of small-area characteristics, there have also been extensive studies on measures of uncertainty, which routinely accompany with the point estimates. A standard measure of uncertainty is the mean squared prediction error (MSPE). There are other measures of uncertainty such as prediction intervals. In terms of estimation of area-specific MSPE, the standard methods include the Prasad-Rao linearization method and resampling methods. See [300] (Chs. 6 & 7).

In their method, the variance components involved in a linear mixed model (LMM; e.g., [173], ch. 1) are estimated using the method of moments (MoM),

TABLE 3.1: (Taken from Buil-Giil (2020)[111]): Small area spatio-temporal model for LADs covariate effects.

	Coefficient Estimate	SE	p-value
Intercept	60.96	2.1	<0.0001
ASS income	1.558	0.8	0.031
Conurbation	0.496	1.1	0.461
Small urban	2.246	1.0	0.025
Percent employed	−0.493	0.8	0.459
Percent white	−0.374	3.3	0.511
Percent Asian	−0.025	2.9	0.593
Mean house price	−1.071	1.1	0.041
Crime rate	−0.543	0.9	0.128
Percent male	0.514	0.8	0.517

also known as the analysis of variance (ANOVA) method. The EBLUP is then obtained with the Prasad-Rao estimators of the variance components. The initial consideration of Prasad and Rao seemed to be simplicity–the ANOVA estimators have closed-form expressions, unlike the ML or REML estimators, which makes it easier to derive and justify a second-order unbiased MSPE estimator. The latter means that the bias of the MSPE estimator is $o(m^{-1})$, where m is the total number of small areas from which data are available. However, there is a "bonus" to the Prasad-Rao method, that is, the ANOVA method requires specification of only up to the second moments of the data; in particular, the normality assumption is not needed. In fact, [210] (RM15) showed that, under the Fay-Herriot model, the Prasad-Rao MSPE estimator is robust to non-normality of the small area-specific random effects although the normality of the sampling errors is still needed.

In terms of resampling methods for MSPE estimation, [185](JLW) proposed a jackknife ([292]) method for estimating the MSPE of EBP. The method is especially convenient to implement under the posterior linearity assumption, which is weaker than assuming that the data are normal, as noted earlier ([108]). It should be noted that the JLW jackknife is not restricted to work under the posterior linearity assumption; the latter just makes the computation easier, because the MSPE of the BP then has an analytic expression. Later, in [183], the authors extended the JLW jackknife to cases where the MSPE of the BP does not have an analytic form. A different approach was taken by [126], who proposed a bootstrap method for the NER model that does not require complete specification of the distribution of the random effects and errors.

In many cases, the data for the outcome variable are binary or counts. In such cases a LMM may not be appropriate; instead, a generalized linear mixed model (GLMM; e.g., [173], ch. 3) may be used (e.g., [109]). In particular, [182] proposed an EBP approach, and extended the Prasad-Rao method of MSPE estimation to SAE with binary data; also see [180]. In those papers, the authors used the MoM estimators of the parameters under a GLMM, instead of the ML estimators which are computationally challenging to obtain (e.g., [173], sec. 4.1). Furthermore, the MoM method relies on weaker assumptions than GLMM. In fact, for the MoM estimators to be consistent, one only requires that the conditional mean function of the response, given the random effects, is correctly specified; an MoM estimator with improved efficiency can be obtained by correctly specifying the conditional first two moments ([191]). It should be noted, however, that the MoM estimator is not robust to misspecification in the distribution of the random effects, unless the GLMM is a LMM (e.g., [186]).

3.5 Bayesian approaches

Linear mixed models are suitable for continuous responses, y, but do not apply for other types of responses – say binary or count data. They can be extended within the framework of generalized linear mixed models which amount to using logistic regression or log linear models with random effects. Estimation procedures are more complicated and computationally expensive than for the linear mixed model case. Inference also relies more heavily on asymptotic approximations to sampling distributions for parameter estimates. Bayesian approaches provide a more unified framework across these different response types. They are generally broken out into empirical Bayes (EB) and hierarchical Bayes (HB) methods. Rao and Molina (2015)[300] given an excellent discussion of this topic.

The EB framework can be described algorithmically as :

1. Obtain the posterior density, $f(\mu|y, \lambda)$, of the small area (random) parameters of interest, μ, given the data y, using the conditional density $f(y|\mu, \lambda_1)$, of y given μ and the density $f(\mu|\lambda_2)$ of μ, with $\lambda = (\lambda_1, \lambda_2)'$ which are the model parameters.

2. Estimate λ from the marginal density of y, namely, $f(y|\lambda)$

3. Use the empirical posterior density, $f(\mu|y, \hat{\lambda})$ to make inferences about μ.

Note that the density on μ is not actually a prior distribution but rather part of the posed model on (y, μ). Thus it can be checked from data. This is in contrast to subjective priors seen in fully Bayesian approaches.

For the basic area-level model, we can re-express it as a two-stage hierarchical model as follows: i) $y_i|\theta_i \sim^{ind} N(\theta_i, D_i)$, ii) $\theta_i \sim^{ind} N(xi'\beta, A), i = 1, \ldots, m$. In a Bayesian framework, the model parameters β and A are treated as random. The pairs (y_i, θ_i) are independent across domains i, conditional on β and A ([197]). Combining these two stages, we get

$$y_i = x_i'\beta + v_i + e_i,$$

where $v_i \sim^{ind} N(0, A)$ and $e_i \sim^{ind} N(0, D_i)$ which involves the area-specific random effects v_i and the direct (design-based) random errors e_i. The best predictor of θ_i is given by the conditional expectation of θ_i given y_i, β, A which is expressed as,

$$\begin{aligned} E(\theta_i|y_i, \beta, A) &= \hat{\theta}_i^B \\ &= \gamma_i y_i + (1 - \gamma_i)x_i'\beta, \end{aligned}$$

where $\gamma_i = A/(A + D_i)$. The reason one can think of this as a best predictor of θ_i is that it results from the posterior distribution without assuming a prior distribution on the model parameters (Rao and Molina 2015).

The estimator $\hat{\theta}_i^B$ can also be considered a Bayes estimator and when the model parameters β and A are estimated from the mixed model for y_i using maximum likelihood (ML) or restricted maximum likelihood (REML), and these estimates plugged in, we obtain the EB estimator of θ_i, namely,

$$\hat{\theta}_i^{EB} = \hat{\gamma}_i y_i + (1 - \hat{\gamma}_i)x_i'\hat{\beta}.$$

Careful inspection of this formula reveals that this exactly coincides with the EBLUP estimator. Rao and Molina (2015)[300] describe in detail various properties of the EB estimator including MSE estimation, EB confidence intervals, and extensions for binary and count data.

Hierarchical Bayes (HB) methods are related to EB but with some important differences. Here, a *subjective* prior distribution $f(\lambda)$ is placed on the model parameters λ. Turning the Bayesian "crank", the posterior distribution $f(\mu|y)$ of the small area parameters of interest μ given the data y is obtained. More specially, $f(y|\mu, \lambda_1)$ and $f(y|\mu, \lambda_2)$ is combined with the subjective prior on $\lambda = (\lambda_1, \lambda_2)'$ using Bayes Theorem. Inferences are focused around the posterior distribution. For instance, μ is estimated by its posterior mean,

$$\hat{\mu} = E(\mu|y),$$

and the posterior variance $var(\mu|y)$ is a measure of precision of the estimator (if finite). The HB method is "exact" but does require specification of a subjective prior. Priors can be diffuse or informative. Informative priors are elicited typically from previous studies relevant to data set y. However, the default very often used is the diffuse prior. However, this choice may not be unique and some diffuse priors can lead to improper posteriors (do not integrate to 1).

Simple calculations show the work flow:

$$f(\mu, \lambda|y) = \frac{f(y, \mu|\lambda)f(\lambda)}{f(y)},$$

and

$$f(y) = \int f(y, \mu|\lambda)f(\lambda)d\mu d\lambda.$$

The posterior density $f(\mu|y)$ is then,

$$\begin{aligned} f(\mu|y) &= \int f(\mu, \lambda)|y)d\lambda \\ &= \int f(\mu|y, \lambda)f(\lambda|y)d\lambda. \end{aligned}$$

Thus the posterior is a mixture of conditional distributions $f(\mu|y, \lambda)$. Since this is also used for EB inferences, sometimes HB is termed Bayes EB. As discussed in Chapter 2, computational approaches like MCMC methods are used to deal with the fact that formal calculation of the above involves multidimensional integration which can become cumbersome for more complex problems (i.e., more complex models and prior specifications).

For the basic area-level model, we assume a prior distribution on the model parameters (β, A). If A is assumed known and a diffuse prior is used for β, then we can write the area-level model as,

$$\begin{aligned} \hat{\theta}_i|\theta_i, \beta, A &\overset{ind}{\sim} N(\theta_i, D_i), i = 1, \ldots, m \\ \theta_i|\beta, A &\overset{ind}{\sim} N(x_i'\beta, b_i^2 A), i = 1, \ldots, m \\ f(\beta) &\propto 1. \end{aligned}$$

Then the HB estimator is $\hat{\theta}_i^{HB} = E(\theta_i|\hat{\theta}, A)$ with A assumed known. The associated posterior variance is used as an estimate of precision. Thus when A is assumed known and a diffuse prior used for β, the HB and BLUP approaches under normality give the same point estimates and measures of variability.

When A is assumed unknown, then the prior on β is replaced by a joint prior on (β, A). Assuming prior independence, $f(\beta, A) = f(\beta)f(A) \propto f(A)$ where $f(A)$ is a prior on A.

Example 3.4 HB analysis of racial disparities in hypertensive disorders of pregnancy in Florida, 2005–2014: Hu *et. al* (2019)[152] attempted to understand the spatio-temporal variations in racial disparities in hypertensive disorders of pregnancy (HDP) in Florida between 2005 and 2014. They used a fully Bayesian analysis to estimate these disparities at the county level. As a comparison, they also fit an HB model that does not account for any spatio-temporal variation. This model can be used to illustrate HB disparity estimation at the county level.

Data records for all registered live births in Florida between 2005 and 2015 were used. Only births for residential Floridians were used. These were then geocoded and duplicated records for women with multiple births were excluded. Finally, women with missing information on HDP or race/ethnicity were excluded from analysis. Diagnosis of HDP was extracted from Birth Records data and gestational hypertension was defined as the development of high blood pressure after 20 weeks of pregnancy. Pre-pregnancy hypertension was excluded from the definition of HDP. Covariates of interest included age groupings, education level, pregnancy smoking status (yes/no) and pre-pregnancy body mass index (BMI).

A county level analysis was conducted in which HDP was treated as a count variable and aggregated at the county level by race/ethnicity, year of conception and covariates. Let y_{ijkl} be the observed number of HDP cases for the ith county, jth year, kth race/ethnicity group and ith covariate pattern. The expected number of cases was then estimated to be $e_{ijkl} = \sum n_{ijkl} \times r_{kl}$ where n_{ijkl} is the total number of women for the ith county, jth year, kth race/ethnicity group and ith covariate pattern and r_{kl} is the average incidence rate for each county from 2005 to 2014. They then assumed that,

$$y_{ijkl}|\theta_{ijkl} \sim Poisson(e_{ijkl} * \theta_{ijkl}),$$

where θ_{ijkl} is the relative risk for the ith county, jth year, kth race/ethnicity group and ith covariate pattern.

The full hierarchical model specification they wrote was,

$$\begin{aligned}
ln(\theta_{ijkl}) &= \alpha + \delta * Race_k + \sum_l x_l'\beta_l + t_j \\
\alpha &\sim U(-inf, inf) \\
\delta &\sim N(0, 0.0001) \\
\beta_l &\sim N(0, 0.0001) \\
t_j &\sim N(0, \tau_j) \\
\tau_j &\sim logGamma(1, 0.0005),
\end{aligned}$$

where α is the intercept, δ measures the racial disparity between Black and non-Black women, $\sum x_l'\beta_l$ is the linear predictor for the four covariates and t_j a random effect for time heterogeneity.

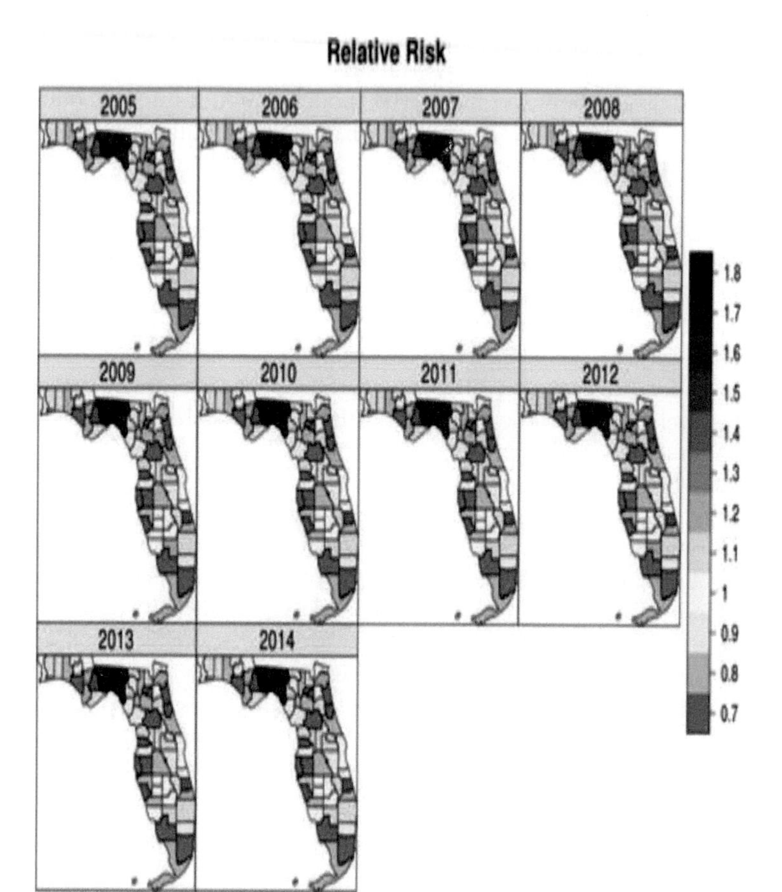

FIGURE 3.3: (Taken from Hu *et al.* (2019)[152]): Estimated county-level relative risk differences for HDP between Black and non-Black women during 2005–2014 in Florida.

Example 3.5 Life expectancy by county, race and ethnicity in the U.S.A., 2000–2019 Dwyer-Lindgren *et al.* (2022)[85] examined the extent to which disparities in life expectancy patterns vary geographically focusing on five racial-ethnic groups in 3110 U.S. counties over a 20 year period. In the end, they used small area estimation methods to describe spatio-temporal variations in life expectance and disparities between racial-ethnic groups.

They focused on death registration data between 2000 and 2019 from the U.S. National Vital Statistics System and population data from the U.S. National Center for Health Statistics to estimate annual sex-specific and age-specific mortality rates stratified by county and racial-ethic group (non-Latino, non-Hispanic White, non-Latino and non-Hispanic Black, non-Latino and non-Hispanic American Indian or Alaska Native (AIAN), non-Latino and non-Hispanic Asian or Pacific Islander (API), and Latino or Hispanic. Mortality rates were adjusted to correct for misreporting of race and ethnicity on death certificates. Modified life tables were then constructed to estimate life expectancy at birth.

The authors built a small area model that specifies the log of the underlying mortality rate as a function of covariates and additional variation by county, year, age and race-ethnicity. Covariates included educational attainment, poverty rate, proportion foreign-born, median household income and population density (all selected based on previously observed associations with mortality). Fixed effects on the county and county-race-ethnicity capture the relationships between each covariate and mortality. For race-ethnicity-specific covariates, the authors included additional random effects to allow for the relationship between the fixed effects and mortality to vary by race-ethnicity. Additional random effects were included to capture additional variation including spatial (between-county) shared across age, year and race-ethnicity; a random effect for variation in mortality by age, time and race-ethnicity group shared across all counties and a random effect to allow for county-specific deviations in mortality patterns by age, time and race-ethnicity. The last random effect incorporated a linear spline in the age and time dimensions to reduce computational complexity.

A fully Bayesian spatio-temporal SAE model at the county and race-ethnicity level was then specified. Graphical posterior predictive checks were done to assess if the observed data are overdispersed and/or zero-inflated relative to the model, linearity checks were done using binned residual plots and model fit was assessed by inspecting plots comparing the estimated time and age trends in mortality to the observed data at the national, state and county level. Further SAE models were built at the county level aggregating across all racial-ethnic groups. The rationale for doing this in order to perform model calibration of the race-ethnicity-specific estimates in order to prevent the race-ethnicity misclassification adjusting from altering the overall mortality rate in a county. Hyper-prior sensitivity analysis was also done followed by full small area model validation using a validation set of county and race-ethnicity pairs. This is a collection of county and race-ethnicity pairs for which the direct mortality rates are a good representation of the underlying rate (stable direct estimates).

Figure 3.4 shows the estimated life expectancies in the U.S. between 2000 and 2009 and demonstrates important differences between racial-ethnic groups. the greatest increases in life expectancy over this period of time were for the Latino population (2.7 years), while the increase for the White population was only 1.7 years over the same period of time and there was no change for the American Indian or Alaska Native population. GBD *et al.* (2022) also noted that the largest gains in life expectance occurred during

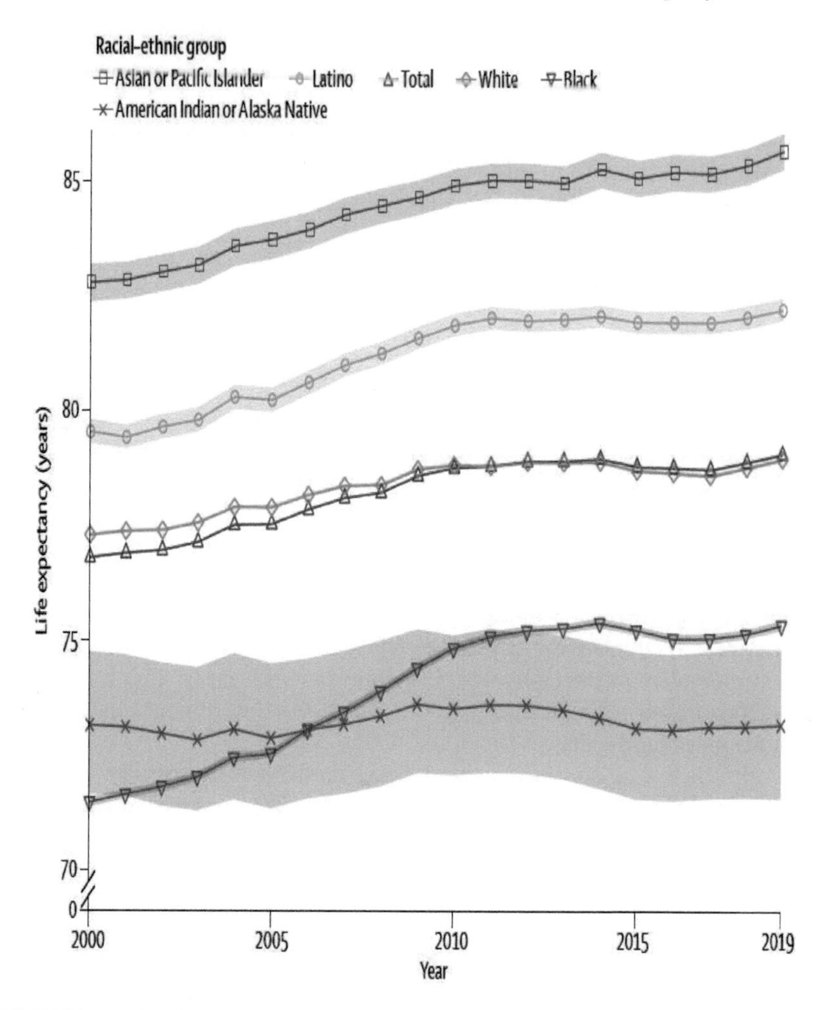

FIGURE 3.4: (Taken from Dywer-Lindgren *et al.* (2022)[85]): Life expectancy estimates (and 95% confidence regions) from birth by racial-ethnic group in the U.S. between 2000 and 2019.

the first 10 year window of the 20 year observation period across most racial-ethnic groups. Figure 3.5 shows that in 2019, there was large variation across all racial-ethnic groups in life expectancy across counties in the U.S. Figure 3.6 shows that differences in life expectancy relative to the White population at the county level were mostly in the same direction as those at the national level across all racial-ethnic groups. Figure 3.7 shows the estimated

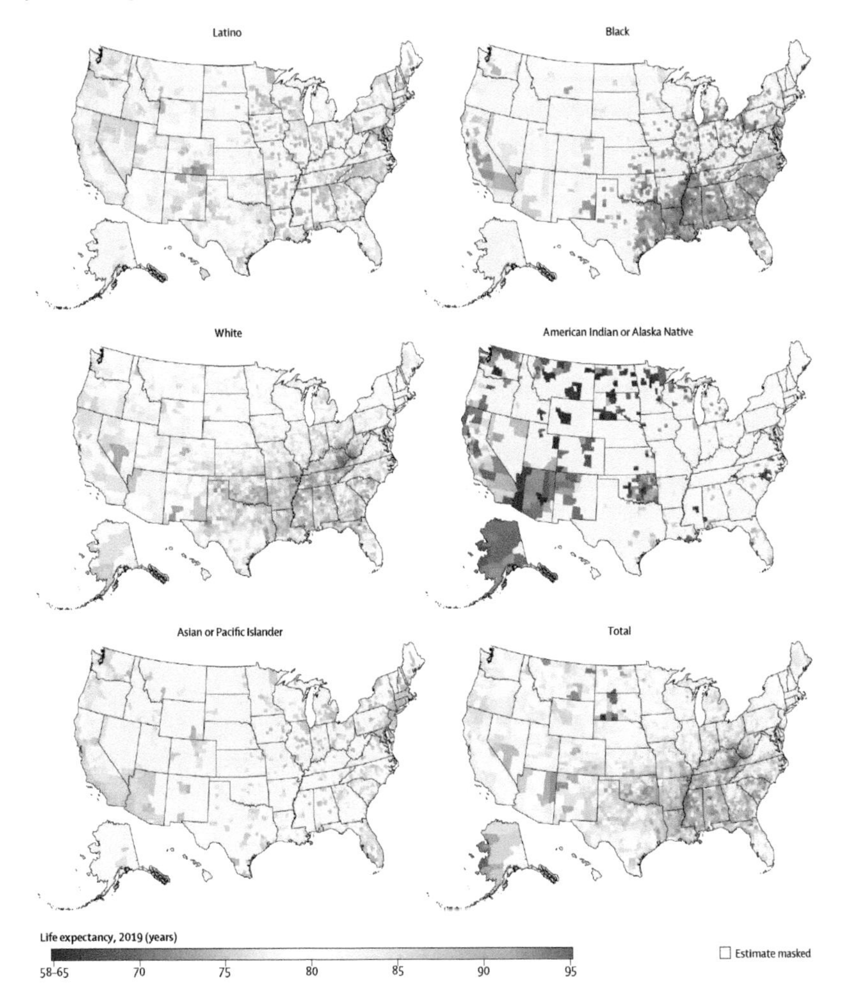

FIGURE 3.5: (Taken from Dywer-Lindgren *et al.* (2022)[85]): Life expectancy estimates by racial-ethnic group across U.S. counties for 2019.

racial-ethnic-specific differences in life expectancy at the county level between 2000 and 2019. Estimated values were masked if the mean annual population was less than 1000 due to the worsening fit of the model and high variability of the estimates. The authors concluded that because they found large variation in life expectancy between the racial-ethnic groups and across locations and time, that this should encourage the collection of comprehensive data at the local level which could help to better understand the drivers of racial-ethnic health disparities ([85]).

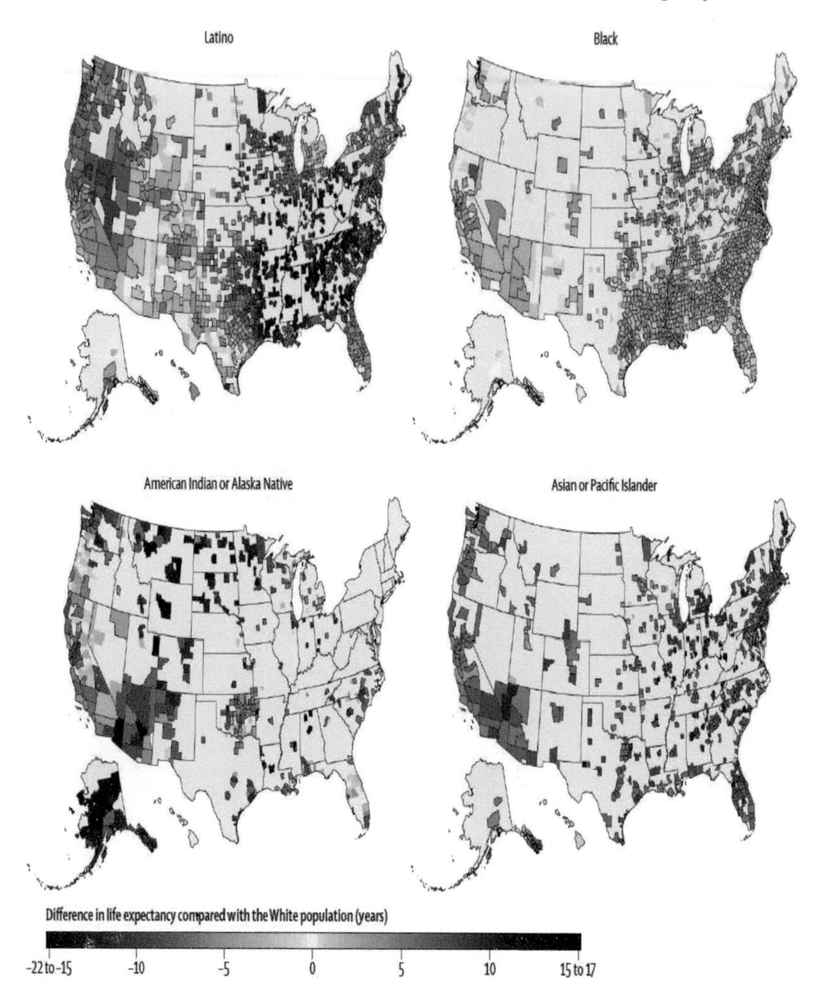

FIGURE 3.6: (Taken from Dywer-Lindgren *et al.* (2022)[85]): (Absolute) differences compared to White population in estimated life expectancies in 2019 across U.S. counties by racial-ethnic group.

3.6 Observed best prediction (OBP)

One advantage of the design-based direct estimates is that they are free of model assumptions, and therefore not affected by model failure. The design-based approach may be inefficient, of course, when sample size for the direct estimate is small, which is the main concern of SAE. It would be nice to combine the advantages of model-based and design-based approaches. Jiang

& Lahiri (2006)[184] attempts to do this by proposing a model-assisted EBP approach. The authors used an assumed mixed effects model, which may be linear or nonlinear, to derive the EBP, and then justified that the EBP is design-consistent in the sense that, when the sample size is large, the EBP is close to the design-based estimator, and this is true whether the assumed model holds or not (the technical term is that, when the sample size n_i for the ith small area goes to ∞, the difference between the EBP and the design-based estimator of the finite population domain mean goes to 0 in probability).

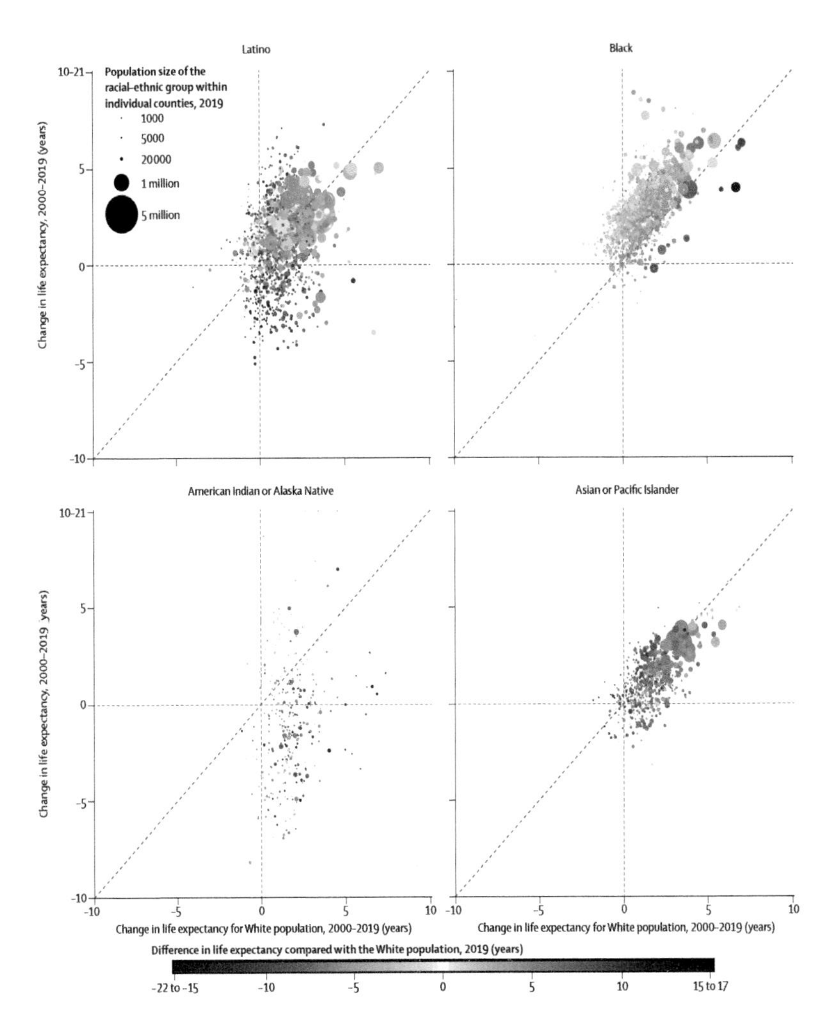

FIGURE 3.7: (Taken from Dywer-Lindgren *et al.* (2022)[85]): (Absolute) life expectancy changes from 2000 to 2019 across U.S. counties by racial-ethnic group.

Since the design-based estimator is known to be accurate when the sample size is large, the EBP is protected from model failure at least for areas with large sample sizes. In practice, due to inhomogeneous of the subpopulation (small area) sizes, some areas do end up with relatively large sample sizes. For example, in a U.S. national survey the sample sizes for California, New York, or Texas are often quite large. Model-assisted methods had been previously used in SAE; see [324], [201], [288], and You & Rao (2003; RM15), among others. An advantage of the Jiang-Lahiri EBP is that an explicit model assumption is not needed for the unobserved units of the finite population. This is in sharp contrast to the pseudo-EBLUP method of [288], who derived a design-consistent estimator assuming that a (super-population) linear mixed model holds for all of the units in the finite population, observed or unobserved. In practice, model assumptions are difficult to check for unobserved units.

However, the model-assisted methods mentioned above are not protected from model failure for areas with small sample sizes. For example, a linear model may be oversimplified that it misrepresents the true small area mean. Of course, one may avoid such model misspecification by carefully choosing the assumed model via a statistical model selection process. On the other hand, there are practical, sometimes even political, reasons that a simple model like LMM is preferred. For example, such a model is simple to use and interpret, and it easily utilizes auxiliary information. Note that the auxiliary data are often collected using taxpayers' money; so it might be "politically incorrect" not to use them, even if that is a result of the model selection.

Equation (3.1) shows that area direct estimate with relatively high sampling variance (or relatively small sample size when the area-level estimate is aggregated from samples within the area) is moved more towards the regression estimator and so is not protected from model misspecification. Observed best prediction (OBP) intends to minimize the impact of such a misspecification. Following [188] and [295], Regardless of potential model misspecification, the true small area means should not be dependent on the assumed model. Note that $\theta_i = \mathrm{E}(y_i|v_i), 1 \le i \le m$. Now suppose that the true underlying model can be expressed as

$$y_i = \mu_i + v_i + e_i, \quad i = 1, \dots, m, \tag{3.2}$$

where μ_i's are unknown means, and v_i's and e_i's are the same as in the Fay-Herriott model. Regardless of the unknown means, $\mathrm{E}(y_i) = \mu_i, 1 \le i \le m$. Therefore, under model (3.2), the small area means can be expressed as

$$\theta_i = \mu_i + v_i = \mathrm{E}(y_i) + v_i, \quad i = 1, \dots, m. \tag{3.3}$$

The last expression in (3.3) does not depend on the assumed model. Note that, hereafter, the notation E (without subscript) represents expectation under the true underlying distribution, which is unknown but not model-dependent.

A well-known precision measure for a predictor is the mean squared prediction error (MSPE; e.g., Prasad & Rao 1990, Das, Jiang & Rao 2004). Jiang *et al.* (2011) considered the vector of the small area means $\theta = (\theta_i)_{1 \le i \le m}$ and its (vector-valued) predictor $\tilde{\theta} = (\tilde{\theta}_i)_{1 \le i \le m}$, the MSPE of the (vector-valued) predictor is defined as

$$\mathrm{MSPE}(\tilde{\theta}) = \mathrm{E}(|\tilde{\theta} - \theta|^2) = \sum_{i=1}^{m} \mathrm{E}(\tilde{\theta}_i - \theta_i)^2. \tag{3.4}$$

Once again, the expectation in (3.4) is with respect to the true underlying distribution (of whatever random quantities that are involved), which is unknown but not model-dependent. Under the MSPE measure, the BP of θ is its conditional expectation, $\tilde{\theta} = \mathrm{E}(\theta|y)$. Under the assumed model Fay-Herriott model, and given the parameters $\psi = (\beta', A)'$, the BP can be expressed as

$$\tilde{\theta}(\psi) = \mathrm{E}_{\mathrm{M},\psi}(\theta|y) = \left[x_i'\beta + \frac{A}{A + D_i}(y_i - x_i'\beta)\right]_{1 \le i \le m}, \tag{3.5}$$

or, componentwisely, $\tilde{\theta}(\psi)_i = \mathbf{x}_i'\beta + B_i(y_i - x_i'\beta), 1 \le i \le m$, where $B_i = A/(A+D_i)$, and $\mathrm{E}_{\mathrm{M},\psi}$ represents (conditional) expectation under the assumed model with ψ being the true parameter vector. Note that $\mathrm{E}_{\mathrm{M},\psi}$ is different from E unless the assumed model is correct, and ψ is the true parameter vector. Also note that the BP is the minimizer of the area-specific MSPE instead of the overall MSPE (3.4). In other words, $\tilde{\theta}_i(\psi) = x_i'\beta + B_i(y_i - x_i'\beta)$ minimizes $\mathrm{E}(\tilde{\theta}_i - \theta_i)^2$ over all predictor $\tilde{\theta}_i$, if the assumed model is correct and ψ is the true parameter vector. For simplicity, let us assume, for now, that A is known. Then, the precision of $\tilde{\theta}(\psi)$, which is now denoted by $\tilde{\theta}(\beta)$, is measured by

$$\mathrm{MSPE}\{\tilde{\theta}(\beta)\} = \sum_{i=1}^{m} \mathrm{E}\{B_i y_i - \theta_i + x_i'\beta(1 - B_i)\}^2 = I_1 + 2I_2 + I_3, \tag{3.6}$$

where $I_1 = \sum_{i=1}^{m} \mathrm{E}(B_i y_i - \theta_i)^2$, $I_2 = \sum_{i=1}^{m} x_i'\beta(1 - B_i)\mathrm{E}(B_i y_i - \theta_i)$, $I_3 = \sum_{i=1}^{m} (x_i'\beta)^2(1 - B_i)^2$. Note that I_1 does not depend on β. As for I_2, by using the expression (3.3), we have $\mathrm{E}(B_i y_i - \theta_i) = (B_i - 1)\mathrm{E}(y_i)$. Thus, we have $I_2 = -\sum_{i=1}^{m}(1 - B_i)^2 x_i'\beta\mathrm{E}(y_i)$. It follows that the left side of (3.6) can be expressed as

$$\mathrm{MSPE}\{\tilde{\theta}(\beta)\} = \mathrm{E}\left\{I_1 + \sum_{i=1}^{m}(1 - B_i)^2(x_i'\beta)^2 - 2\sum_{i=1}^{m}(1 - B_i)^2 x_i'\beta y_i\right\}. \tag{3.7}$$

The right side of (3.7) suggests a natural estimator of β, by minimizing the expression inside the expectation, which is equivalent to minimizing

$$Q(\beta) = \sum_{i=1}^{m}(1 - B_i)^2(x_i'\beta)^2 - 2\sum_{i=1}^{m}(1 - B_i)^2 x_i'\beta y_i = \beta'X'\Gamma^2 X\beta - 2y'\Gamma^2 X\beta, \tag{3.8}$$

where $X = (x_i')_{1\le i\le m}$, $y = (y_i)_{1\le i\le m}$ and $\Gamma = \text{diag}(1 - B_i, 1 \le i \le m)$. A closed-form solution of the minimizer is obtained as

$$\tilde{\beta} = (X'\Gamma^2 X)^{-1} X'\Gamma^2 y = \left\{\sum_{i=1}^{m}(1 - B_i)^2 x_i x_i'\right\}^{-1} \sum_{i=1}^{m}(1 - B_i)^2 x_i y_i. \quad (3.9)$$

Here we assume, without loss of generality, that X is of full column rank. Note that $\tilde{\beta}$ minimizes the "observed" MSPE which is the expression inside the expectation on the right side of (3.7). Jiang *et al.* (2011)[188] called $\tilde{\beta}$ given by (3.9) the *best predictive estimator*, or BPE, of β. A predictor of the mixed effects θ is then obtained by replacing β in the BP (3.5) by its BPE (note that here A is assumed known). This predictor is known as the *observed best predictor*, or OBP.

Let us now refer back to the Fay-Herriot model but with A unknown. Again, we begin with the left side of (3.4), and note that the expectations involved are with respect to the true underlying distribution that is unknown, but not model-dependent. By (3.5), we have, in matrix expression, $\tilde{\theta}(\psi) = y - \Gamma(\mathbf{y} - X\beta)$, where Γ is defined below (3.8). By (3.2) and (3.3), it can be shown that

$$\text{MSPE}\{\tilde{\theta}(\psi)\} = \text{E}\{(\mathbf{y} - X\beta)'\Gamma^2(y - X\beta) + 2A\text{tr}(\Gamma) - \text{tr}(D)\}, (3.10)$$

where $D = \text{diag}(D_i, 1 \le i \le m)$. The BPE of $\psi = (\beta', A)'$ is obtained by minimizing the expression inside the E on the right side of (3.10), which is equivalent to minimizing

$$Q(\psi) = (y - X\beta)'\Gamma^2(y - X\beta) + 2A\text{tr}(\Gamma). \quad (3.11)$$

Let $\tilde{Q}(A)$ be $Q(\psi)$ with $\beta = \tilde{\beta}$ given by (3.9). It can be shown that $\tilde{Q}(A) = \mathbf{y}'\Gamma P_{(\Gamma X)^{\perp}}\mathbf{\Gamma} y + 2A\text{tr}(\Gamma)$, where for any matrix M, $P_{M^{\perp}} = I - P_M$ with $P_M = M(M'M)^{-1}M'$ (assuming nonsingularity of $M'M$), hence, $P_{(\Gamma X)^{\perp}} = I_m - \Gamma X(X'\Gamma^2 X)^{-1}X'\Gamma$ and I_m is the m-dimensional identity matrix. The BPE of A is the minimizer of $\tilde{Q}(A)$ with respect to $A \ge 0$, denoted by $\tilde{A}$. Once $\tilde{A}$ is obtained, the BPE of β is given by (3.9) with A replaced by $\tilde{A}$. Given the BPE of ψ, $\tilde{\psi} = (\tilde{\beta}', \tilde{A})'$, the OBP of θ is given by the BP (3.5) with $\psi = \tilde{\psi}$.

Essentially, what OBP does is entertain two models, one is the assumed model and the other is a broader model. The assumed model is used to derive the BP of the small area mean, which is no longer the BP when the assumed model fails. The broader model, on the other hand, is only used to derive a criterion for estimating the parameters under the assumed model, and the criterion is not model-dependent. The parameter estimator obtained by minimizing the observed MSPE is called the best predictive estimator (BPE). Because OBP estimates the parameters under an objective criterion that is unaffected by model misspecification, it is not surprising that OBP is more robust against model failure than EBLUP in terms of predictive performance.

The latter was demonstrated both theoretically and empirically in Jiang *et al.* (2011) and subsequent work ([177, 55, 17]).

Example 3.6 OBP estimation for hospital data: Ganesh (2009)[102] proposed a Fay-Herriot model as $y_i = \beta_0 + \beta_1 x_i + v_i + e_i$ to fit the data. However, an inspection of the scatter plot (see Figure 3, right plot) suggests some nonlinear trend. In fact, it appears that a quadratic model would fit the data well except for a potential "outlier" at the upper right corner.

The question is what to do in this situation. One option would be to look for a more complex model that fits the data better. This approach will be explored later. Another option is to stay with the relatively simple quadratic model, but take into account the potential model misspecification. This would also avoid overfitting, especially given the small sample size. Following the latter approach, the quadratic model, expressed as

$$y_i = \beta_0 + \beta_1 x_i + \beta_2 x_i^2 + v_i + e_i, \quad i = 1, \dots, 23, \tag{3.12}$$

is fitted using the OBP method, which is known to be more robust to model misspecification than the EBLUP method. The OBP is based on the BPE of the model parameters, rather than based on the ML, REML or Prasad-Rao estimators. To illustrate the difference, let us assume, for now, that A is known. Under the general expression of the Fay-Herriot model, the BPE of β has the expression

$$\hat{\beta} = \left\{ \sum_{i=1}^{m} \left(\frac{D_i}{A + D_i} \right)^2 x_i x_i' \right\}^{-1} \sum_{i=1}^{m} \left(\frac{D_i}{A + D_i} \right)^2 x_i y_i. \tag{3.13}$$

In comparison, the MLE of β has the expression

$$\tilde{\beta} = \left(\sum_{i=1}^{m} \frac{x_i x_i'}{A + D_i} \right)^{-1} \sum_{i=1}^{m} \frac{x_i y_i}{A + D_i}. \tag{3.14}$$

Comparing (3.13) and (3.14), it is seen that both estimators are weighted averages of the data; the only difference being how the weights are assigned.

This seems to be intuitive when recalling the expression of the BP, which is (3.5) with $\hat{\beta}, \hat{A}$ replaced by the true β, A, respectively. In other words, the BP is a weighted average of the direct estimator, y_i, and model-based estimator, $x_i'\beta$ (assuming that β is known), and the model part is more relevant to area with larger D_i. Jiang (2017,p. 45)[181] wrote the following in interpreting the difference between BPE and MLE: "Imagine that there is a meeting of representatives from the different small areas to discuss what estimate of β is to be used in the BP. The areas with larger D_i think that their 'voice' should be heard more (i.e., they should receive more weights), because the BP is more relevant to their business. Their request is reasonable (although,

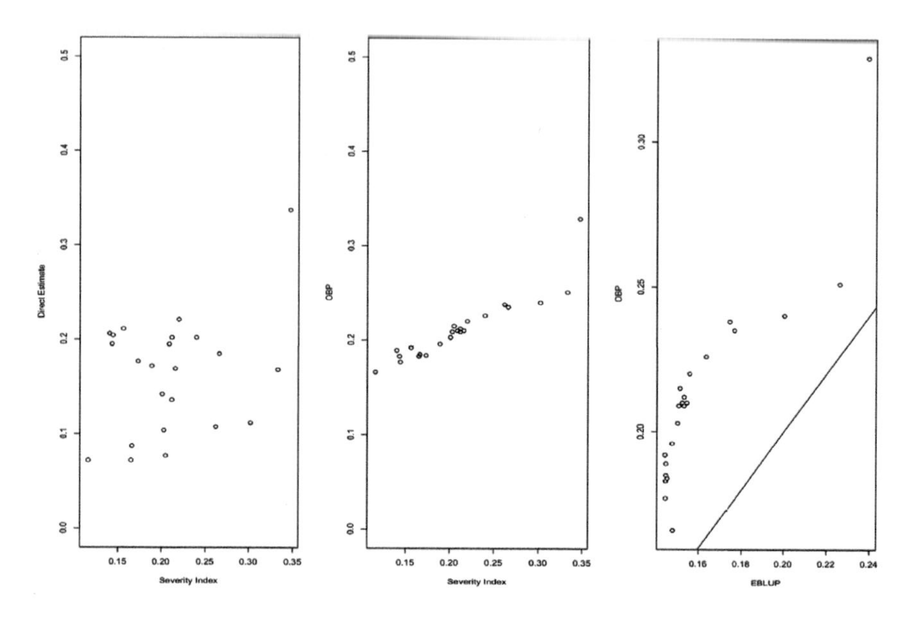

FIGURE 3.8: (Taken from Jiang and Rao, (2020)[189]): *Trio of plots from the hospital dataset showing i) the direct estimates vs the severity index, ii) the OBP vs the severity index (notice the smoothing effect produced) and iii) the OBP vs the EBLUP estimates. The last plot reflects the effect the differential weighting of hospitals to estimate the BPE vs the MLE of β. The line of identity is overlayed.*

politically, this may not work ...)". It should be noted that it is the BP, not the OBP, who determines how to assign weights to the direct and model-based estimators; the OBP only finds a way to estimate the parameters involved in the BP, namely β and A, to minimize the potential damage in case the model is misspecified. The EBLUP, on the other hand, finds a different way to estimate the parameters, typically via ML, REML or MoM estimators, which are different than the BPE. For the hospital data, in particular, the BPE under model (3.12) are given by $\hat{\beta}_0 = 0.280$, $\hat{\beta}_1 = -0.989$, $\hat{\beta}_2 = 3.261$, and $\hat{A} = 2.099 \times 10^{-4}$. A trio of plots of the direct estimates and resulting OBPs and EBLUPs are presented in Figure 3.8. The effect of differential weighting of hospitals is clearly evident in the rightmost plot which compares the OBPs to the EBLUPs (the line of identity is overlayed). In this case, using the BPE estimates forces the OBPs to be systematically larger in magnitude then their EBLUP counterparts.

3.6.0.1 OBP versus the BLUP

Write the assumed model as

$$y = X\beta + Zv + e, \tag{3.15}$$

where X, Z are known matrices; β is a vector of fixed effects; v, e are vectors of random effects and errors, respectively, such that $v \sim N(0, G)$, $e \sim N(0, \Sigma)$, and v, e are uncorrelated. Now let the true underlying model be

$$y = \mu + Zv + e, \tag{3.16}$$

where $\mu = \mathrm{E}(y)$. The focus is on prediction of a vector of mixed effects which we express as,

$$\theta = F'\mu + R'v, \tag{3.17}$$

where F, R are known matrices. Suppose that G, Σ are known. Then, the BP of θ, under the assumed model is given by $\mathrm{E_M}(\theta|y) = F'\mu + R'\mathrm{E_M}(v|y) = F'X\beta + R'GZ'\mathbf{V}^{-1}(y - X\beta)$, where $\mathrm{E_M}$ denotes expectation under the assumed model, $V = \mathrm{Var}(y) = \Sigma + ZGZ'$ and β is the true vector of fixed effects, under the assumed model. Now if we can write $B = R'GZ'V^{-1}$ and $\Gamma = F' - B$, then the BP can be expressed in as

$$\mathrm{E_M}(\theta|y) = F'y - \Gamma(y - X\beta). \tag{3.18}$$

Now let $\breve{\theta}$ denote the right side of (3.18) with a fixed, but arbitrary β. Then, by (3.16) and (3.17), we have $\breve{\theta} - \theta = H'v + F'e - \Gamma(y - X\beta)$, where $H = Z'F - R$. Thus, we have $\mathrm{MSPE}(\breve{\theta}) = \mathrm{E}(|\breve{\theta} - \theta|^2) = \mathrm{E}(|H'v + F'e|^2) - 2\mathrm{E}\{(v'H + e'F)\Gamma(y - X\beta)\} + \mathrm{E}\{(y - X\beta)'\Gamma'\Gamma(y - X\beta)\} = I_1 - 2I_2 + I_3$. It is understood that the I's here are different from those in (3.6). Clearly, I_1 does not depend on β. Also, I_2 does not depend on β either. Thus, we can write the MSPE as

$$\mathrm{MSPE}(\breve{\theta}) = \mathrm{E}\{I_1 - 2I_2 + (y - X\beta)'\Gamma'\Gamma(y - X\beta)\}. \tag{3.19}$$

The BPE of β is obtained by minimizing the expression inside the expectation which gives

$$\tilde{\beta} = (X'\Gamma'\Gamma X)^{-1}X'\Gamma'\Gamma y, \tag{3.20}$$

assuming that $\Gamma'\Gamma$ is nonsingular and X is full rank. Once the BPE is obtained, the OBP of θ is given by the right side of (3.18) with β replaced by $\tilde{\beta}$. Now we turn our focus to the MLE of β which is given by

$$\hat{\beta} = (X'V^{-1}X)^{-1}X'V^{-1}y. \tag{3.21}$$

Thus, the BLUP of θ is given by the right side of (3.18) with β replaced by $\hat{\beta}$. We now look at the comparison of the MSPE of the OBP and BLUP. First, consider a class of empirical best predictors (EBPs) that can be written as

$$\breve{\theta} = F'y - \Gamma(y - X\breve{\beta}), \tag{3.22}$$

where $\breve{\beta}$ is a weighted least squares (WLS) estimator of β expressed as

$$\breve{\beta} = (X'WX)^{-1}X'Wy, \tag{3.23}$$

and W is a positive definite weighting matrix.

It is now becomes clear that the BPE and MLE are special cases of the WLS, hence the OBP and BLUP are special cases of the EBP. Then, $\breve{\theta} = [F' - \Gamma\{I - X(X'WX)^{-1}X'W\}]y \equiv Ly$. By (3.16) and (3.17), it can be shown that

$$\begin{aligned}\text{MSPE}(\breve{\theta}) &= \text{tr}\{R'(G - GZ'V^{-1}ZG)R\} \\ &\quad +\mu'\{I - X(X'WX)^{-1}X'W\}'\Gamma'\Gamma\{I - X(X'WX)^{-1}X'W\}\mu \\ &\quad +\text{tr}\{(L - B)V(L - B)'\}. \end{aligned}\tag{3.24}$$

The first term on the right side of (3.24) does not depend W. As for the second term, [188] show that it can be bounded from below and that the lower bound is achieved by the OBP. Similarly they show that the third term can be bounded from below and that the lower bound is achieved by the BLUP.

This then leads to the following theorem:

Theorem 3.1 Jiang *et al.* **(2011)[188]:** *The MSPE of the EBP (3.22)–(3.23) can be expressed as*

$$\text{MSPE}(\breve{\theta}) = a_0 + \mu' A_1(W)\mu + \text{tr}\{A_2(W)\}, \tag{3.25}$$

where $a_0 \geq 0$ *is a constant that does not depend on the EBP;* $A_1(W), A_2(W) \geq 0$ *and depend on* W*, hence the EBP.* $\mu' A_1(W)\mu$ *is minimized by the OBP, which has* $W = \Gamma'\Gamma$*;* $\text{tr}\{A_2(W)\}$ *is minimized by the BLUP, which has* $\mathbf{W} = V^{-1}$.

It is clear that that the second term disappears when the mean of y is correctly specified. Now suppose that the mean of y is misspecified. Then, it can be shown that $\mu' A_1(W)\mu \geq \lambda_{\min}(\Gamma'\Gamma)|P_{X^\perp}\mu|^2$, where $\lambda_{\min}$ denotes the smallest eigenvalue. Thus, provided that $\lambda_{\min}(\Gamma'\Gamma)$ has a positive lower bound, the second term has the order $O(|P_{X^\perp}\mu|^2)$. On the other hand, the third term is usually $O(1)$. Thus, the difference in their second terms is $O(|P_{X^\perp}\mu|^2)$ in favor of the OBP, while the difference in their third terms is $O(1)$ in favor of the BLUP.

What this means is that if $|P_{X^\perp}\mu|^2 \to \infty$, the OBP can have lower MSPE than the BLUP but even if the mean of y is correctly specified, the ratio of the MSPEs of the OBP and BLUP goes to one as the sample size increases ([188]).

3.6.1 Nonparametric/semi-parametric small area estimation

Using the work of [175], a non-parametric area-level model, extending the Fay-Herriot model, can be expressed as

$$y_i = f(x_i) + v_i + e_i, \quad i = 1, \ldots, m, \tag{3.26}$$

where the assumptions about v_i and e_i are the same as in the Fay-Herriot model, but $f(\cdot)$ is an unknown function. Opsomer *et al.* (2008)[272] used a penalized spline (P-spline) approximation to $f(\cdot)$. Specifically, the P-spline is in the form of

$$\tilde{f}(x) = \beta_0 + \beta_1 x + \cdots + \beta_p x^p + \gamma_1 (x - \kappa_1)_+^p + \cdots + \gamma_q (x - \kappa_q)_+^p, \tag{3.27}$$

where p is the degree of the spline, q is the number of knots, κ_j, $1 \leq j \leq q$ are the knots, and $x_+ = x 1_{(x>0)}$. Opsomer *et al.* (2008)[272] assumed that the γ coefficients are random; this leads to the well-known connection between P-spline fitting and LMM (e.g., [362]) that is used to determine the penalty parameter. Jiang, Nguyen and Rao (2010)[175] considered model selection in choosing the degree of the spline, p, and number of knots, q, using fence methods, a class of strategies for model selection that is particularly suitable for non-conventional problems (e.g., [179]). Rao, Sinha & Dumitrescu (2014)[301] considered a similar P-spline approach to SAE under semi-parametric mixed models.

Mendez and Lohr (2011)[249] noted that for spline-based approaches, one needed to have the x_{ij} for population units, not just $\bar{X}_i$, the population mean of the x's. In addition, much of the auxillary data are categorical instead of continuous; as a result, the mean function may not be smooth. They took the approach of subsetting and interactions instead and extending [248], who developed tree-based approaches to model dependent data, [249] extended the proposed tree-based models to SAE. This recognized earlier work on using classification and regression trees for survey data (see [116, 325, 354, 355]). Mendez and Lohr (2011)[249] developed tree growing and pruning approaches. They then went a step further and proposed random forests (RF) ([35]) for SAE which they called mixed RFs to allow random effects. More details on tree-based methods and random forests are described in Chapter 5.

Datta, Delaigle, Hall & Wang (2018)[71] noted that measurements of auxiliary variables used in SAE are often subject to measurement errors. Ignoring such error-in-variable can lead to estimators that perform even worse than the direct survey estimators. The authors proposed a semi-parametric approach based on the Fay-Herriot model to produce reliable prediction intervals for small-area characteristics of interest. The approach is semi-parametric because it is assumed that the distribution of the auxiliary variable without error, X, which is unobserved, is completely unknown; other parts of random variables, such as the area-specific random effects, the sampling errors, and the measurement errors corresponding to X, follow either parametric or known distributions.

3.6.2 Model selection and diagnostics

Model selection is an important relatively new topic in SAE which was noted earlier in [24] and [110], among others. Datta & Lahiri (2001)[70] used a Bayes factor in choosing between a fixed effects model and a random effects model. Meza & Lahiri (2005)[253] demonstrated limitations of Mallow's C_p in selecting the fixed covariates in a NER model. Vaida & Blanchard (2005)[357] proposed a conditional AIC method that is applicable to selection among NER models. We discuss here though in more detail the work of [179] who proposed the fence methods, that are especially suitable to nonconventional model selection problems, such as mixed model selection.

We start out by defining $Q_M = Q_M(y, \theta_M)$ to be a measure of lack-of-fit, where y represents the vector of observations, M indicates a candidate model, and θ_M denotes the vector of parameters under M. Q_M only satisfies the basic requirement that $\mathrm{E}(Q_M)$ is minimized when M is a true model, and θ_M the true parameter vector under M. Then, one can construct a statistical *fence* or barrier and declare and a candidate model M inside the fence if

$$\hat{Q}_M \quad \leq \quad \hat{Q}_{\tilde{M}} + c\hat{\sigma}_{M,\tilde{M}}, \tag{3.28}$$

where $\hat{Q}_M = \inf_{\theta_M \in \Theta_M} Q_M$, Θ_M being the parameter space under M, $\tilde{M}$ is a model that minimizes $\hat{Q}_M$ among $M \in \mathcal{M}$, the set of candidate models, and $\hat{\sigma}_{M,\tilde{M}}$ is an estimate of the standard deviation of $\hat{Q}_M - \hat{Q}_{\tilde{M}}$. The constant c on the right side of (3.28) can be fixed (e.g., $c = 1$) or adaptively chosen. The calculation of $\hat{Q}_M$ is usually straightforward. For example, in many cases Q_M can be chosen as the negative log-likelihood, or residual sum of squares. On the other hand, the computation of $\hat{\sigma}_{M,\tilde{M}}$ can be quite challenging. Jiang, Nguyen and Rao (2010)[187] proposed a simplified procedure that avoids the calculation of $\hat{\sigma}_{M,\tilde{M}}$.

3.6.2.1 A simplified adaptive fence procedure

We assume that $\mathcal{M}$ contains a full model, M_{f}, of which each candidate model is a submodel. It follows that $\tilde{M} = M_{\mathrm{f}}$. The new procedure declares the term a model is in the fence if

$$\hat{Q}_M - \hat{Q}_{M_{\mathrm{f}}} \quad \leq \quad c, \tag{3.29}$$

where c is chosen adaptively as follows. For each $M \in \mathcal{M}$, let $p^*(M) = \mathrm{P}^*\{M_0(c) = M\}$ be the empirical probability of selection for M, where $M_0(c)$ denotes the model selected by the fence procedure based on (3.29) with the given c, and P^* is is obtained by bootstrapping under M_{f}. If B such bootstrap samples are drawn, then let $p^*(M)$ be the proportion of times that M is selected by the fence procedure corresponding to (3.29) with the given c. Now simply let $p^* = \max_{M \in \mathcal{M}} p^*(M)$. Since p^* depends on c, one can define c^* to be the c that maximizes p^*.

Typically the optimal model is neither M_{f} nor M_*, the minimal model (dimensionwise; e.g., a model with only the intercept). However, these two extreme cases are handled using the baseline adjustment and threshold checking

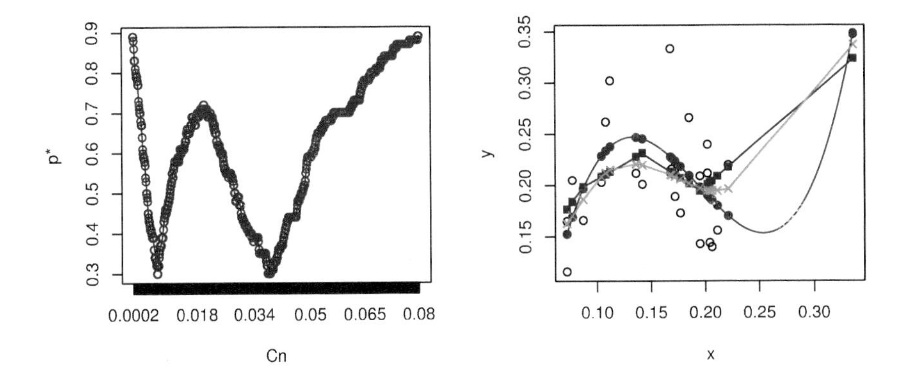

FIGURE 3.9: (Taken from Jiang and Rao (2020)[189]): Left: A plot of p^* against c_n from the search over the full model space. Right: Raw data and the fitted values and curves; red dots and curve—the cubic function resulted from the full model search; blue squares and lines—the linear spline with 4 knots from the restricted model search; green X's and lines—the GAM fits.

methods developed by [179]. The baseline adjustment is done by generating an additional vector of covariates, say, X_{a}, so that it is unrelated to the data. Then, define the model M_{f}^* as M_{f} plus X_{a}, and replace M_{f} in (3.29) by M_{f}^*, but let $\mathcal{M}$ remain unchanged. This way one knows for sure that the new full model, M_{f}^*, is not an optimal model (because it is not a candidate model). The threshold checking inequality is given by $\hat{Q}_{M_*} - \hat{Q}_{M_{\mathrm{f}}^*} > d_*$, where d_* is the maximum of the left side of the threshold inequality computed under the bootstrap samples generated under M_*. In case the threshold inequality holds, we ignore the right tail of the plot of p^* against c that eventually goes up and stays at one Figure 3.9 shows a plot of this.

Another minor adjustment can also be made. Since p^* is a sample proportion, we can construct a (large sample) lower confidence bound,

$$p^* - 1.96\sqrt{p^*(1-p^*)/B} \tag{3.30}$$

where B is the bootstrap sample size. When selecting c that maximizes p^* we take (3.30) into account. More specifically, suppose that there are two peaks in the plot of p^* against c located at c_1 and c_2 such that $c_1 < c_2$. Let p_1^* and p_2^* be the heights of the peaks corresponding to c_1 and c_2. As long as p_1^* is greater than the confidence lower bound at p_2^*, that is, (3.30) with $p^* = p_2^*$, we choose c_1 over c_2.

Example 3.7 Model selection for the hospital data: The model is the same as that described before with $x_i'\beta = \beta_0 + \beta_1 x_i$, where x_i is the severity index, defined as the average fraction of females, Blacks, children and extremely ill kidney recipients at hospital i. However, we suspect one potential outlier (at the upper right corner) when the linear model is fitted; see the right figure of Figure 3.9. Jiang *et al.* (2010)[187] used the fence method to identify the optimal model in this case, which led to a cubic model corresponding to the smooth curve in the figure. Specifically, consider a spline-based nonparametric area-level model, and use the fence method to select the degree of polynomial, p, and the number of knots, q, for the spline. The fence method has selected the model $p = 3$ and $q = 0$, that is, a cubic function with no knots, as the optimal model. This analysis was repeated 100 times each time using different bootstrap samples, and all results led to the same model. The left figure of Figure 3.9 shows the plot of p^* against c $(= c_n)$ in the fence model selection. This and other model fits are also on the same figure – namely i) fence with a full model search (red), ii) fence but with a more restricted space of candidate models, namely, the linear splines only (i.e., $p = 1$). In this case, the fence method selected a linear spline with four knots (i.e., $q = 4$) as the optimal model (blue) and iii) generalized additive models with the BRUTO procedure ([133]) which augments the class of models to look at a null fit and a linear fit for the spline function, and embeds the resulting model selection (i.e., null, linear or smooth fits) into a weighted back-fitting algorithm using generalized cross-validation for computational efficiency (green). The red curve clearly appears to fit the data the best.

4

Causality, Moderation, and Mediation

4.1 Socioecological framework for health disparities

Social ecology posits that disease ensues from the complex interplay of determinants operating across multiple levels of influence, including the individual level and the community level. On the individual level, variables of interest often reflect key constructs from theories/frameworks of health promotion, such as the Health Belief Model. However, biological indicators of clinical prognosis and outcome also merit inclusion, when available (see Figure 4.1). On the community level, key variables of interest include, though are not limited to neighborhood poverty, educational attainment, racial composition, and employment. These social determinants have consistently been found to influence individual health, above and beyond known individual risk factors for an outcome of interest. Perhaps more importantly, they are differentially distributed by race/ethnicity in the United States, and many individual-level variables. This logic reflects the tenets of social ecology, and the inherent complexity in the etiology of health disparity.

4.2 Causal inference in health disparities

Identifying the causes of health disparities is important to developing strategies to reducing or eliminating them. This could be at the policy level and the individual level. But in health disparities analysis, identification of such causal drivers is challenging because causal factors can interact or lie along causal chains that make it difficult to tease apart the causal versus non-causal effects. Causal mechanisms can operate at different levels as illustrated in Figure 4.1 each of which can involve unique approaches for conceptualization and measurement ([171]).

Causal effects are typically derived using a potential outcomes approach arising from different treatments or exposures (i.e., potential causal health disparity driver). However, since only the outcome associated with the "assigned" exposure is observed, the other not provided is termed "counterfactual".

DOI: 10.1201/9781003119449-4

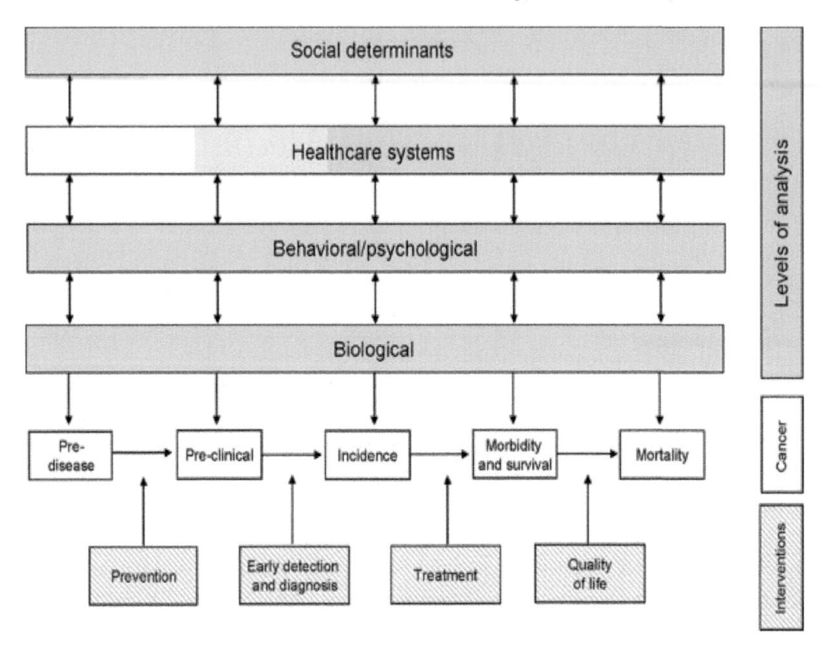

FIGURE 4.1: (Taken from Hiatt and Breen (2008)[143]): Conceptualization of multilevel interactions along the cancer continuum. Healthcare systems are less likely to influence cancer incidence than mortality and are lightly shaded in the preclinical phase of the continuum.

4.2.1 Experimental versus observational studies

Randomized (or experimental) studies provide an ideal setting for evaluating causality. When feasible, then exposures are under the control of a random process, thus mitigating the bias the estimates of treatment effect that might result from other factors that might also affect outcomes – also known as confounders. In health disparity research, experimental studies face two particular challenges: i) it may be infeasible to randomize causal factors of interest (e.g., exposure to racism, neighborhood walkability), and ii) it's not clear how generalizable the effects will be when applied to other populations and situations. As a result, observational studies are much more commonly encountered in health disparity research.

In such studies, one cannot control the treatment or exposure variable directly. As a result, other variables could be correlated with the exposure that also contribute to the outcome. Adjusting for this type of confounding requires the development of specialized estimation and inferential procedures.

4.2.2 Challenges with certain variables to be treated causal factors

As discussed in Chapter 1, race/ethnicity as an analytical variable requires additional thought. Typically thought of as a man-made construct, race/ethnicity is thought to operate thought pathways related to differential treatment, social isolation, and structural racism ([26]). In addition, the ancestry component through genetic analysis can also be quantified (and teased apart from the self-identified component [6]).

Still, race/ethnicity is a very common analytic factor often (incorrectly) analyzed for a causal interpretation. Under the potential outcomes framework, race/ethnicity can easily violate some of the basic underlying assumptions (discussed in detail in the next section). First, randomized experiments which can guarantee exchangeability (counterfactual outcome and actual observed outcome are independent) are not feasible because race/ethnicity cannot be assigned at the time of randomization. Positivity, which requires that individuals in each stratum of the covariates have a non-zero probability of being in the exposed group and of being in the unexposed group is often violated in race/ethnicity studies of health disparities ([26]). For example, [252] showed that areas with little data in their analyses were related to co-occurrence of racial segregation and poverty. Lastly, the consistency assumption which requires that all exposed individuals receive the same version of the treatment (sometimes called the stable unit treatment value assumption (SUTVA)) that also requires no interference between treated and control groups. It has been shown that this assumption is commonly violated when using variables like race/ethnicity but also with variables like education or income. As a result, direct assessment of race/ethnicity as a causal factor requires very specific analytical tools if viewed only through the lens of traditional causal inference. These will not be discussed here but interested readers can consult [360] for instance.

As a counter to these arguments is a large body of work from the health and social sciences to the humanities that have addressed the above counterfactual assertions not just for variables like race but also for consideration of the conceptualization of variables like gender (see, for instance, [206, 207, 198, 205]). Alternatively, these types of variables can more directly be viewed through the lens of causal mediation or moderation.

4.3 Average treatment effects

There has been a large amount of theoretical work focused in estimating average treatment effects (ATEs) under various assumptions. Much of this has come from the world of economics where causal probing into things like active labor market programs like job assistance or classroom teaching programs has been of interest. Examples include [141] and [32].

The simplest set up which will be discussed here is the case of estimating ATE under a binary treatment under the assumption that the treatment satisfies exogeneity. As mentioned above, different versions of this assumption are named unconfoundeness ([312]), selection of observables ([19]) or conditional independence ([214]).

The estimation methods can be grouped as follows: i) regression-based methods (e.g., [125]), ii) matching on covariates (e.g., [4]), iii) propensity score blocking and weighting (e.g., [313]), iv) combinations of these (e.g., [308]) and v) Bayesian methods (e.g., [320]). The discussion here will focus on the first three and readers are encouraged to consult the referenced articles for more detail about the other two methods.

4.3.1 What are we trying to estimate and are these identifiable?

Using the potential outcomes notation, assume that n units indexed by $i = 1, \ldots, n$ are drawn randomly from a large population. Associated with each unit are the potential outcome pair $(y_i(0), y_i(1))$ where 1 and 0 indicate active treatment or control, respectively. In addition, each unit has a vector of covariates (exogenous variables) c_i. These are assumed not to be affected by the treatment and often their values are taken prior to treatment assignment but this is not sufficient ([157]). Treatment assignments are indexed by $t_i = 0$ (control) or $t_i = 1$ (treatment). Thus the observable quantities are (t_i, t_i, c_i), where y_i is either $y_i(0)$ or $y_i(1)$.

The average treatment effect (ATE) is then defined as

$$ATE = E(y(1) - y(0)).$$

Sometimes it's of interest to focus on the average treatment effect for the treated (ATT) defined as,

$$ATT = E(y(1) - y(0)|t = 1).$$

A typical example where ATT is of more direct interest would be the examination of policy programs that are directed at individuals disadvantaged in some way.

Sample versions of ATE and ATT can easily be defined as, $SATE = \frac{1}{n}\sum_i (y_i(1) - y_i(0))$ and $SATT = \frac{1}{n_T}\sum_{i:t_i=1}(y_i(1) - y_i(0))$, where $n_T = \sum_i t_i$. Abadie and Imbens (2004)[4] also introduce conditional versions of ATE and ATT where the focus is conditional on the distribution of the covariates.

We now expand on the assumptions of identifiability which previously introduced.

Assumption 1 *Unconfoundedness :* $(y(0), y(1)) \perp t|c$.

Originally termed “ignorable treatment assignment" by [312], it has also been termed conditional independence by [214]. Barnow et al. (1980)[19] called this “selection on observables" in a regression framework. The second major assumption involves the joint distribution of the treatments and covariates:

Assumption 2 *Overlap:* $0 < P(t = 1|c) < 1$.

Additional regularity conditions involving smoothness. on the conditional regression functions and the propensity score (discussed later) are needed to establish more formal theoretical results ([157]).

Given these two main assumptions, one can identify ATEs. This follows because given unconfoundedness,

$$E(y(t)|c) = E(y(t)|t, c) = E(y|t, c).$$

Thus, one can estimate ATE by first estimating the ATE for the subpopulation with covariates x followed by averaging over the distribution of c. Here, we need to be able to estimate $E(y|c, t)$ for all values of t and c. If the overlap assumption is violated, then we could not estimate these because at those values of c there would be only treated or control units. Imbens (2004)[157] discusses the use of weaker assumptions including mean independence or unconfoundedness for controls and weak overlap.

An important result that extends on the unconfoundedness assumption demonstrates that one does not need to condition simultaneously on all covariates but rather conditioning could be done solely on the so-called propensity score ([312]). The propensity score is defined as the conditional probability of receiving the treatment,

$$e(c) = P(t = 1|c) = E(t|c).$$

Propensity scores can be estimated in many ways but simple parametric models include logistic regression. Then the following assumption can be stated:

Assumption 3 *Unconfoundedness given the propensity score: Under unconfoundedness, then* $(y(1), y(0) \perp t|e(c))$.

This result follows because one can show under unconfoundedness that $P(t = 1|y(0), y(1), e(c))$ and that $P(t = 1|e(c))$.

4.3.2 Estimation of ATE and related quantities

Most research has focused on methods for ATE estimation that can fall into one of 5 buckets: i) regression estimators which are methods that rely on consistent estimation of regression functions $\mu_0(c)$ and $\mu_1(c)$ under control and treatment, respectively; ii) matching estimators which compare outcomes across pairs of matched treated and control units with each unit matched to a fixed number of observations with the opposite treatment. The matching is done with respect to covariates x; iii) propensity score methods which include weighting, blocking, and matching on the propensity score; iv) combination methods which are generally motivated by the consideration that combining two approaches may lead to more robust inference and v) Bayesian methods. We will now dedicate some space to discuss each in turn.

4.3.2.1 Regression estimators

We can designate a regression estimators $\mu_t(c)$ for $t = 0, 1$. Given these functions, ATE can be estimated by,

$$\widehat{ATE}_{reg} = \frac{1}{n}\sum_i(\hat{\mu}_1(c_i) - \hat{\mu}_0(c_i)).$$

If $\sum_i t_i\hat{\mu}_1(c_i) = \sum_i t_i y_i$ and if this also holds for the controls, then $\widehat{ATE}_{reg}$ can be expressed also as,

$$\widehat{ATE}_{reg} = \frac{1}{n}\sum_i t_i(y_i - \hat{\mu}_0(c_i)) + (1 - t_i)(\hat{\mu}_1(c_i) - y_i).$$

For ATT estimation, only the control regression function needs to be estimated from which the outcomes for the treated units can then be predicted. The estimator then averages the difference between the actual outcomes for the treated and their predicted values under the control model,

$$\widehat{ATT}_{reg} = \frac{1}{n_T}\sum_i t_i(y_i - \hat{\mu}_0(c_i)).$$

It's common to use parametric regression functions to estimate these regression functions from sample data. This includes linear regression where the regression function is specified as,

$$y_i = \alpha + \mu_t(c_i) + \tau t_i + e_i = \alpha + x_i'\beta + \tau t_i + e_i$$

with $E(e_i) = 0$ and $var(e_i) = \sigma^2$ typically assumed. Or one can specify separate regression functions for the two treatment conditions. If this is the case, one can estimate two regression functions separately on the two subsamples and then substitute the predicted values into the equation for $\widehat{ATE}_{reg}$.

Regression estimators, however, can be very sensitive to differences in the covariate distributions between treated and control units. Consider the case where $\mu_0(c)$ is used to predict the missing outcomes for the treated. With a linear regression function, the average prediction is $\bar{y}_{0+(\bar{c}_1-\bar{c}_0)'\hat{\beta}}$. Thus when the two covariate vector averages are very close, the precise specification of the regression function is not very influential but when they differ, the predictions can be sensitive to these differences and thus the specification of the linear regression models.

Many other approaches that fall under the regression estimator idea have been proposed including nonparametric estimators ([125]) who proposed using series methods that incorporate propensity scores or [145] who also showed how using series methods could be simplified to eliminating the need to estimate propensity scores. Heckman *et al.* (1997, 1998)[140, 139] used kernel estimators (non-parametric regression). More details can be found in the cited references. Of note is that with each of these more flexible methods, there is a notion of choice of a tuning or smoothing parameter which is typically done via predictive considerations and using something like a cross-validation-type criterion.

4.3.2.2 Matching estimators

Regression estimators predict missing potential outcomes using the estimated regression function. Thus if $t_i = 1$, then $y_i(0)$ is imputed using a consistent estimator $\hat{\mu}_0(c_i)$. Matching estimators also do a type of imputation but only use the outcomes of closest neighbors from the opposite treatment group. In a way, this makes matching estimators more similar to nonparametric regression estimators which have a local averaging quality built into the construction.

Given a matching metric, only the number of matches to a given unit needs to be specified. Using one-to-one matching leads to the least bias but highest variance (low smoothing) but can make the matching estimator easy to use. Most matching estimators are applied in settings with the following qualities: i) interest is in ATT and ii) there are many controls available for matching. Then given a matched set (of size 1 or more) of controls to each treated unit, the ATT estimator is obtained by calculating the difference between two sample means. Any remaining bias is typically ignored.

Given a sample consisting of triples taking the form $(y(t_i), c_i, t_i), i = 1, \ldots, n$, defined the imputed potential outcomes,

$$y_i(0) = \begin{cases} y_i & \text{if } t_i = 0 \\ \frac{1}{M}\sum_{J_M(i)} y_j & \text{if } t_i = 1, \end{cases}$$

and

$$y_i(1) = \begin{cases} \frac{1}{M}\sum_{J_M(i)} y_j & \text{if } t_i = 0 \\ y_i & \text{if } t_i = 1. \end{cases}$$

where $J(M)$ are the M matches of unit i. Then Abadie and Imbens (2002) defined the simple matching estimator as,

$$\widehat{ATE}_M = \frac{1}{n}\sum_i (y_i(1) - y_i(0)).$$

They demonstrated that the bias of this estimator is $O(n^{-1/k})$ where k is the dimension of the covariates. Abadie and Imbens (2002)[4] further go on to clarify that it is only continuous covariates that should be counted in the dimension k since with discrete covariates, matching will be exact in large samples, thus not contributing to the order of the bias. Also, if one matches only the treated units and the number of controls is much larger than the number of treated units, then this bias can be ignored ([4]).

Matching estimators require a distance metric in choosing the optimal matches. The standard approach is a Euclidean metric defined as $d(c, c') = (c - c')'(c - c')$ where c and c' indicate two different covariate vectors (not the transpose of one another). It's also common practice to remove scaling effects and standardize the covariates first. This can be done by defining the distance as $d(c, c') = (c - c')'\Sigma_c^{-1}(c - c')$ where Σ_c is the variance-covariance matrix of the covariates. One particular example is the Mahalanobis distance which use the Σ_c of the pre-treatment variables. Other interesting alternatives can be found in [375]. Imbens (2004)[157] discusses the optimality of a given metric in terms of minimizing expected squared bias.

4.3.2.3 Propensity score methods

Propensity score methods date back to seminal work by [312] where interest is in adjusting for differences in the propensity score which is the conditional probability of receiving the treatment. This can be done in a number of different ways. One can weight observations using the propensity scores to create balance between treated and control units in the weighted sample. Another popular strategy is to stratify on binned ranges of the propensity score, a technique known as blocking. Finally, one can introduce the propensity score as a covariate directly into a regression model.

If the propensity score is known to the researcher apriori (and does not have to be estimated from the data), then any one of these methods is effective at eliminating confounder bias in ATE estimation. However, it's more common to have to estimate the propensity score from the data in which case, the bias reduction gains are sometimes less clear. The propensity score model specification becomes an issue as does potentially dealing with high dimensional covariates. In practice, it has been found that the performance will depend on the smoothness of the propensity score and whether additional information is available to help anchor the model.

The differences in average outcomes for treated and controls are defined as,

$$\frac{\sum_i t_i y_i}{\sum_i t_i} - \frac{\sum_i (1-t_i) y_i}{\sum_i 1-t_i},$$

is not unbiased for ATE because conditional on the treatment indicator, the distribution of the covariates differ. However, by weighting units by the reciprocal of the propensity score, one can undo this imbalance.

This relies on the following equalities:

$$E(\frac{ty}{e(c)}) = E(\frac{ty(1)}{e(c)}) = E(E(\frac{ty(1)}{e(c)}|c)) = E(\frac{e(c)E(y(1)|x)}{e(c)}) = E(y(1)),$$

using unconfoundedness to get the result. Similarly,

$$E(\frac{(1-t)y}{1-e(c)}) = E(y(0)).$$

This then implies that,

$$ATE = E(\frac{ty}{e(c)} - \frac{(1-t)y}{1-e(c)}).$$

Simple plug-in estimation yields the sample estimator,

$$\tilde{ATE}_{ps} = 1/n \sum_i (\frac{t_i y_i}{e(c_i)} - \frac{(1-t_i)y_i}{1-e(c_i)}).$$

As clean as this formula is, one problem is that the weights do not sum to 1. Thus normalized versions of the propensity scores can be used in order to have this effect. One example can be found in [145]. Implementation often requires the estimation of the propensity scores indicated by $\hat{e}(x)$. As these are plugged in, we get the operationalized estimate of ATE labeled $\widehat{ATE}_{ps}$.

In [312], they suggest blocking on $e(x)$ by dividing the sample into M blocks with approximately the same $e(x)$ values. Then given these blocks (strata), estimate within each block the ATE as if random assignment held, then accrue these across the blocks. Optimality results have been obtained assuming known propensity scores but not with estimated ones ([157]). Questions arise regarding what value should M take (number of blocks). The classical rule of thumb approach based on early work by [62] is to take $M = 5$ which was shown to remove at least 95% of the bias in the case of a single covariate. For more general situations, this continues to be an active area of research. Blocking can be thought of as a type of non-parametric regression adjustment where the unknown adjustment function is approximated by a step function with fixed jump points.

4.3.2.4 Combination methods

There have been a number of attempts to combine two of the three previously described methods in order to add coherence. For instance, neither matching nor propensity scoring directly address the correlation between the outcome and the covariates. Furthermore, [307] discuss the idea of double robustness where as long as the parametric model for either the regression function or the propensity score is correctly specified, the resulting estimator of ATE is consistent. Another example is matching which can lead to consistent estimators without additional assumptions. Hence, methods that combine matching and regression are robust against misspecification of the regression function. Imbens (2004)[157] discusses a number of combination methods including i) weighting and regression, ii) blocking and regression, and ii) matching and regression.

4.3.2.5 Bayesian methods

Rubin (1978)[320] introduced a general approach for estimating ATE and distributional treatment effects from a Bayesian paradigm. However, as Imbens (2004) points out, there is little literature on estimating ATE under unconfoundedness either for the whole population or for just the treated. It is also less clear how Bayesian methods would be used with pairwise matching.

Within the regression setting, Bayesian approaches may be useful however. In the presence of many covariates, Bayesian variable selection approaches could be employed using appropriate priors (e.g., spike and slab regression – [255]; [106]; [165]). Another reason to consider the use of Bayesian methods is that the estimation of unobserved outcomes has a similar flavor to missing data under the missing at random (MAR) assumption. In these areas, Bayesian methods are used widely. A prominent example is that of multiple imputation ([318]). The main unique aspect that would have to be considered is that in causal inference applications, the amount of missingness would be at 50% which could add complications in implementation.

4.3.2.6 Uncertainty estimation for ATE estimators

Imbens (2004)[157] provides a detailed discussion of estimating variances for ATE estimators. He discusses brute force methods that would appeal to asymptotic arguments, methods for cases where the regression functions or propensity scores are estimated using series or sieves and finally bootstrapping ([90]). For matching estimators, subsampling ([286]) is advocated to deal with the ties produced by matching algorithms that can lead in additional discreteness in the sampling distribution of the ATE estimator.

4.3.3 Assessing the assumptions

The unconfoundedness assumption is not directly testable. Recall, that it states that the conditional distribution of $y(0)$ given receipt of the active treatment is identical to the distribution of $y(0)$ given receipt of the control treatment and given covariates, and similarly for $y(1)$. But since we do not observe all of these potential outcomes, only indirect tests can be constructed (for example, [138, 311]). The idea behind these indirect tests is to focus on estimating a causal effect that is known equal to zero. If the test suggests an effect different than zero, the unconfoundedness assumption is suspect. One approach to do this was developed by Rosenbaum (1987)[311] which relies on having multiple control groups in hand (e.g., ineligible participants and eligible nonparticipants). Comparing these two groups should yield a zero treatment effect difference. Nonrejection of the test in the case where the two control groups are likely to have different potential biases makes it more likely that the unconfoundedness assumption holds.

The choice of the covariates is also a consideration. There may be some covariates that should not be adjusted for. In other cases, the removal of some covariates with weak correlation with the treatment variable and the outcome can reduce variance. This is more observed as a finite sample result rather than something related to asymptotic precision ([157]). With regards to the first issue, the unconfoundedness assumption may apply with one set of covariates but not on an expanded set. As [157] discusses, a particular case occurs with covariates that are themselves intermediate outcomes.

The second main assumption in estimating ATEs requires that the propensity score is strictly between zero and 1 (the overlap assumption). In principle this is testable but the issue is to detect a lack of overlap in covariate distributions and then what to do if such an overlap does not exist. Various strategies for this assessment include plotting covariate distributions by treatment groups. For high dimensional data, one can inspect pairs of marginal distributions by treatment status or inspecting the distribution of the propensity score in both treatment groups. However, misspecification of the propensity score model may lead to failure to detect a lack of overlap. Another strategy is to look a the quality of the worst matching in a matching procedure. If the worst matching distance is large relative to the standard deviation of the covariates, there is some reason for concern.

If a lack of overlap is suspected, one can conclude that the ATE cannot be estimated with sufficient precision or one can decide to focus on an ATE that is estimable with greater precision. This might involve removing units with propensity scores below some threshold.

Example 4.1 The effect of wealth on health and child development in Swedish lottery players: The impact of indicators of socioeconomic status on health has been well established. As [50] summarize, these relationships begin early in life where children from low-income households experience a greater probability of premature birth and other chronic health conditions as they age (see, for example, [69]). These early challenges are correlated with adult socioeconomic status where higher incomes are associated with better health outcomes (see, for example, [74]).

In an effort to try and establish a causal relationship between the two, [50] exploited the essentially random assignment of prizes in three samples of Swedish lottery players and then estimated the causal effect of wealth on the individual's health as well as the health of their children. The authors noted that their study allowed them to observe the factors conditional on which the assignment was made. Next, the prize winnings were substantial (almost $1 billion in total) which would increase the signal of the effect of interest. Finally, the authors had access to very high-quality administrative data from which they could track a host of health outcomes in excess of 20 years post lottery.

Two primary analyses were carried out – one for adults and one they termed an intergenerational analysis. For the former, they focused on all-cause and cause-specific mortality as well as outcomes related to hospitalizations and drug prescriptions. For the latter, they examined children's academic achievement and cognitive and non-cognitive skills. Interestingly, for the adult analyses, the authors found that the causal effect of wealth on mortality and healthcare utilization was essentially zero (i.e., their confidence intervals as calculated using clustered data analysis techniques from [221] were tight around zero). This finding held up when conducting stratified analyses by age, income, sex, health, and education. In the latter analyses, again, the authors found non-significant causal effects. The only outcomes which showed potential causality was in the adult analysis, wealth was causally associated with a small decrease in the usage of anti-anxiety and sleeping medications. In the intergenerational analysis, the authors found that lottery wealth was causally related to increases in a child's risk of hospitalization and is also causally related to a decrease in risk for obesity near the end of the teenage years.

As [198] notes in his interest commentary, while this study is a clever way to minimize confounding effects when studying a difficult-to-assess causal relationship, it does have significant limitations in that the generalization of the conclusions to the broader Swedish population can be dubious. In fact, as [50] themselves note, the average difference between the lottery players' age in a winning year and a randomly chosen Swedish adult was about 10 years. Other factors they studied seemed relatively balanced between the two groups of individuals (including education, marital status, income, retirement status, and hospitalizations for a variety of conditions).

4.4 Use of instrumental variables

When exposures or treatments are randomly assigned, this ensures that both measured and unmeasured confounders are on average equally distributed across assignment groups. Non-compliance could complicate analyses based on the actual treatment received if non-compliance is related to the outcome.

The random assignment mechanism can be used as an *instrument* which can be used to estimate the ATE as if everyone complied. So when discussing the use of instrumental variables (IV, definition to follow) for the analysis of observational studies, we will follow the interesting exposition of [226], where the method and the underlying assumptions are framed against the gold standard of random assignment.

An IV is one that predicts the exposure, but conditional on the exposure, does not predict the outcome. In other words, the IV affects the outcome only through the exposure. Random assignment is an idealized IV but there may be naturally occurring IVs that could be used in observational studies provided they meet necessary assumptions. Notationally, for a randomized experiment, we will follow [226] and represent the IV as z, the exposure as x, the outcome as y, and confounders as c. The IV z can be seen to satisfy the following assumptions:

1. Relevance: z causes x.

2. Exclusion: z predicts y through x.

3. Exchangeability: z shares no confounders with y.

These assumptions are depicted in the directed acyclic graph (DAG) in Figure 4.2. So why does z satisfy these assumptions? For relevance, randomization happens automatically because assignment determines x (assuming

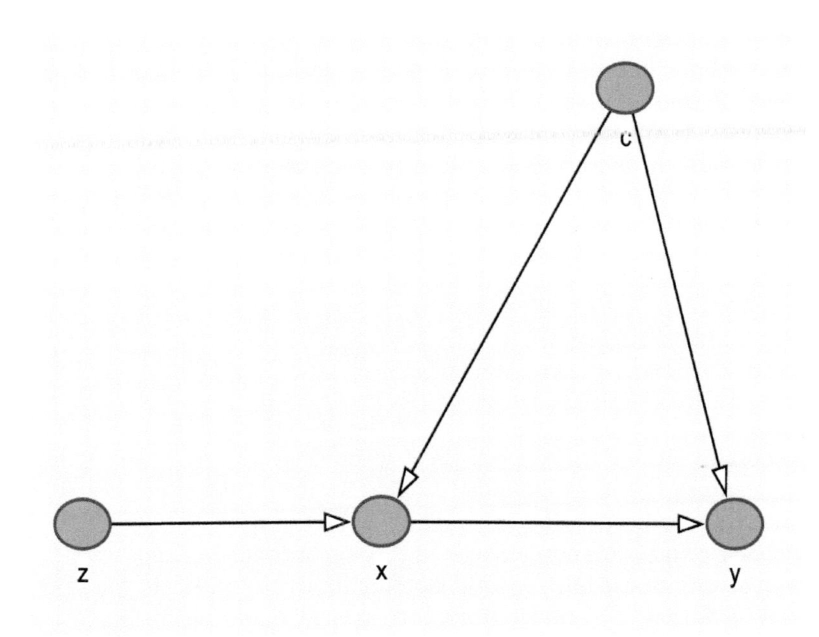

FIGURE 4.2: (Adapted from Lousdal (2018) [226]): Directed acyclic graph a random assignment as an IV.

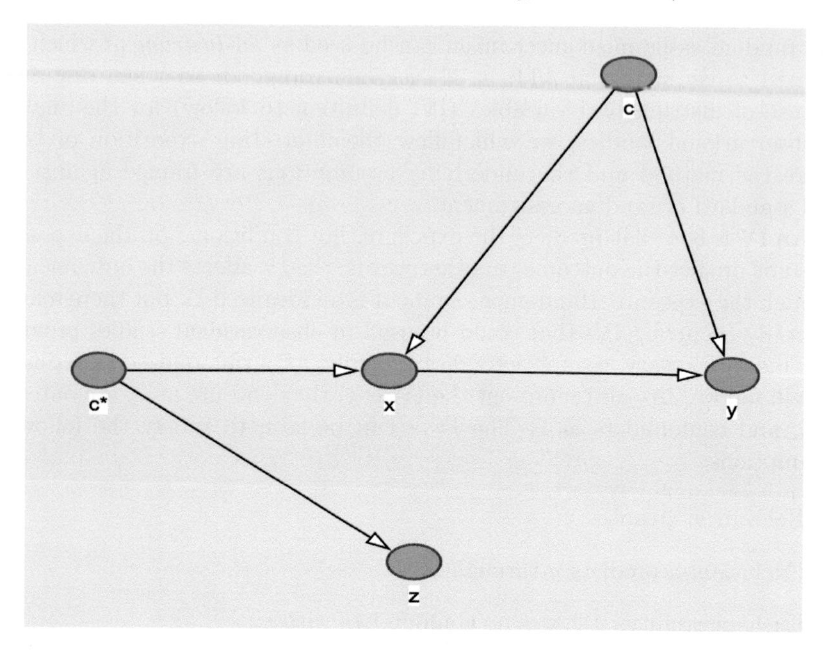

FIGURE 4.3: (Adapted from Lousdal (2018) [226]): Directed acyclic graph an IV in an observational study.

no non-compliance). Double-blindedness can ensure exclusion holds. Finally, randomization is known to lead to equally distributed confounders across assignment groups.

Then the average effect of x on y can be calculated from the average effects of z on y and z on x. Specifically, for a binary exposure, this is

$$\frac{E(y|z=1)-E(y|z=0)}{E(x|z=1)-E(x|z=0)}.$$

Continuous treatments can also be handled as the numerator and denominator turn into covariances rather than expected differences ([226]). The numerator is the intent-to-treat effect. The denominator measures compliance. With non-compliance, the denominator shrinks and the ratio then increases – essentially in an effort to estimate the causal effect when there was no non-compliance.

One can use IVs in an extended fashion in observational studies. The assumptions above need to be generalized as in the new DAG in Figure 4.3. Specifically, x and z are now associated through a common exposure c^*. Some common examples used are genetic factors, access to treatment based on geographic variation, and preference for treatment based on facility variation ([226]).

Martens *et al.* (2006) [237] describe a useful hierarchy of instruments. First, the most valid one is a variable that is controlled by design (e.g., randomized prevention strategies to discourage risky behaviors). Next, examples of natural randomization processes can sometimes be identified. For instance, with Mendelian randomization, alleles are allocated at random in offspring. Finally, when neither of these is available, one can select a source of natural variation that only produces a weak association between x and z.

Even with these three assumptions, confidence intervals for the causal effect of interest can be too wide to be of much use. Thus a fourth assumption has been proposed in order to obtain better point estimates and inferences. This relates to effect homogeneity. In the limit, this would mean that the effect of x on y should be constant across individuals. A weaker version would be that there is no effect modification/moderation (discussed later) on the x to y relationship. In practice though, it's likely that some of the confounders c will be effect modifiers. So an alternative weaker fourth assumption is that of monotonicity which when used, does constrain the degree of generalizability a study will confer ([226]).

4.4.1 Verifying the assumptions

The relevance assumption can be empirically verified by examining the F-statistic associated with the regression fit of z on x. The exclusion assumption cannot be directly empirically assessed but requires subject-matter knowledge instead. Random assignment with double blinding ensures this holds. Exchangeability is only partially testable from the data using measured covariates but confounding from unmeasured variables cannot be ruled out. Again, randomization ensures this is not an issue. The fourth (weaker) assumption of monotonicity is ruled out by design with randomization but requires subject matter knowledge in observational studies. Violation of assumptions can lead to biased causal effect estimation (discussed next).

4.4.2 Estimation

The simplest IV estimation technique is a two-stage least squares approach wherein the first stage consists of fitting a regression line of x on z and the second stage involves fitting a regression line of y on the fitted values from the first stage. The regression parameter associated with stage-one fitted values is the IV point estimate. Other covariates can be added at either stage. Doing so will relax the assumption of exchangeability from a marginal one to a conditional one ([226]). The underlying idea here is that the predicted values from stage one are unaffected by the common unmeasured confounders c and thus will produce a less biased estimate of the causal effect of interest.

Example 4.2 Estimating the causal effect of ending SNAP subsidies for sugar-sweetened drink consumption: Lawmakers in the United States have proposed a national policy which would modify existing benefits from the Supplemental Nutrition Assistance Program (SNAP) in an effort to promote healthier food consumption. One of the proposed modifications is to ban SNAP dollars from being used to purchase sugar-sweetened drinks since earlier research uncovered an association between participation in the program and increased consumption of sugar-sweetened drinks [217]. There might be then reason to believe a connection to increased likelihood of downstream deleterious health effects including type 2 diabetes and obesity.

The ideal approach of conducting a randomized clinical trial was deemed unethical since it would result in some low-income Americans not being randomized to the food subsidy program. So instead, [23] conducted an IV analysis where the IV was chosen to be whether an individual lived in a state with a fingerprinting requirement for participation in the program. This IV was thought to be related to the exposure variable of program participation in terms of either encouraging or discouraging participation and should not be related to the outcome of interest (amount of sugar-sweetened drink consumption).

This is an example of using IV analysis to study the causal impact of changes in public policies on health outcomes. In fact, in a recent review article, [22] uncovered 22 studies that used IV analysis to estimate policy causal effects.

4.5 Traditional mediation versus causal mediation

Mediation analysis asks if the effect of a binary exposure x (now defined more generally than treatment assignment) on an outcome y involves changing an intermediate variable M. The idea can be dated back to work by [371] and the seminal paper by [20] which greatly popularized mediation analysis in the social sciences. This intermediate variable is known as a mediator. A directed acyclic graph (DAG) of such a relationship is presented in Figure 4.4. In this figure are also represented the roles of confounding variables C_{xy} and C_{My}. These confounders were not included in the [20] paper but were in fact discussed in an earlier paper by [194].

In order to answer the question of whether mediation is present or not, the traditional approach uses a model-based definition. It consists of formulating two linear regression models,

$$M = \alpha_M x + \beta M C_{xy} + e_M,$$

and,

$$y = \alpha_y x + \beta_y C_{xy} + \gamma_y M + e_y,$$

where e_M and e_y are model errors that follow the usual assumptions of having zero mean and constant variance. Subscripts on the regression parameters track the particular response the corresponding predictor is linked to.

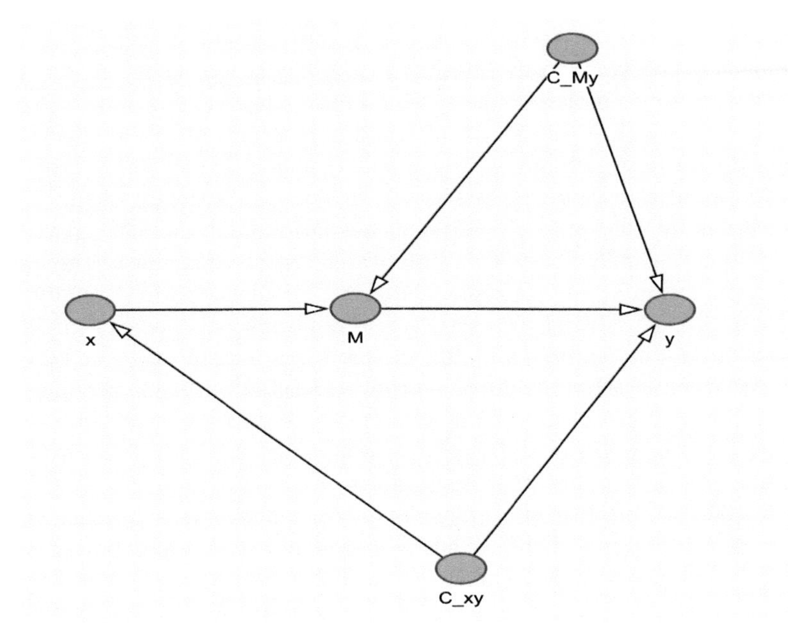

FIGURE 4.4: (Adapted from Naimi et al. 2015)[262]: A directed acyclic graph depicting causal mediation.

The indirect effect of x on y is defined as $\alpha_M \gamma_y$ which is the product of the coefficient of x in the mediator model with the coefficient of M in the outcome model. This represents the effect of x on M and the effect of M on y, and thus their product represents the effect of x on y through M. In contrast, the direct effect is captured in α_y of the outcome model. When originally developed, [20] assumed a continuous mediator and continuous outcome. These assumptions were relaxed to accommodate a number of other scenarios including non-continuous mediators or outcomes, multiple mediators, and multi-level mediators and outcomes ([229, 137]).

While simple to construct, the traditional approach to mediation analysis ignores the inherent directionality of the links between effects in the DAG (i.e., the arrows). Hence the estimated effects are measuring only conditional associations. But this directionality actually implies causality. The arrows drawn from x to M and y and from M to y imply that these variables affect one another in the directions displayed. Hence the analysis should be done in a way that justifies such an interpretation ([267]). This conceptual difference has also been noted by many other authors ([229, 290]). So while mediation analysis is inherently about estimating causal effects, it's not immediately obvious how to do this in the mediation setting. Typically, in non-mediation settings with the exposure at two settings, this would be done using randomization to where we would observe the outcome in both settings. Randomization would remove confounding on average and thus it is reasonable to simply compare outcomes in the two exposure groups. In the mediation setting however, for either the direct or indirect effects, we no longer have two observable conditions to compare that correspond to usual perceptions of causal effects. But using explicit causal thinking paves the way to speak directly about the causal effects we want to explore and assess whether we can estimate them.

Additionally, the simpler traditional mediation analysis makes particular assumptions that may not hold in practice. These are inherent to the model-based formulation of the concept. These include identification assumptions, additivity (i.e., no x by M interaction) and uniformity of effects (x on M and M on y) across individuals. Finally, the models are assumed to be correctly specified. Some of these assumptions can be relaxed but some are more difficult to address. For instance, the assumption of no x M interaction is very restrictive as there are many situations where such an interaction would be expected ([230]). Note also that if non-linear models are used instead of linear models, then the product of coefficients may not be on the same scale as the causal effect of interest ([267]). Thus it makes more sense to define effects in a more model-free way. An explicit causal inference approach allows this. It does not however remove the need for assumptions at the estimation step. It does however allow examination of what models to use based on the data at hand. This will result in the use of more flexible models that make fewer assumptions.

4.5.1 Effect identification

To answer the question of how much (if any) of the effect of x on y goes through M, we can develop natural direct and indirect effects within a causal paradigm. In order to do so, we need to first define the individual total effect. Each individual i has two potential outcomes, $y_i(1)$ and $y_i(0)$ where 1 and 0 indicate if individual i experienced the exposure condition x or not. Then the individual total effect TE_i is defined as, $TE_i = y_i(1) = y_i(0)$ and the average total effect is defined as $TE = E(y(1)) - E(y(0))$ where the expectation is taken over the population distribution.

In reality, we do not observe individual effects since we never observe both potential outcomes for the same individual. Instead, we observed the realized outcome which is one of the two potential outcomes. Now consider the DAGs presented in Figure 4.5 which presents two parallel worlds for the same individual. Here, everything is kept the same except that in one world the exposure is set to 1 and 0 in the other world. Since x is then a fixed value for everyone, there is no longer a causal link between C_{xy} and x.

Now we will split the individual total effect TE_i into two contrasts using the mediator M – one contrast representing the mediated effect and the other a direct effect for the individual. The potential outcome now should represent a hypothetical world where x is set to one condition but M is set to its value under the other exposure condition. Notationally, we will represent

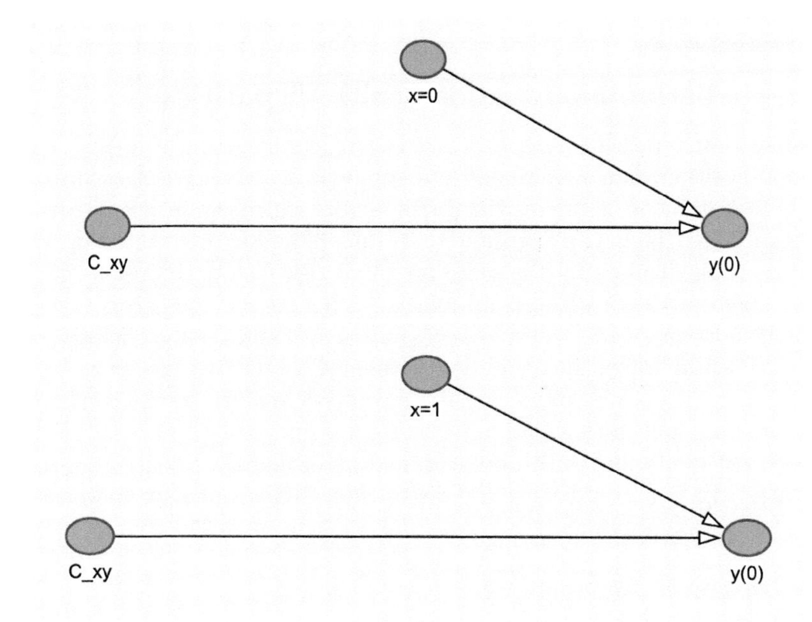

FIGURE 4.5: (Adapted from Nguyen et al. 2020)[267]: DAGs for total effect. Here x is set to a value that breaks the causal link between C_{xy} and x.

this as $y(x, M(x'))$ where x and x' represent the two different exposure conditions. Now consider a situation where $x_i = 1$ but the mediator is set for the individual to $M_i(0)$.

Then TE_i can be split into two parts: i) a shift from $y_i(0, M_i(0))$ to $y_i(1, M_i(0))$ and ii) a shift from $y_i(1, M_i(0))$ to $y_i(1, M_i(1))$. Part i) is termed the natural direct effect (NDE) and part ii) is termed the natural indirect effect (NIE). NEI represents the effect of switching the mediator from $M_i(0)$ to $M_i(1)$ while the exposure if actually fixed so there is no direct effect component here. This decomposition is called the direct-indirect decomposition ([267]) based on the order of the component effects. We could just as easily do it the other way and split the total effect into NIE followed by NDE which is called the indirect-direct decomposition. The average natural direct and indirect effects then similarly decompose the average total effect.

So then to answer the question of whether there is a mediated effect, [267] recommend using the direct-indirect decomposition. Their rationale is that under this decomposition, they are not questioning the existence of a direct effect but are considering the possibility of a mediated effect in addition to the direct effect. If no mediated effect exists, then the total effect is the same as the natural direct effect. Interestingly, if the question of interest is in addition to the mediated effect, is there a direct effect, then [267] recommend the indirect-direct decomposition since if there is no direct effect, then the total effect is the same as the natural indirect effect.

4.6 Mediation analysis for health disparities

Variables that represent more abstract constructs like race/ethnicity, socioeconomic position or neighborhood environment are thought of as upstream factors that influence more proximal risk factors which can lead to health disparities ([263]). Thus there is interest in understanding how these upstream variables are explained by the more proximal risk factors. Examples include cancer stage at diagnosis and its relationship between socioeconomic position and mortality ([153]), serum potassium levels and their association with upstream self-identified race and downstream diabetes ([53]).

This naturally leads one to consider mediation analysis methods. However, traditional methods for mediation posit strict assumptions for causal inference that are not easily met with upstream factors of interest ([262]) from health disparities studies. To estimate the direct causal effects of x on y, we require the following assumptions:

A0: No uncontrolled exposure-outcome confounding.

A1: No uncontrolled mediator-outcome confounding.

A2: No mediator-outcome confounders affected by the exposure.

A3: No exposure-mediator interaction.

A1-A3 are shown in Figure 4.4. If in addition the so-called stable unit treatment value assumption ([321]) is also met, then standard mediation methods can be used. These include the difference method and the generalized product method (discussion following). However if A4 does not hold, then the difference method is no longer valid and if A3 does not hold then neither standard method will yield valid causal inferences.

In health disparity studies, these assumptions are likely to be violated, and thus approaches with fewer assumptions have been proposed ([262]). One such approach is to define and estimate a counterfactual disparity measure (CDM) ([262]) as,

$$CDM(M = 1) = E(y(M = 1)|x = 1) - E(y(M = 1)|x = 0),$$

where $M = 1$ denotes the presence of the mediator variable and x is assumed to be a two-level factor exposure (yes if $x = 1$, no otherwise). This equation represents the magnitude of exposure disparity that would be observed in the presence of mediation. To estimate $CDM(M = 1)$, notice that fewer assumptions are required for the upstream exposure but are still required for the mediator. Assumption A1 is not required because part of the association between exposure x and outcome y may be due to exposure-outcome confounding. In fact, many health disparity upstream factors do not have counterfactual interpretations and thus C_{xy} cannot represent confounders in the usual causal sense ([358]). One option is to standardize $CDM(M = 1)$ by the distribution of certain covariates that are associated with both x and y. Finally, the way in which M relates to x determines whether standard approaches or more general approaches should be used to estimate $CDM(M = 1)$.

4.7 Traditional moderation versus causal moderation

Moderation occurs when the relationship between two variables depends on a third variable which is called a moderator. The effect of a moderator can be characterized statistically as an interaction estimated (usually) within a linear regression model ([20]). However, there is a growing literature on the estimation of more general forms of interactions like non-linear interactions using modern machine learning techniques ([322, 356, 368], etc).

Causal moderation refers to situations where interest lies in estimating conditional treatment effects. That is, investigation will involve estimating whether the effect of a treatment t on an outcome y is conditional upon the value of a moderator variable s ([18]). If such evidence is found, then the interpretation of this conditionality must follow. If a difference in treatment effect across different values of S is found, then this reflects treatment effect heterogeneity. However, what cannot immediately be established if whether the heterogeneity is caused by s. This further claim is known as causal moderation. This implies that counterfactual intervention upon s would alter the treatment effect. The magnitude of this effect would imply a degree of stability or influence to the manipulation of s thereby providing insights into the generalizability of the treatment effect ([18]). Causal moderation can be an important finding in disparity research as it can open up new strategies for disparity reduction strategies ([304]).

To further illustrate this distinction, consider first the goal of finding treatment effect heterogeneity. For ease of discussion, we will consider binary versions of the treatment and moderator and the outcome will be represented at $y(t, s)$ where t and s take on separate values of t and s at a time. Also, suppose that a random sample of size n is drawn from a population of interest. Units are indexed by $i = 1, \ldots, n$ and are randomly assigned to $t = 1$ or $t = 0$. In addition to observing the value of S_i, we also observe a vector of other covariates x_i assumed to be collected pre-treatment. Now consider the following quantity which captures treatment effect heterogeneity,

$$E[y_i(1,1) - y_i(0,1)|s_i = 1] - E[y_i(1,0) - y_i(0,0)|s_i = 0],$$

where the expectations are taken with respect to the distribution of potential outcomes from the population from which the samples are drawn ([18]). This quantity captures the average treatment effect (ATE) of t for units where $t = 1$ and the ATE for units where $T = 0$. Since the expectation is taken conditional on s, the moderator is treated as observational with no causal component of its own measured ([18]).

To estimate causal moderation effects, one must go further. Thus one can define the average treatment moderation effect (ATME) given by δ as,

$$\delta = E[y_i(1,1) - y_i(0,1) - y_i(1,0) - y_i(0,0],$$

where the expectation is taken over the population distribution.

4.7.1 Parallel estimation framework

Bansak (2021) details five assumptions necessary for the identification of ATME from the observables in the sample. These are,

1. SUTVA (Stable Unit Treatment Value Assumption): each individual has only one potential outcome under each exposure condition which here must encompass the treatment and the moderator. If $t_i = t'_i$ and $s_i = s'_i$ then $y_i(\bar{t}, \bar{s}) = y_i(\bar{t}', \bar{s}')$ where $\bar{t}$ and $\bar{s}$ are the full treatment and moderator vectors across all subjects.

2. Complete randomization of the treatment

3. Pre-treatment moderator and confounders: this means that the moderator s and a set of confounders x are pre-treatment and hence the treatment can have no effect on either of them. That is, given randomization of the treatment, $(y_i(1,1), y_i(0,1), y_i(1,0), y_i(0,0), s_i, x_i) \perp t_i$.

4. Moderator conditional independence: this is conditional independence between the potential outcomes and the moderator. This is written as $(y_i(1,1), y_i(0,1), y_i(1,0), y_i(0,0) \perp s_i|x_i$.

5. Moderator common support which is written as $0 < P(s_i = 1|xi) < 1$.

Given assumptions 1-5, [18] showed that,

$$\delta = E_x[E[y_i|y_i = 1, s_i = 1, x_i] - E[y_i|t_i = 0, s_i = 0, x_i] - E[y_i|t_i = 1, s_i = 0, x_i] \\ + E[y_i|t_i = 0, si = 0, x_i]].$$

Under assumption 3, $F(x|t) = F(x)$ for all x and t where $F(x)$ is the joint distribution of x and $F(x|t)$ is the conditional distribution of x given t. Therefore we can write,

$$E_x[E[y_i|t_i = t, s_i = s, x_i]] = E_{x|t}[E[y_i|t_i = t, s_i = s, x_i]|t_i = t].$$

Writing things out this way shows that δ can be re-expressed by subsetting the data by the treatment level and then proceeding to apply covariate-adjustment strategies separately for the treated and untreated units. This is equivalent to holding t constant and estimating the causal effect of S on y. Commonly used methods like regression, matching, and propensity score weighting can be used. Bansak (2021)[18] calls this the parallel estimation framework. Matching, in particular, is made easier using this approach and as [18] shows, developing statistical inferential procedures is made more straightforward.
Remark: (Linear) regression approaches to estimating causal effects rely upon specific model assumptions which can include linearity and constant error variances. These may not always hold in practice where estimation results could be sensitive to the functional form of the model and other model specifications. Non-parametric approaches could be employed at the price of increased computational burden and tuning. Another nice alternative would be to use parallel within-treatment subset matching methods. Here, matching on the covariates X would be done, and then within each matched sub-sample (i.e., treated and controls), the effect of the estimate of s on y can be estimated.

4.7.2 Causal moderation without randomized treatments

In health disparity estimation, it's of course not common to have randomization of the focus variable and hence the above methods do not immediately generalize. Dong *et al.* (2022)[80] considers identification and estimation of causal moderation in the more general case without explicitly considering if the variables (including the focus variable) have been randomized or not.

The main differences from above arise in the assumptions for identification which need to be made more stringent. The SUTVA assumption is still required. Ignorability of the exposure/treatment and moderator given the covariates is required. This implies that $(y(0,0), y(0,1), y(1,0), y(1,1)) \perp (t,s)|x$. In non-randomized studies, this necessitates that both the treatment and moderator assignment is independent of the potential outcomes conditional upon the observed covariates. Next, independence of treatment and moderator given the covariates. This assumption holds in all randomized studies however in non-randomized studies, this necessitates that treatment assignment is independent of the moderator conditional on the observed covariates. Next, we now need treatment-by-moderator common support: $0 < P(t,s|x) < 1$. This assumption may not automatically hold in situations where only the treatment has been randomized. Thus the assumption is necessary in both types of studies.

Dong *et al.* (2022)[80] then define their version of ATME and go even further, defining other quantities of interest including average moderated treatment effect on the treated (AMTT) and average moderated treatment effect on targeted subgroups (AMTS) which focuses on the difference among the potential outcomes for a specific subgroup defined by s and t.

For estimation of ATME, [80] develop a generalized propensity score method. Recall when the treatment variable is dichotomous, the propensity score is the probability of being in the treatment group given covariates. The generalization here is to extend it to treatments with multiple categories. This is often estimated using logistic or multinomial regression and weights taken to be the inverse of the propensity scores.

Example: Estimating the moderated effect of preschool. Dong *et al.* (2022)[80] analyzed data from the Early Childhood Longitudinal Study Kindergarten Class (ECLS-K) from 1998-99. A sample of 22,666 children attending kindergarten during the 1998-99 academic year was generated. Academic achievement measures on math and reading were the focus and assessed in the Fall of kindergarten to the Spring of grade 8. Additional data on child and family characteristics were also collected at entry into the study.

The sample consisted of two groups being compared: a preschool group (7367 children) and a parental care group (3150 children). The outcome variable was an Item Response Theory (IRT) scale score of the child's math achievement in Fall of kindergarten taken on a z-score transformed scale. Identification of causal moderation by speaking English at home of disparity in IRT between the two pre-K entry groups was the focus of the study.

Covariates used to estimate generalized propensity scores included race, weight, age at kindergarten entry, parents' educational level, income, composite SES, household structure (number of parents and siblings), and whether the child lived in a rural or urban environment. The following protocol was used for estimating ATME:

1. Generate a new set of groupings based on treatment-by-moderator groupings. With a treatment having two levels and a moderator having two levels (English-speaking home or not), this resulted in 4 groups.

2. Estimate generalized propensity scores using multinomial logistic regression for each child.

3. Generated inverse propensity score weights.

4. Dong et al. (2022) also assessed the overlap in generalized propensity scores and covariate balance by fitting kernel densities among the four subgroups.

5. Use the approach in [80] to estimate ATME using a general linear model including weights and controlling for covariates (for added robustness).

Figure 4.6 shows a graphical summary of various ATME estimates taken from the Dong et al. (2022) paper along with their 95% confidence intervals. Note that ATMS estimates (i.e., average moderated treatment effect on targeted subgroups) are also included but not of interest here. The ATME analysis with added covariates produced slightly smaller estimates than without controlling for covariates. Interestingly, the method in [80] produced slightly larger point estimates of ATME than conventional moderation analysis after controlling for covariates.

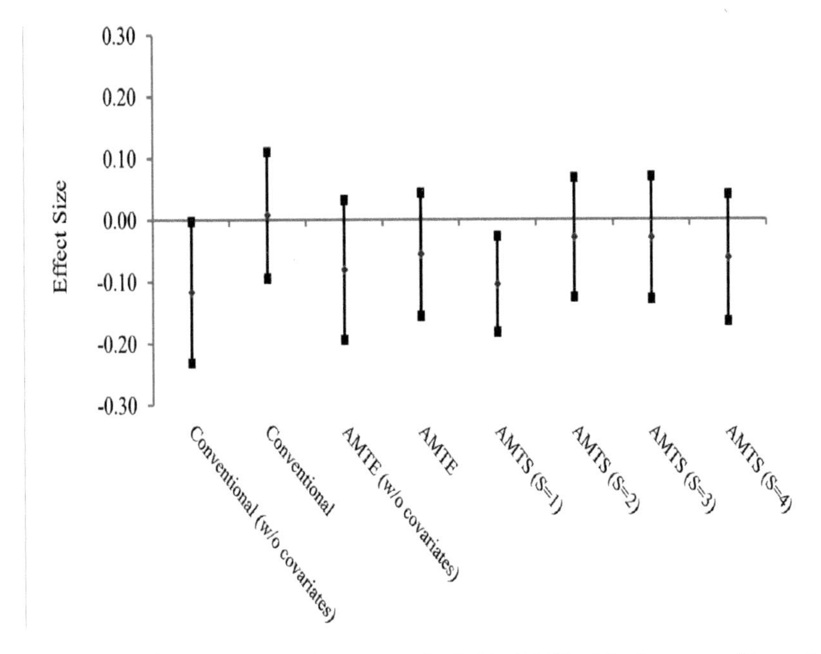

FIGURE 4.6: (Taken from Dong et al. (2022)[80]): Moderator effect sizes (how preschool IRT is moderated by English speaking in the home) with corresponding 95% confidence intervals.

5

Machine Learning Based Approaches to Disparity Estimation

5.1 What is machine learning (ML)?

The focus of this chapter is to explore some more algorithmic approaches to HDE where the focus may be prediction from labeled data, the discovery of previously unknown patterns in data without pre-existing labels, or some hybrid of the two. There has been much effort by the research community devoted to try and distinguish between the various modeling cultures of generative (or statistical) modeling and algorithmic (or predictive) modeling ([37]; [81]). According to Breiman, statistical modeling looks to put forward "stochastic models which fit the data and then make inferences about the data-generating mechanism based on the structure of those models", whereas predictive modeling (often termed machine learning (ML)) is, "effectively silent about the underlying data generating mechanism", and thus proceeds via an algorithmic approach allowing for many competing algorithms but focusing on the accuracy of predictions made on new datasets. The rise of algorithmic modeling is often attributed to the influence of the big data revolution, something that the health disparity community is also experiencing (reference). The reason that this connection exists is that big datasets (both tall and wide) afford the opportunity to fit more complex model structures (which may result in more accurate predictions conditional on sufficient computing power and memory) whose functional form is unknown apriori and must be discovered from data.

Given the workup presented to this point, ML may appear to be less than useful for HDE. However, this is not the case because i) HDE can sometimes be formulated from a predictive point of view, or, ii) statistical modeling has expanded its scope to allow for much more complex structures inferred from big, complex datasets while still focusing on the underlying data generating mechanism and, iii) there are new types of disparity estimation problems that fall nicely under the machine learning umbrella.

5.1.1 Supervised versus unsupervised machine learning

Machine learning approaches are broadly classified into supervised and unsupervised categories. What distinguishes these two is the presence of a health

DOI: 10.1201/9781003119449-5

outcome to which a predictive model using potentially related covariates is built. Supervised methods assume outcomes are available. On the other hand, unsupervised methods are presented typically only with covariate data and their goal is to uncover new trends or patterns or estimate the joint distribution of the covariates. Examples include clustering or bump/mode hunting ([99]). A partial overlap between these two broad categories is also possible and methods that operate under this paradigm are termed semi-supervised. Examples of this for health disparity research will be discussed in Chapter 6.

5.1.2 Why is ML relevant for health disparity research?

Most of the big data sources for the study of disparities (and more broadly public health), can be classified into one of five categories. According to [258], these are a) information about underlying biology like genomic data, b) contextual information like geospatial data, c) administratively collected medical record data, d) wearable device data like global positioning system (GPS) or continuous monitoring devices like activity monitors, e) electronic data like social media postings, search terms, or cell phone records.

For example, [374] discusses big data issues around minority health and health disparities. They identify various opportunities to move disparity research forward. In particular, they see the types of big datasets described above as providing opportunities to incorporate social determinants of health and to better understand disparity etiology and thus guide interventions to reduce disparities. Various big data challenges are also identified with specific attention being given to unique issues that pertain to disparity research. These include ethical issues and data access. Other authors have noted that big data can have unintended consequences and actually exacerbate disparities at times. Take for example, genomic data which is notoriously non-diverse racially, ethnically, and along multiple other axes ([211, 94, 232]). In fact, this was one of the motivating factors for the All Of Us study of NIH ([270]).

It's not uncommon to want to integrate data sources from multiple categories as well resulting in multilevel data. The scale of data collection continues to accelerate adding to the complexity of health disparity research. As a result, ML approaches can be useful here as well. As noted by [258], public health surveillance systems that monitor trends in disease incidence, health behaviors, and environmental conditions have proven to be areas where ML approaches have been adopted since the focus is often on prediction or hypothesis generation.

5.2 Tree-based models

Following [166], a decision tree is a graphical model describing decisions and their possible outcomes.

In many settings, the decision maker may not know what the decision rule is and thus this needs to be discovered by modeling data. The trees are formulated dependent on the nature of the response variable. When the outcome y is a classification label (class-valued outcome), a classification tree is constructed. These can include things like the disease status of a patient. Here the goal would be to build a tree that predicts (on external validation data) the outcome using covariates x from training data. Not only should this decision rule be accurate with respect to predictions, but it should also be understandable. That is, it should not be so complex that the decision maker is left with a black box.

The use of tree methods for classification has a history that dates back at least 40 years. Much of the early work emanated from the area of social sciences, starting in the late 1960s, and computational algorithms for the automatic construction of classification trees began as early as the 1970s. Algorithms such as the THAID program developed at the Institute for Social Research, University of Michigan, laid the groundwork for recursive partitioning algorithms, the predominate algorithm used by modern-day tree classifiers, such as Classification and Regression Tree (CART).

Classification trees are decision trees derived using recursive partitioning data algorithms that classify each incoming x-data point (case) into one of the class labels for the outcome. A classification tree consists of three types of nodes

1. Root node: The top node of the tree comprising all the data.
2. Splitting node: A node that assigns data to a subgroup.
3. Terminal node: Final decision (outcome).

In general, recursive partitioning works as follows. The classification tree is grown starting at the root node. The root node is split into two daughter nodes: a left and a right daughter node. In turn, each daughter node is split, with each split giving rise to left and right daughters. The process is repeated in a recursive fashion until the tree cannot be partitioned further due to lack of data or some stopping criterion is reached, resulting in a collection of terminal nodes. The terminal nodes represent a partition of the predictor space into a collection of rectangular regions that do not overlap. This is referred to as a binary recursive partitioned tree. Alternative splitting strategies include multiway splits producing multiple daughter nodes although there is not much evidence indicating that their predictive performance is better than the simpler trees.

A good split is in terms of an impurity function to measure the decrease in tree impurity for a split. The purity of a tree is a measure of how similar observations in the leaves are to one another. The best split for a node is found by searching over all possible variables and all possible split values and choosing that variable and split point that reduces impurity the most. There are several impurity functions used. These include the twoing criterion, the entropy criterion, and the gini index. The gini index is arguably the most popular. When the outcome has two class labels (the so-called two-class problem), the gini index corresponds to the variance of the outcome if the class labels are recoded as being 0 and 1.

The size of the tree is crucial to the accuracy of the classifier. Too shallow and the terminal nodes will not be pure, and the accuracy of the classifier will suffer due to high bias. Too deep (too many splits), and the predicted class label will have high variance. To determine the optimal size of a tree, the tree is grown to full size (i.e., until all data are spent) and then pruned back. The optimal size is determined using a complexity measure that balances the accuracy of the tree as measured by cost complexity and by the size of the tree.

Decision trees can also be used in regression settings where y is a continuous measurement (such as age, blood pressure, ejection fraction for the heart, etc.). These can be written succinctly as,

$$y = h(x) + e = \sum_{k=1}^{K} c_k I(x \in R_k) + e,$$

with usual regression assumptions on the model errors. Here, R_k represents the distinct partitions of the predictor space along the coordinate axes and the number of partitions (K) determined by the growing and pruning algorithm. Regression trees can be constructed using recursive partitioning similar to classification trees. Impurity is measured using mean-square error. The terminal node values (c_k) in a regression tree are defined as the mean value (average) of outcomes for patients within the terminal node. This is the predicted value for the outcome.

There is a longer history of work on regression trees that employ different strategies. The first published regression tree algorithm is AID proposed by Morgan and Sonquist [259] which uses as a measure of node impurity the distribution of the observed y values in the node. AID finds binary splits that most reduce the node impurity being the sum of squared deviations about the mean and cases with missing values are excluded. Another algorithm is $M5'$ proposed by Quinlan [293], which constructs piecewise linear models. It first constructs a piecewise constant tree and then fits a linear regression model to the data in each leaf node. $GUIDE$ proposed by Wei-Yin Loh ([225]) yields unbiased splits by employing chi-square analysis of residuals and bootstrap calibration of significance probabilities. The predominant algorithm used now is $CART$, proposed by Breiman, Friedman, Olshen and Stone in 1984 ([38])

Tree-based models have also been developed for time-to-event data. Here the focus is on understanding how time-to-event varies in terms of different variables that might be collected for a patient. Examples include time to death from a certain disease, time until recurrence (for cancer), time until first occurrence of a symptom, or simple all-cause mortality. The analysis of time-to-event data is often complicated by the presence of censoring. Decision trees can be used to analyze right-censored survival data ([213]). Such trees are referred to as survival trees. Survival trees can be constructed using recursive partitioning. One impurity measure uses the log-rank test. In the case of a survival tree, terminal nodes are composed of patients with similar survival. The terminal node value in a survival tree is the survival function and is estimated using those patients within the terminal node.

5.2.0.1 Understanding the decision boundary

By following the path as a case moves down the tree to its terminal node, the *decision rule* for that case can be read directly off the tree. Such a rule is simple to understand as it is nothing more than a sequence of simple rules strung together.

The *decision boundary* on the other hand is a more abstract concept. These are estimated by a collection of decision rules for cases taken together—or in the case of decision trees, the boundary produced in the predictor space between classes by the decision tree. Unlike decision rules, decision boundaries are difficult to visualize and interpret for data involving more than one or two variables. However, when the data involves only a few variables the decision boundary is a powerful way to visualize a classifier and to study its performance.

Ishwaran and Rao [159] developed an analysis depicted in Figure 5.1. The outcome is presence or absence of prostate cancer and the independent variables are prostate specific antigent (PSA) and tumor volume, both having been transformed on the log-scale. On the left-hand side is the classification tree for a prostate cancer data set. Each case in the data is classified uniquely depending on the value of these two variables. Terminal node values are assigned by majority voting.

The right-hand side of Figure 5.1 displays the decision boundary for the tree. The blue region is the space of all values for PSA and tumor volume that would be classified as non-diseased, whereas the red region are those values classified as diseased. Superimposed on the figure using white and green dots are the observed data points from the original data. Green points are truly diseased patients, whereas white points are truly non-diseased patients. Clearly, the classifier is classifying a large fraction of the data correctly. Some data points are misclassified though. The misclassified data points in the center of the decision space are especially troublesome. These points are misclassified because the decision space for the tree is rectangular. If the decision boundary were smoother, then these points would not be misclassified. The non-smooth nature of the decision boundary is a well-known deficiency of classification trees and can seriously degrade performance, especially in complex decision problems involving many variables.

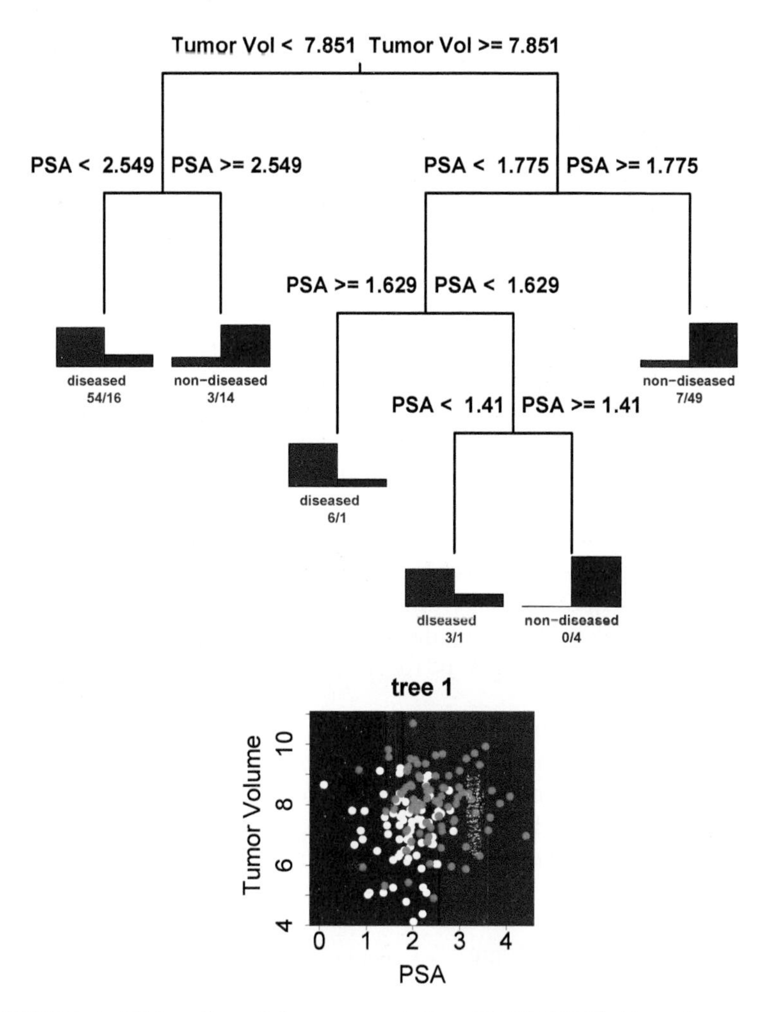

FIGURE 5.1: (Taken from Ishwaran and Rao (2009) [159]): Decision tree (left-hand side) and decision boundary (right-hand side) for prostate cancer data with PSA and tumor volume as independent variables (both transformed on the log-scale). Barplots under terminal nodes of the decision tree indicate the proportion of cases classified as diseased or non-diseased, with the predicted class label is determined by majority voting. Decision boundary shows how the tree classifies a new patient based on PSA and tumor volume. Green points identify diseased patients and white points non-diseased patients from the data.

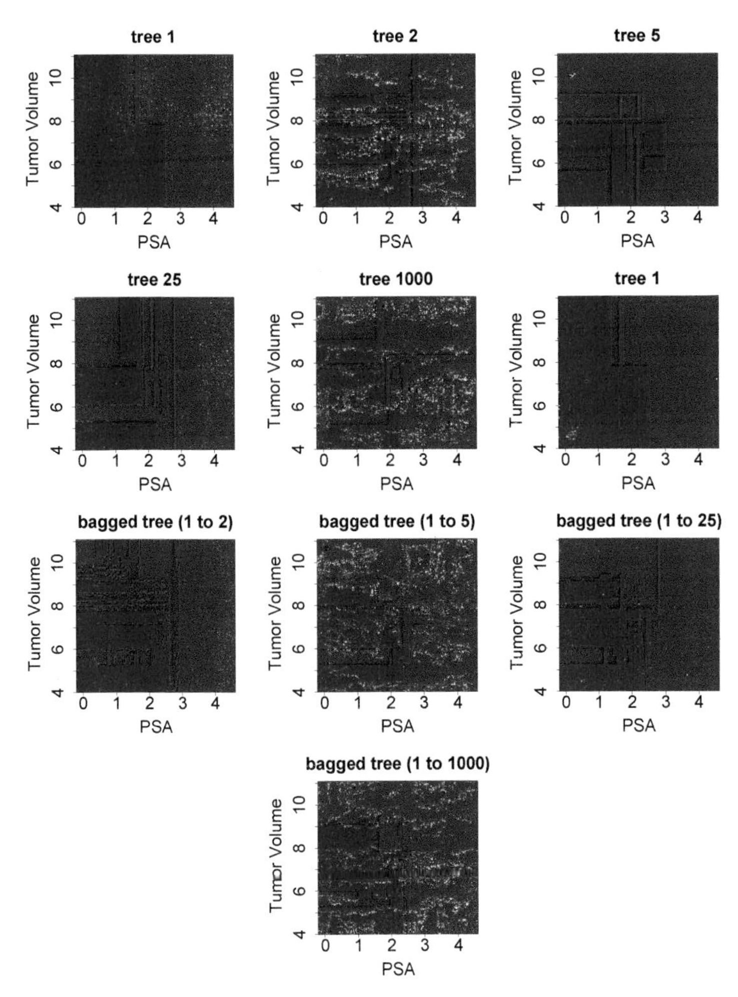

FIGURE 5.2: (Taken from Ishwaran and Rao (2009)[159]): Top row shows decision boundary for a specific bootstrapped tree (1000 trees used in total). Bottom plot shows different aggregated (bagged) decision trees.

5.2.0.2 Bagging trees

If the original data set is perturbed in some way, then the classifier constructed from the altered data can be surprisingly different than the original classifier. This is an undesirable property, especially if small perturbations to the data lead to substantial differences.

This property can be demonstrated using the prostate data set of Figure 5.1. Here bootstrap resampling ([90]) is used to perturb the data. One thousand bootstrap samples of the prostate data were drawn. A classification tree was calculated for each of these samples. The top panel of plots in Figure 5.2 shows decision boundaries for four of these trees (bootstrap samples 2, 5, 25, and 1000; note that tree 1 is the classification tree from Figure 5.1 based on the original data). One can see quite clearly that the decision spaces differ quite substantially—thus providing clear evidence of the instability. However, trees constructed from different perturbations of the original data can produce decision boundaries that in some instances have better behavior than the original decision space (over certain regions). Thus, one can capitalize on the inherent instability using aggregation to produce more accurate classifiers.

This idea in fact is the basis for a powerful method referred to as "bootstrap aggregation", or simply "bagging". Bagging can be used for many kinds of predictors, not just decision trees. The basic premise for bagging is that if the underlying predictor is unstable, then aggregating the predictor over multiple bootstrap samples will produce a more accurate, and more stable, procedure that can produce more accurate predictions.

To bag a classification tree, the procedure is as follows (bagging can be applied to regression trees and survival trees in a similar fashion):

1. Draw a bootstrap sample of the original data.

2. Construct a classification tree using data from Step 1.

3. Repeat Steps 1-2 many times, independently.

4. Calculate an aggregated classifier using the trees formed in Steps 1-3. Use majority voting to classify a case. Thus to determine the predicted outcome for a case, take the majority vote over the predicted outcomes from each tree in Steps 1-3.

The bottom panel of plots in Figure 5.2 shows the decision boundary for the bagged classifier as a function of the number of trees. This plot was invented and designated a classification aggregation tablet (CAT scan) by [296]. The first plot is the original classifier based on all the data (tree 1). The second plot is the bagged classifier comprised of tree 1 and the bootstrap tree derived using the first bootstrap sample, the third plot is the bagged classifier using tree 1 and the first four bootstrap trees, and so forth. As the number of trees increases, the bagged classifier becomes more refined. By 1000 trees (last plot) the bagged classifier's decision boundary is fully defined.

5.2.1 Tree-based models for health disparity research

Disparity estimation using trees can be seen as a non-parametric extension to regression (or GLM) based modeling in that the tree model generates a more flexible and local estimate of the functional $h(x)$ whose form can vary depending on the type of outcome (see next section for more details). However, doing so would require a departure from traditional tree building towards what is known as treed regression ([9]) where a local linear fit within each terminal node is fit. This local linear fit could include the focus variable f for which disparity estimates across its levels are of interest. This type of approach will be explored in more detail in Chapter 6. In what follows, is an example of an approach for HDE that is more directly tied to usual tree construction.

Example 5.1 Classification trees for examining gender disparities in the timing of angiography in patients with acute coronary syndrome: Beirman *et al.* [29] combined data from the Discharge Abstract Database (DAD) created by the Canadian Institute for Health Information with Statistic Canada's Canadian Community Health Survey (CCHS) by linking at the patient level. The DAD provides information on admission and discharge dates, diagnostic codes, age, sex, postal code and discharge information. The CCHS provides information on demographic metrics including language, ethnicity, cultural group, geographical region (urban versus rural), marital status, education, residence type, and household income among other variables. Their primary outcome variable of interest was the delay to procedure defined as the difference in days between the date of admission to an acute care facility and the date of angiography procedure (defined as a 0/1 binary outcome based on a cutoff of 1 day.

Beirman *et al.* (2015)[29] built a classification tree using Gini impurity as the splitting criterion during recursive partitioning, followed by a cross-validated pruning algorithm. Their strategy was to build the tree using the clinical variables and both sexes combined and then add in the sociodemographic variables for further splitting – see Figure 5.3. Once the tree was built, then in order to assess disparities in the outcome, they fed the women and men separately down the tree and examined which terminal nodes they fell in. They then estimated delay rates by sex and then fit socioeconomic adjusted Lorenz curves of delays and compared these to the line of identity (see Figure 5.4).

5.3 Tree-based models for complex survey data

Toth and Eltinge (2011)[355] describe the use of regression trees for the analysis of complex survey data. Their problem of interest was to use auxiliary information to estimate finite population parameters of interest however the functional form of the relationship between the auxiliary variables and finite population parameter is flexible enough to entertain complex interaction effects. As [355] state, previous methods that aimed to do that (references) largely ignored the sampling design (selection probabilities) and had no real theoretical justification. In their work, [355] devised a recursive partitioning

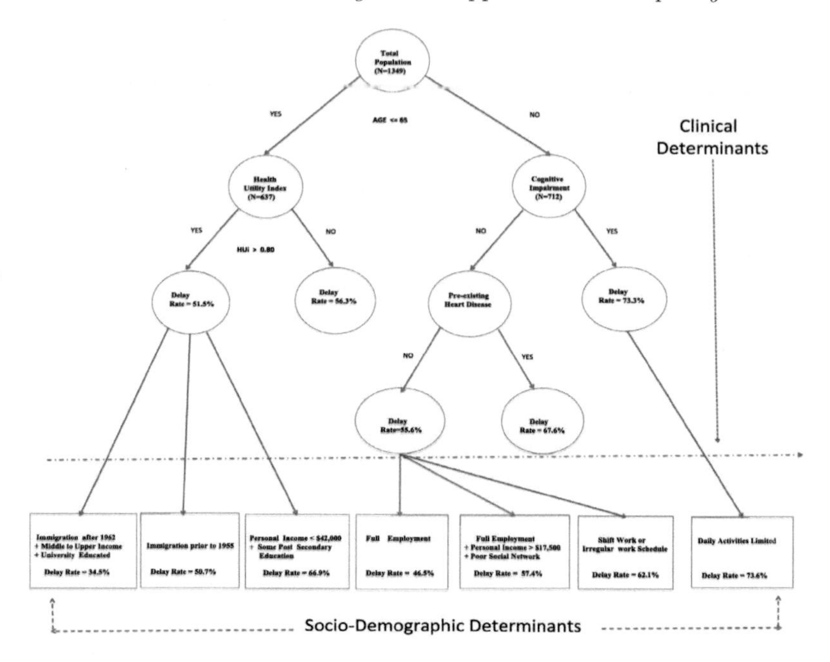

FIGURE 5.3: (Taken from Bierman et al. (2015)[29]): Fitted tree-based model showing gender disparities in the timing of angiography.

scheme that incorporated sampling probabilities and was shown to give design consistent estimators of finite populations totals. Importantly, since the total estimates would be derived from partitions of the predictor space discovered by recursive partitioning on the same data, the theory had to acknowledge this fact. Their theory provided conditions on the sampling design and the recursive partitioning algorithm itself. They required that the population estimator based on sample data partitions were L^p consistent with respect to the superpopulation model and that the estimator based on the sample data be L^2 consistent with respect to the design as an estimator for the finite population parameter defined using the same partition.

Toth and Eltinge (2011)[355] considered the following setup: a population of elements $(y_i, x_i, z_i); i = 1, \ldots, N$. The finite population is assumed to be generated i.i.d. from a superpopulation model. Here y_i is the outcome and x_i are the covariates of interest. The z_i are known characteristics of the population elements that are used in the sample design but not of direct interest. So in other words, (y_i, x_i) are known for only the sampled elements and z_i is known for each population unit. They then defined survey-weighted versions of recursive partitions and the so-called boxes containing sampled observations in them.

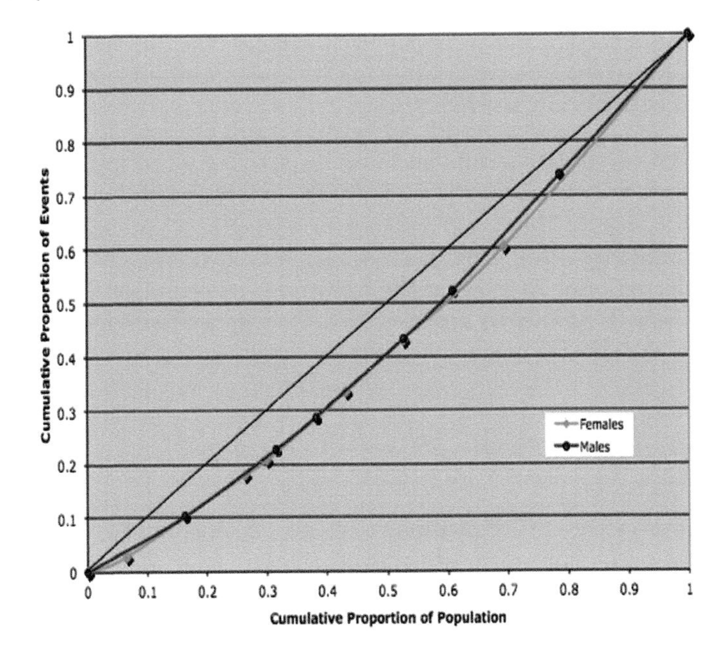

FIGURE 5.4: (Taken from Bierman et al. (2015)[29]): Fitted Lorenz curves by race. Data points are subgroups identified by the tree.

5.4 Random forests

Random forests (RF) are ensembles models which aggregate many individual models (base learners) each of which is constructed from different realizations of data. There are a number of different versions of RF in the literature but exposition is most easily developed under the RF that can be thought of as an extension to bagging. For RF, we will follow the notation developed in [162]. We will assume we have a response y, and x a $p-$ dimensional feature. The response y can be continuous, binary, categorical, or survival, and x can be continuous or discrete. We assume the underlying problem involves a nonparametric regression framework where the goal is to estimate a functional $h(x)$ at x. Estimation is based on learning or training data $\mathscr{L} = [(x_1, y_1), \ldots, (x_n, y_n)]$, where (x_i, y_i) are independently distributed with the same distribution F. Examples of $h(x)$ are the:

1. The conditional mean $h(x) = E(y|x)$ in regression.

2. The conditional class probabilities $h(x) = (p_1(x), ..., p_K(x))$ in a $K-$ multiclass problem,where $p_k(x) = P(y = k|x)$.

3. In survival analysis, $h(x) = P(T > t|x)$. Here $h(x)$ is the survival function and (y, δ) are the observed data pairs with $y = min(T, C)$ where C is the censoring time and $\delta = 1I(T \leq C)$.

As in [35], we define a random forest as a collection of randomized tree predictors $[h(., \Theta_m, \mathscr{L}), m = 1, \ldots, M]$. This notation denotes the mth random tree predictor of $h(x)$ and Θ_m are independent identically distributed random quantities encoding the randomization needed for constructing a tree that are selected prior to growing the tree and is independent of the learning data, $\mathscr{L}$. The tree predictors are combined to form the finite forest estimator of $h(x)$,

$$h(x, \Theta_1, \ldots, \Theta_M, \mathscr{L}) = \frac{1}{M} \sum_m h(x, \Theta_m, \mathscr{L}). \tag{5.1}$$

Theoretical properties of RF continue to evolve. Breiman (2001)[35] produced a bound for prediction error (generalization error) for a RF that involved a trade-off between the number of variables randomly selected for splitting and the correlation between trees. Specifically, he showed that as the number of variables increases, individual tree accuracy improves but the correlation between trees also grows which impedes performance of the RF. Meinhaussen (2006)[247] proved consistency of the RF for quantile regression situations and [27] proved consistency of the RF for classification under an assumption of random splitting and [161] proved consistency of RF for survival outcomes under a counting process formulation.

5.4.1 Hypothesis testing for feature significance

In 5.1 we showed how to estimate a health disparity for levels of a focus variable f using tree-based models and a predictive point of view. Here we describe methodology that allows more traditional hypothesis testing for feature significance with random forests (and thus naturally extends to tree-based models as well). Mentch and Hooker (2016)[250] develop a subsampling approach for creating supervised ensembles like random forests. They showed that by controlling the subsampling growth rate, that individual predictions from the random forests are asymptotically normal. Using this fact, they developed a formal hypothesis testing framework for features significance which if formulated around the focus variable f amounts to testing if a disparity exists or not with regards to levels of f. The authors focused on a simple scenario: take just two covariates x_1 and x_2 and fit a random forest model to outcome y. This relationship can be represented generically as $y = f(x_1, x_2) + e$ for random errors e. To test the significance of variable x_2, they make use of a test set of size n_{test} consisting of covariates x_{test}. They then build two random forests from the training data – one using both x_1 and x_2 which can be labelled $\hat{f}_{12}$, and the other using only x_1 which can be labelled $\hat{f}_1$. Predictions at each point in x_{test} are then made using each random forest ensemble and the vector of differences was shown to have multivariate normal limiting distribution with mean μ and covariance matrix Σ by [250]. Thus using consistent estimators of these, $\hat{\mu}'\hat{\Sigma}^{-1}\hat{\mu} \sim \chi^2_{n_{test}}$. This test statistic can thus be used to formally test the hypothesis,

$$H_0 : f_{12} = f_1 \forall (x_1, x_2) \in x_{test} \qquad H_1 : f_{12} \neq f_1 \quad forsome(x_1, x_2) \in x_{test}.$$

In the work of [251], they further showed by imposing additional structure on the test set allows them to avoid training an additional random forest as well as perform testing for additivity.

Remark 1 Variable importance: There is a growing literature on variable importance measures for trees and random forests (e.g., [35, 224, 160, 122]). While these are useful as interpretive tools to extract more model structure from what otherwise might look like black-box predictors, these variable importance measures do not focus on the notion of health disparity estimation. For this reason, we will not be discussing them here but rather refer interested readers to the relevant references.

Example 5.2 Random forests for defining obesogenic and obesoprotetctive environments: Nau *et al.* (2015)[264] used random forests to identify community characteristics that together predict obesity at an ecological level. Specifically, they used a variation of random forests called conditional random forest (CRF). They defined obesogenic environments for children as those communities that fell into the highest quartile of community-level body mass index (BMI) z-score and obesoprotective communities as those falling into the lowest quartile. So the goal was to use a CRF as a classifier based on community-level variables.

Their data came from electronic health record data of measured height and weight on children geocoded to a diverse set of 1288 communities in Pennsylvania. Community features came from secondary data that have been linked to obesity before resulting in 44 community characteristics of interest that include social factors, food availability, and physical activity features. In total, their dataset has 22,497 individual children between the ages of 10-18. Geocoding was restricted to those children between 2 and 18. Standardized BMI z-scores were calculated using CDC growth charts.

CRFs are a version of RFs designed to handled highly correlated predictors such as would be expected in this study. Figure 5.5 shows the resulting fit from a single tree. The data plotted in each terminal node represent the distribution of obesogenic and obesoprotective communities falling into that node. CRFs use an ensemble of trees and then can generate variable importance measures similar to those found in usual RFs.

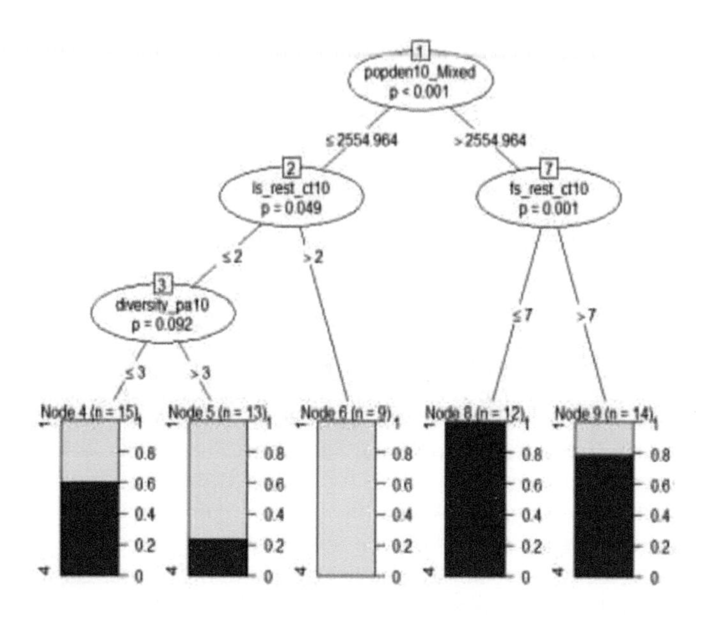

FIGURE 5.5: (Taken from Nau et al. (2015)[264]): Single conditional random forest (CRF) for identifying community factors that discriminate obesogenic versus obesoprotetctive communities.

Example 5.3 Random forests for assessing the relative importance of race versus healthcare and social factors on prostate cancer mortality: Hanson *et al.* (2019). Journal of Urology.

Black men have an increased prostate cancer mortality versus their White counterparts. Hanson *et al.* (2019)[129] conducted a study where they sought to assess the relative importance of race versus healthcare and social factors on prostate cancer-specific mortality. They used data from the Surveillance, Epidemiology, and End Results (SEER) database focusing on men diagnosed with prostate cancer older than 40 years of age between 2004 and 2012. They stratified patients matching Black and White patients by birth year, stage of cancer at diagnosis, and age at diagnosis. They then applied random forests focusing on variable importance measures and compared variables broadly categorized into four categories – tumor characteristics, race, healthcare factors, and social factors. They compared an analysis using the matched cohort versus the overall cohort.

Their analysis found that race did not, in fact, dominate healthcare and social factors and that in fact, tumor characteristics at the time of diagnosis were the markedly most important variables associated with prostate cancer-specific mortality. More specifically, for many strata, healthcare, and social

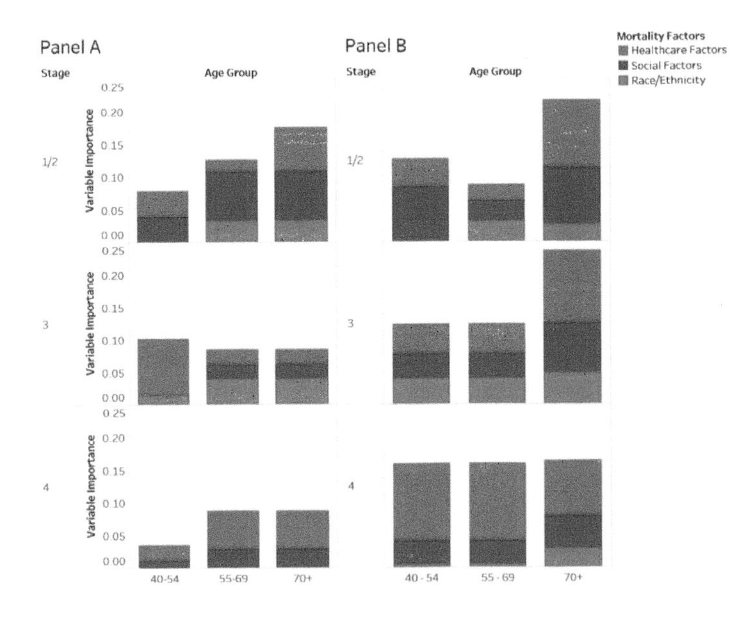

FIGURE 5.6: (Taken from Hanson et al. (2019)[129]): Random forest relative variable importance for three groups of factors – race, social and healthcare. Panel A is the analysis for the matched cohort. Panel B is analysis for the full cohort.

factors were more important than race (see Figure 5.6) for both the matched cohort and the full cohort. They concluded that all three groups of factors deserved attention if disparity reduction was to be achieved.

Example 5.4 Contextualizing COVID-19 spread: a county level analysis, urban versus rural, and implications for preparing for future waves: Rao, Zhang and Mantero (2020)[298] looked at applying RF methodology to understand the determinants of difference in COVID-19 infection rates between rural (populations $< 50,000$) and urban counties (populations $\geq 50,000$) in the U.S. To that end, recently [199] designed a dataset containing a machine-readable file with demographic, socioeconomic, healthcare, and education data for each county in the 50 states and Washington, D.C. organized by FIPS codes which are unique county code identifiers. This data was cobbled together from 10 governmental and academic sources at the county level. The resulting dataset contains more than 300 contextual county-level variables. They then merged this contextual data with county-level time series data from the JHS CSSE COVID-19 dashboard [79] which gives continuously updated confirmed infection and death counts over time.
Detailed description of the data COVID-19 infection volume time series came from the Johns Hopkins University CSSE COVID-19 Tracking Project

and Dashboard which when the data was pulled ranged from 01/22/2020 until 04/12/2020. Climate data came from NOAA. County-level demographic data were extracted from the U.S. Census Bureau and the USDA. Healthcare capacity-related data came from the Kaiser Family Foundation. Traffic score information came from the Center for Neighborhood Technology. ICU bed information came from Kaiser Health Network. Additional COVID-19 case information came from USAfacts. Physician workforce data came from AAMC.

Many of the variables were not usable in their original forms, many involved counts within a county but did not take into account the overall size of the county itself. This would make it impossible to directly compare between counties. Therefore [298] did the following: all count variables were standardized by their totals, for example, counts of racial and gender groups were divided by the total population of the county, and household counts were divided by the total number of households in the county. State-level variables were excluded in the analysis since the analysis wanted to group counties that experienced similar increases in infection rates using the forests. Any variables with a missingness rate of over 45% were removed as well as highly correlated variables were removed. This resulted in a final set of 186 variables that were analyzed. Missing values were imputed using random forest imputation ([347]).

Some counties had to be omitted from the analysis and this was mostly due to poor fit in the `growthcurver` procedure (described next). Either the model was not estimable or the estimated midpoint time was much farther out than the data that was available at the time of analysis. This resulted in a loss of 16.8% of the counties. Also, for any counties that continued to have zero infections although the model could not be fit, the slopes were assumed to be zero.

County-specific confirmed infections growth curve fitting and growth rate estimation

The infections time series county-level data was obtained from [199] that updated on Apr 13, 2020. The counts of infection in each county were standardized by the corresponding county population and then fit into the growth curve model. The growth curves for each county was estimated based on logistic equation which is commonly used in population ecology [339, 68, 309] utilizing R package `growthcurver` [338]:

$$N_i(t) = \left(\frac{K_i}{1 + \frac{(K_i - n_i)e^{-r_i t}}{n_i}} \right) + \epsilon_i(t),$$

where $N_i(t)$ represents the proportion of infected people at time t for a given county i, n_i as the size of initial infection proportion, K_i as the carrying capacity, r_i is the growth rate with respect to the infection proportion, and $\epsilon_i(t)$ the model errors assumed to have zero mean and constant variance. Nonlinear least squares is used to estimate model parameters.

The growth curve slopes were obtained by taking the derivative of $N_i(t)$ with respect to t for each county as:

$$\text{slope}_i = \frac{\partial N_i(t)}{\partial t} = \frac{\hat{K}_i \hat{n}_i \hat{r}_i (\hat{K}_i - \hat{n}_i) e^{\hat{r}_i t}}{\left(\hat{K}_i + \hat{n}_i \left(e^{\hat{r}_i t} - 1\right)\right)^2},$$

where estimated parameter values are indicated by a hat sign. Then to calculate the maximal slope, the midpoint of time for t was plugged in which for this type of function represents when the change in the outcome is greatest.

Random forest fitting Growth curve slope estimates were treated as responses (y) and the 186 contextual variables described above as county level predictors ($x_j; j = 1, \ldots, 186$). Separate forests were fit for rural and urban counties. Visualization of RF fits was done using parallel coordinate plots and multi-variable co-plots. These are created based on clusters that were determined with the PAM method using random forest distances as described in [233]. Random forest distances work similarly to random forest proximity but are more sensitive to the tree topology therefore able to provide better clusters. Like random forest proximity, a pair of points are considered highly proximal if they are in the same terminal node, but unlike proximity, instead of simply assigning zero if they are not in the same terminal node, a number between 0 and 1 is used depending on how far down the tree the two points became disjoint.

In order to attempt to ascertain potential differences in how rates of infection increase relate to the contextual variables between urban and rural settings, rural county data was dropped down the RF trained on urban data, and urban county data was dropped down the RF trained on rural data. For this type of reverse prediction, the resulting errors were calculated and 95% confidence intervals determined.

Figure 5.7 shows the estimates growth curve slopes versus $\log_{10}$(population) based on 2018 census population values or all counties in the U.S. Blue coloring indicates rural counties and red coloring urban. While the majority of estimated slopes are not large, it is clear that there are a mixture of urban and rural counties with large slope estimates.

Random forests were fit separately to urban and rural counties. For the urban forest, the % variance explained was 32.26% and 32.56% for the rural forest. This demonstrated good model validation for both forests. In order to better visualize the fitted random forests, [298] categorized counties by slope estimate groupings as determined by the fitted forests. Parallel coordinate plots are shown in Figure 5.8 and Figure 5.9 for urban and rural counties, respectively. Each group is represented by lines moving horizontally and each variable by a vertical line (whose range of values is above and below the vertical line). Lines connect the mean values of each variable for that group. The mean value of the slope for the group is shown in the first vertical line. The variables are sorted according to relative variable importance.

It's clear that there are clusters of variables that clearly separate slope groups and that the variables differ for the urban versus rural random forest.

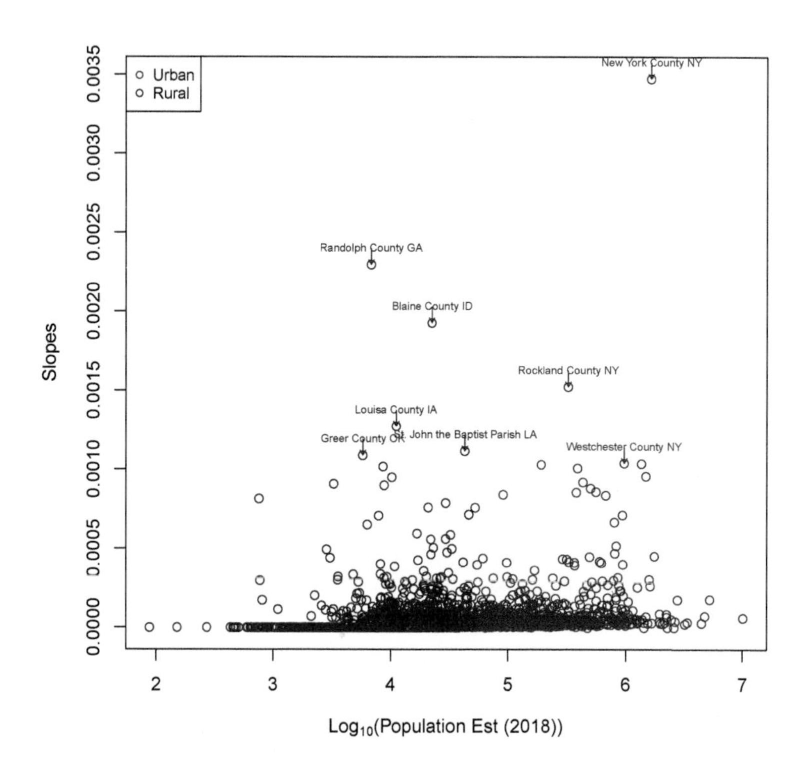

FIGURE 5.7: (Taken from Rao, Zhang and Mantero (2020)[298]): County-specific growth rate estimates (slopes) versus $log_{10}(population)$ based on 2018 census numbers. Coloring by rural or urban status.

For the urban parallel coordinate plot, such variables included the percentage of Hispanic, Black or African American male and female (HBA_FEMALE, HBA_MALE), international migration (INTERNATIONAL_MIG_2018), housing density, population density and May 2018 average and maximum temperature values in degrees F. For rural counties, such variables included percentage of non-Hispanic, Black or African American male and female (NHBAC_FEMALE, NHBAC_MALE, NHBA_MALE, NHBA_ FEMALE), 2018 and percent poverty as estimated in 2018. Other variables of rural importance also included age – specifically the percentage of the population that were elderly.

Figure 5.10 and Figure 5.11 show co-plots focusing on these key variables. This allows a closer inspection of how the growth curve slope estimates continuously change as a function of other variables. In particular, each co-plot showed co-dependence on 4 other variables. For the urban co-plot, variables

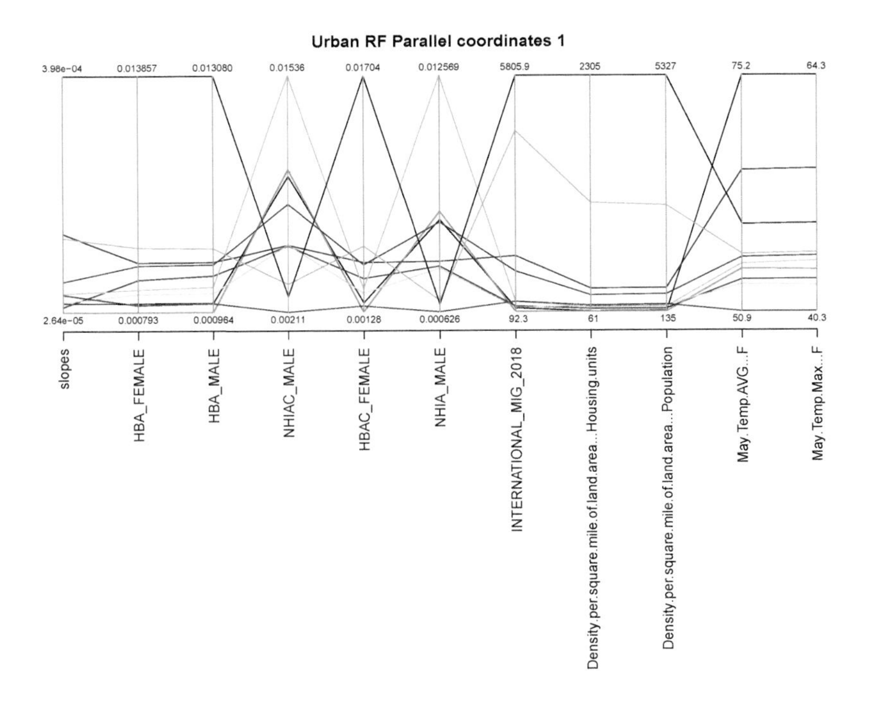

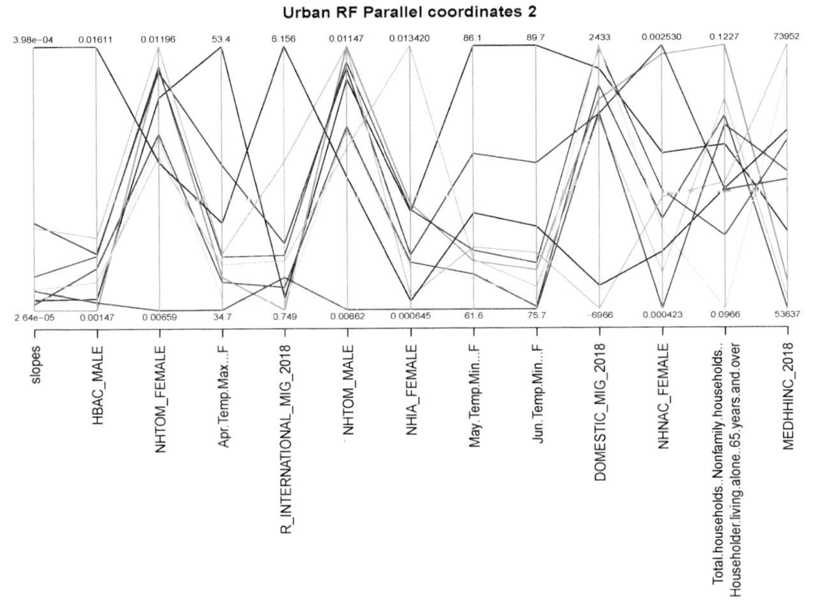

FIGURE 5.8: (Taken from Rao, Zhang and Mantero (2020)[298]): Parallel coordinate plots for urban counties.

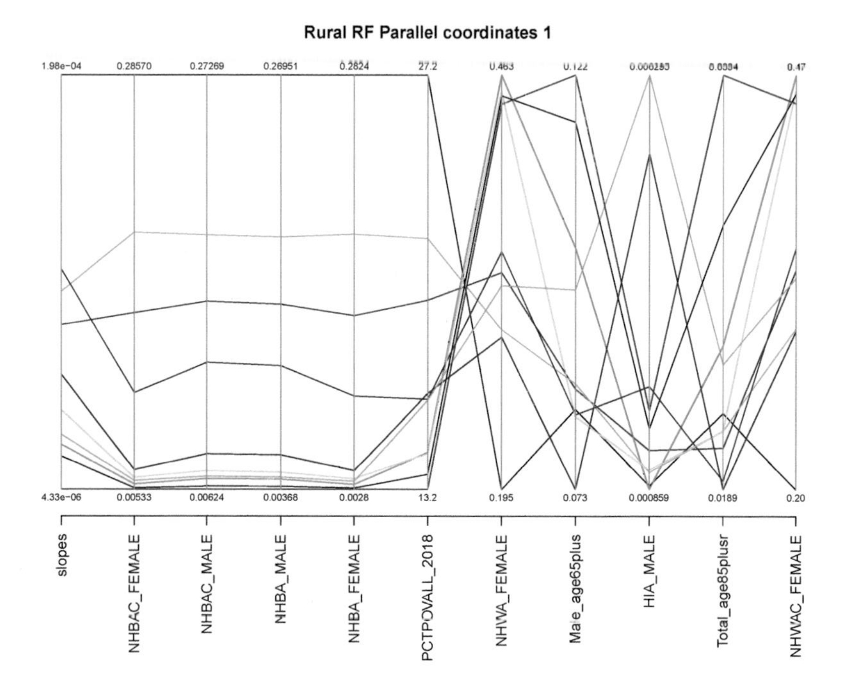

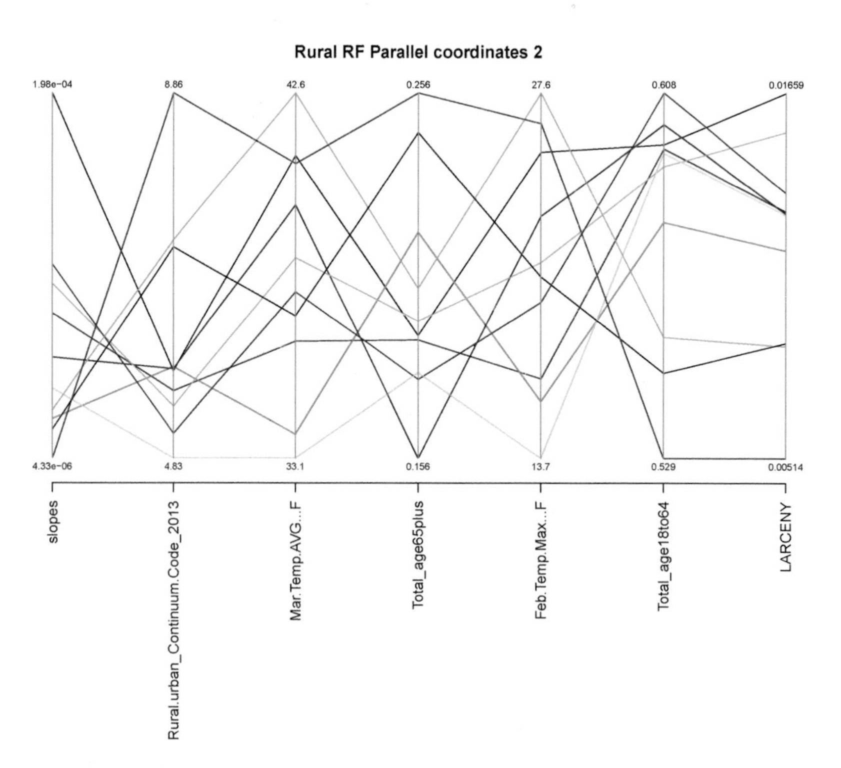

FIGURE 5.9: (Taken from Rao, Zhang and Mantero (2020)[298]): Parallel coordinate plots for rural counties.

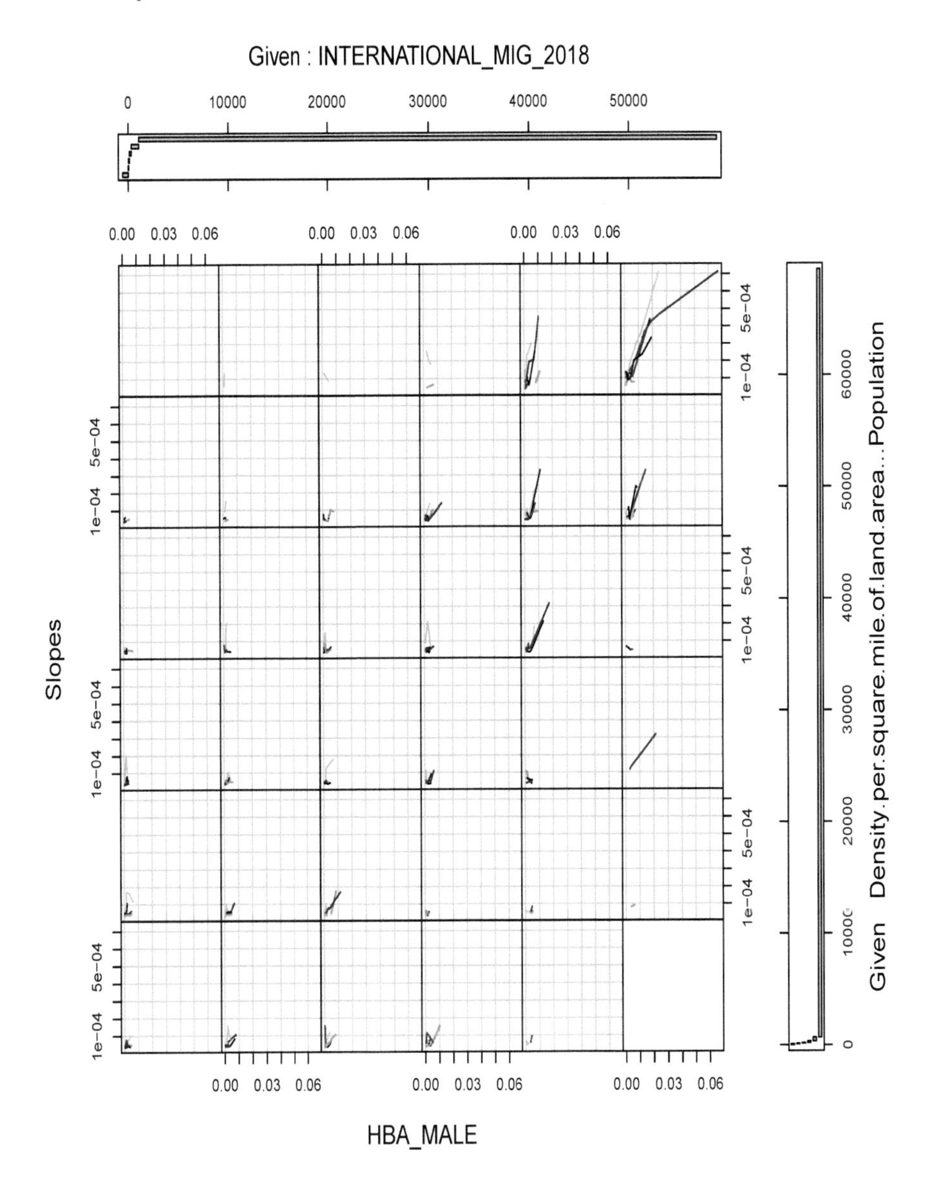

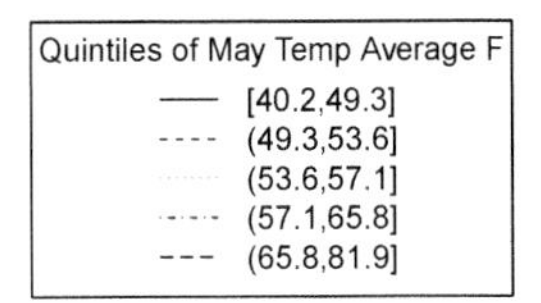

FIGURE 5.10: (Taken from Rao, Zhang and Mantero (2020)[298]): Co-plot for urban counties.

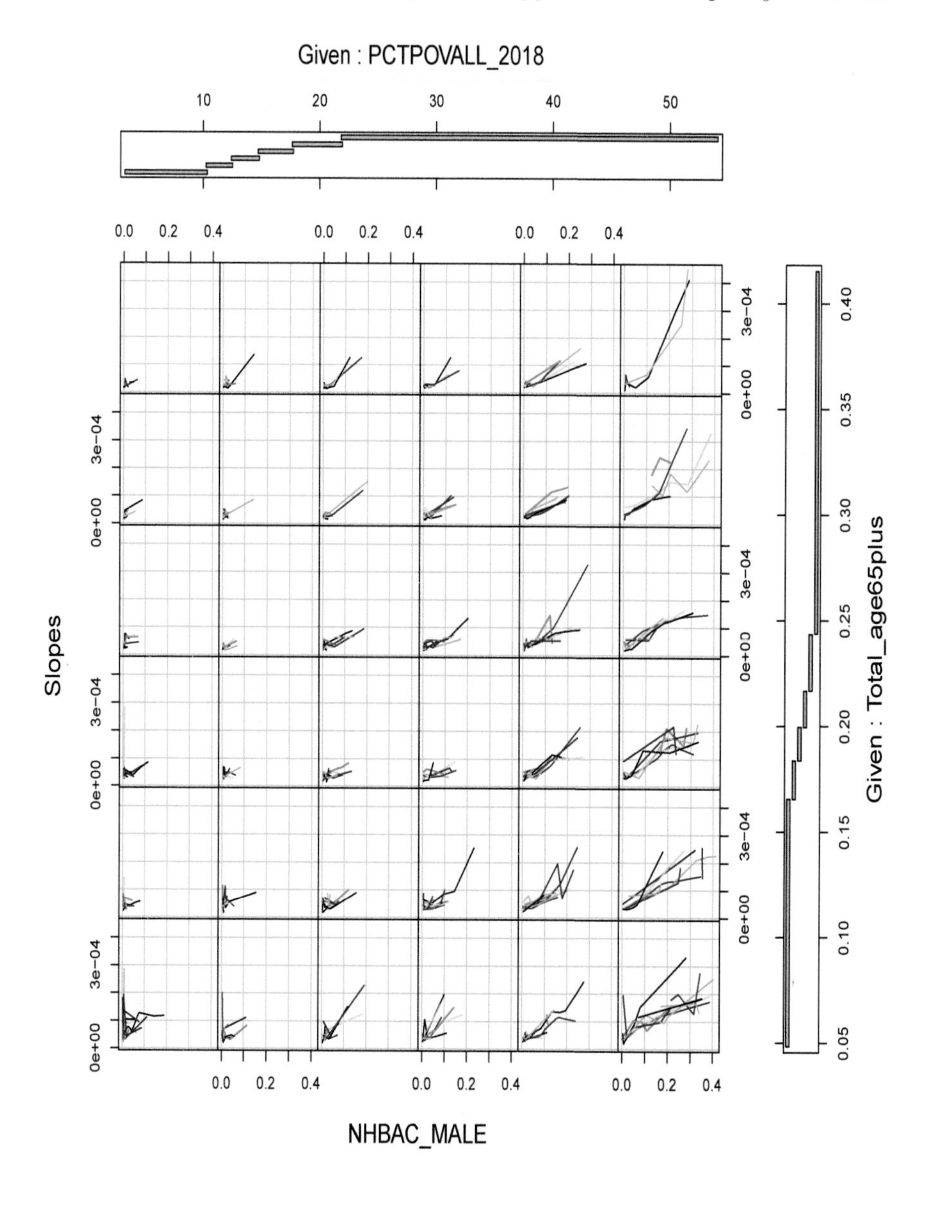

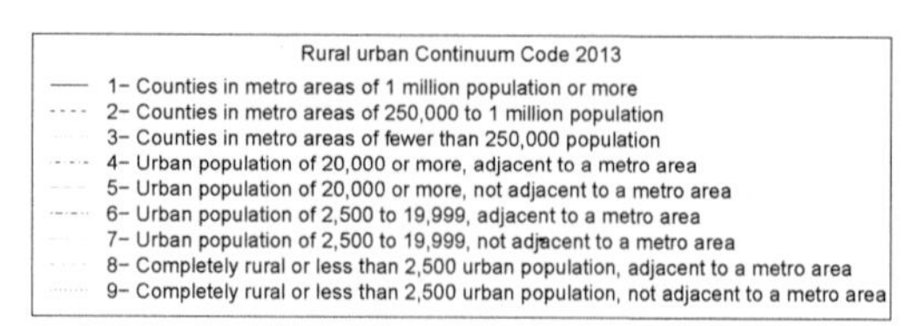

FIGURE 5.11: (Taken from Rao, Zhang and Mantero (2020)[298]): Co-plot for rural counties.

plotted include HBA_MALE, population density, and 2018 international migration numbers. Each line is shown with a different color and plotting character. As the legend indicates, they represent quintiles of the 2018 average May temperature. There are some clearly interesting patterns where slopes are seen to rise dramatically. For instance, the top right panel indicates that for counties with higher average 2018 May temperatures, higher percent Black male populations, and higher degrees of international migration, COVID-19 spread much more dramatically than in other urban counties.

Contrast this with the rural co-plot. There are multiple interesting panels here but focus again on the top right panel. Here each line represents a group of counties classified by rural-urban continuum codes in 2013 with larger numbers indicating smaller population counties either adjacent or not adjacent to a metro area. Smaller, (and also more isolated) counties saw a much more rapid increase in COVID-19 spread when accompanied by having a proportionately more Black, older population who also had a higher percentage of their population in 2018 living in poverty.

Reverse predictions for urban counties were generated from the rural forest and for rural counties from the urban forest. Absolute error 95% confidence intervals were $\left[4.967 \times 10^{-5}, 5.513 \times 10^{-5}\right]$ and $\left[7.224 \times 10^{-5}, 8.535 \times 10^{-5}\right]$, respectively. The non-overlap further confirms some differences in county-level structure being captured by both forests.

5.5 Shrinkage estimation

With tree-based models, we demonstrated how more flexible, non-parametric modeling structures could be formulated. These models are tailored more naturally to modeling complex interactions between predictors and can also produce highly interpretable models. We also demonstrated that more accurate predictions using trees could be achieved by using tree ensembles and that predictive inferences could be used to estimate disparities.

We will now go back and assume a more familiar regression setting where disparity estimates are part of the regression parameter estimation except now we entertain shrinkage methods designed to address more complex tasks – namely i) variable selection (i.e., sparsity), ii) dealing with correlated predictors and iii) estimation with high dimensionality (i.e., large numbers of predictors). For HDE with big data, all of these things are potentially at play.

5.5.1 Generalized Ridge Regression (GRR)

We will start with a response vector $y \in \mathbb{R}^n$ and a set of predictors where $X = (X_{(1)}, \ldots, X_{(p)})$ is an $n \times p$ design matrix, where specifically, $X_{(k)} = (x_{k,1}, \ldots, x_{k,n})^T$ denotes the kth column of X. We assume that the relationship between y and the predictors follows

$$y = X\beta + \varepsilon, \tag{5.2}$$

where $\varepsilon = (\varepsilon_1, \ldots, \varepsilon_n)^T$ are independent measurement errors such that $\mathbb{E}(\varepsilon_i) = 0$ and $\mathbb{E}(\varepsilon_i^2) = \sigma_0^2 > 0$. The true value for the coefficient vector $\beta = (\beta_1, \ldots, \beta_p)^T \in \mathbb{R}^p$ is an unknown value $\beta_0 = (\beta_{0,1}, \ldots, \beta_{0,p})^T$ where a number of the true coefficients may be zero.

When the number of predictors dominates the sample size, we are in the "big-p small-n problem" which poses unique challenges to estimating β_0. One issue, which is often under-appreciated, is multicollinearity. With very large p, significant sample correlation between predictor variables can occur as a pure artifact of the dimensionality; even when the true design matrix is orthogonal (see [45, 93] for an excellent discussion). Groups of variables become highly correlated with other groups of variables sporadically [93]. This is on top of other true correlations that might be present due to issues around the technology that generated the data or the science itself.

Hoerl and Kennard proposed generalized ridge regression (GRR) over 50 years ago. This is a method specifically designed for correlated and ill-conditioned settings [147, 146]. Although Hoerl and Kennard never considered using GRR in problems where p could be magnitudes larger than n, it can in fact be applied effectively in such contexts.

We start by going back to the definition of GRR. Let $\Lambda = \text{diag}\{\lambda_k\}_{k=1}^p$ be a $p \times p$ diagonal matrix with diagonal entries $\lambda_k > 0$. The GRR estimator with ridge matrix Λ is then defined by the equation

$$\hat{\beta}_\text{G} = (Q + \Lambda)^{-1} X^T y,$$

where $Q = X^T X$. An important property of $\hat{\beta}_\text{G}$ is that it exists whether Q is invertible or not. An alternate useful representation for $\hat{\beta}_\text{G}$ recasts GRR as an ℓ_2-penalization problem:

$$\hat{\beta}_\text{G} = \underset{\beta \in \mathbb{R}^p}{\arg\min} \left\{ ||y - X\beta||_2^2 + \sum_{k=1}^{p} \lambda_k \beta_k^2 \right\}, \tag{5.3}$$

where $||\cdot||_2$ is the ℓ_2-norm. In the special case when $\Lambda = \lambda I_p$, where I_p is the $p \times p$ identity matrix, one obtains the ridge estimator

$$\hat{\beta}_\text{R} = (Q + \lambda I_p)^{-1} X^T y.$$

The parameter $\lambda > 0$ is referred to as the ridge parameter. Setting $\lambda = 0$, and assuming that Q is invertible, yields the OLS (ordinary least squares) estimator $\hat{\beta}_\text{OLS} = Q^{-1} X^T y$.

5.5.1.1 Geometrical and theoretical properties of the GRR estimator in high dimensions

In the classical setting when $n > p$, GRR can be described as a constrained optimization problem involving the contours of an ellipsoid centered at the

OLS estimator. This geometrical interpretation still holds when $p \geq n$, but requires replacing the OLS by its generalization, the minimum least squares (MLS) estimator.

The following lemma is helpful.

Lemma 1 *(From Ishwaran and Rao (204)[168]): Let $p \geq n$ and let $X = UDV^T$ be the singular value decomposition (SVD) of X, where $U(n \times n)$ and $V(p \times n)$ are column orthonormal matrices ($UU^T = U^TU = V^TV = I_n$) and $D(n \times n)$ is a diagonal matrix with entries $d_1 \geq d_2 \geq \cdots \geq d_n \geq 0$. Let $A = V^T(Q + \lambda I_p)$. Then for any $\lambda > 0$,*

$$A^+ = VS_\lambda^{-1}, \tag{5.4}$$

where $S_\lambda = \text{diag}\{d_i^2 + \lambda\}_{i=1}^n$ is an $n \times n$ diagonal matrix and A^+ denotes the Moore-Penrose [278] generalized inverse of A. Furthermore, $AA^+ = I_n$.

This is useful because Lemma 1 allows one to re-write $\hat{\beta}_G$ in a more insightful manner. We first recast $\hat{\beta}_G$ as a rescaled ridge estimator. Let $X_* = X\Lambda^{-1/2}$ and $Q_* = X_*^T X_*$ (hereafter we use a subscript "$*$" to indicate a term mapped under the transformation $X\Lambda^{-1/2}$). Then

$$\begin{aligned} \hat{\beta}_G &= \Lambda^{-1/2}(\Lambda^{-1/2}Q\Lambda^{-1/2} + I_p)^{-1}\Lambda^{-1/2}X^Ty \\ &= \Lambda^{-1/2}(Q_* + I_p)^{-1}X_*^Ty \\ &= \Lambda^{-1/2}\hat{\beta}_R^*, \end{aligned} \tag{5.5}$$

where $\hat{\beta}_R^* = (Q_* + I_p)^{-1}X_*^Ty$ is the ridge estimator for the design matrix X_* with ridge parameter $\lambda = 1$. Let $X_* = U_*D_*V_*^T$ be the SVD for X_*. Let $d_{1,*} \geq \cdots \geq d_{n,*} \geq 0$ denote the diagonal elements of D_*. Using Lemma 1, [168] proved the following.

Theorem 5.1 *(From Ishwaran and Rao (204)[168]): If $p \geq n$, then for any $\lambda_k > 0$ for $k = 1, \ldots, p$,*

$$\hat{\beta}_G = \Lambda^{-1/2}V_*S_{*1}^{-1}R_*^Ty, \tag{5.6}$$

where $S_{*1} = \text{diag}\{d_{i,*}^2 + 1\}_{i=1}^n$ and $R_* = U_*D_*$. Moreover (5.6) can be calculated in $O(pn^2)$ operations.

It should be noted that the ridge estimator is a special case of the (5.6),

$$\hat{\beta}_R = VS_\lambda^{-1}R^Ty, \tag{5.7}$$

where $R = UD$. Thus the ridge estimator can also be computed in $O(pn^2)$ operations.

They then focused on describing a geometrical interpretation for $\hat{\beta}_G$. As they showed, the MLS estimator plays a vital role. For this, and all other results, we hereafter assume that $p \geq n$ and that $\lambda_k > 0$ and $\lambda > 0$, unless otherwise stated. For notational convenience, we often suppress dependence on n.

Definition 5.1 *Call any vector $\beta \in \mathbb{R}^p$ a least squares solution if $||y-X\beta||_2^2 \leq ||y - X\theta||_2^2$ for all $\theta \in \mathbb{R}^p$. A vector β is called a MLS solution if β is a least squares solution and $||\beta||_2^2 < ||\theta||_2^2$ for all other least squares solutions θ.*

We can then state a famous result due to to [279], which states that the MLS estimator exists, and it is the unique estimator

$$\hat{\beta}_{\text{MLS}} = X^+ y = \lim_{\lambda \to 0} \hat{\beta}_{\text{R}} = V S_0^+ R^T y,$$

where $S_0^+ = \text{diag}\{s_{0i}^+\}_{i=1}^n$ is the Moore-Penrose generalized inverse of S_0, defined by

$$s_{0i}^+ = \begin{cases} 1/d_i^2 & \text{if } d_i > 0 \\ 0 & \text{otherwise.} \end{cases}$$

Ishwaran and Rao's (2014) [168] result was based on the modified MLS estimator derived using the transformed design matrix X_*. The modified MLS estimator is defined as

$$\hat{\beta}^*_{\text{MLS}} = \Lambda^{-1/2} V_* S_{*0}^+ R_*^T y.$$

It should be noted that when $\Lambda = \lambda I_p$ that $\hat{\beta}^*_{\text{MLS}} = \hat{\beta}_{\text{MLS}}$. Then [168] derived the following geometrical interpretation for GRR.

Theorem 5.2 *(From Ishwaran and Rao (204)[168]): $\hat{\beta}_G$ is the solution to the following optimization problem:*

$$\underset{\beta \in \mathbb{R}^p}{\text{minimize}}\ \mathbb{Q}(\beta, \hat{\beta}^*_{MLS}) \quad \text{subject to} \quad \beta^T \Lambda \beta \leq L, \tag{5.8}$$

for some $L > 0$, where

$$\mathbb{Q}(\beta, \hat{\beta}^*_{MLS}) = (\beta - \hat{\beta}^*_{MLS})^T Q (\beta - \hat{\beta}^*_{MLS})$$

and $\mathbb{Q}(\cdot, \hat{\beta}^*_{MLS})$ is an ellipsoid with contours $\mathbb{S}(c) = \{\beta : \mathbb{Q}(\beta, \hat{\beta}^*_{MLS}) = c^2\}$ centered at $\hat{\beta}^*_{MLS}$.

Theorem 5.2 shows that the GRR estimator is the solution to a constrained optimization problem involving the contours of an ellipsoid centered at the modified MLS. This represents a generalization of the traditional setting from an optimization problem involving the OLS to one involving the MLS. The constraint region is also generalized. For GRR, the constraint region is an ellipsoid that depends upon Λ, as opposed to a spherical constraint region. Another important difference is that the dimension of the subspace that $\hat{\beta}_G$ lies in depends upon n, and not p (see Figure 5.12).

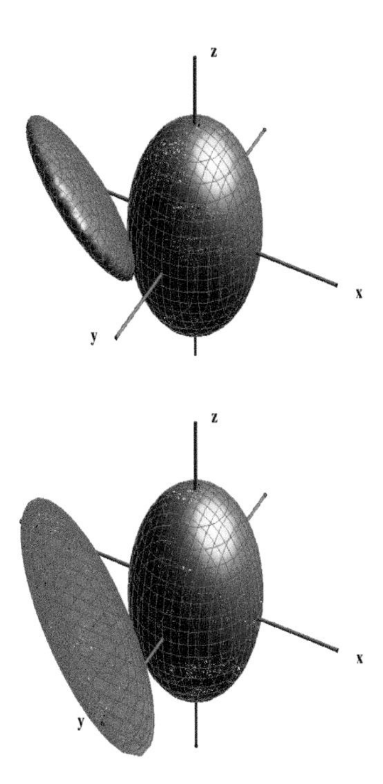

FIGURE 5.12: (Taken from Ishwaran and Rao (2014)[168]): Top figure corresponds to GRR with $\lambda_k = \infty$ for $k \geq 4$ using a simulation where $p = 100, n = 25$ and $\beta_{0,k} = 0$ for $k \geq 3$. Only the first 3 coordinates of $\hat{\beta}_{\mathrm{G}}$ are nonzero and these equal the point where the ellipsoid first touches the elliptical constraint region. Bottom figure is $\lambda_k = \infty$ for $k \geq 3$. Now only the first two coordinates of $\hat{\beta}_{\mathrm{G}}$ are nonzero.

5.5.2 Ideal variable selection for GRR

We will now follow the development shown in [167] to study how to do variable selection using the GRR. Theorem 3 of [168] showed that the GRR lies within the subspace $\Lambda(\mathscr{V}_*)$ containing the modified MLS; its exact orientation being heavily determined by its ridge parameters. As we showed, this orientation plays a crucial role in the properties of the GRR. By using very large ridge parameters we showed that the modified MLS, and hence the GRR, is capable of non-uniformly decorrelating variables. The following result builds on this idea and will help motivate the concept of ideal variable selection.

Theorem 5.3 *Define $\mathbb{J}_k = (0, \ldots, 0, 1, 0, \ldots, 0)^T$ to be the p-dimensional vector with a 1 in coordinate k and 0's elsewhere. If $\lambda_k \to \infty$, then $\mathscr{V}_\infty \perp \mathbb{J}_k$ where $\mathscr{V}_\infty$ is the limit of $\mathscr{V}_*$. Furthermore, the kth coefficient of $\hat{\beta}_G$ in the limit is zero and its remaining coefficients equal the GRR estimator restricted to the design matrix obtained by removing the kth column of X. Likewise, these results extend to the case when $r > 1$ ridge parameters converge to ∞.*

Theorem 5.3 shows that if $\lambda_k = \infty$ when $\beta_{0,k} = 0$, then $\hat{\beta}_G$ will be orthogonal to the kth coordinate axes (see Figure 5.12 for illustration). If p_0 equals the number of nonzero coefficients of β_0, then it is clear that by setting $\lambda_k = \infty$ for the $n - p_0$ zero coefficients, that a GRR estimator can be constructed so that it equals zero for the truly zero coefficients. Clearly, this ideal estimator has perfect accuracy over the zero coefficients. However, we would also like this estimator to accurately estimate the nonzero coefficients. To do so we need to set the ridge parameters for these coefficients accordingly, but what are these constraints, and can they always be satisfied?

To study this, we introduce the following measure:

$$\mathbb{D}(\Lambda; \beta_0) = \left\| \left(I_p - \Lambda^{-1/2} V_* D_* (\Lambda^{-1/2} V_* D_*)^+ \right) \beta_0 \right\|_2^2 \Big/ \|\beta_0\|_2^2.$$

This value can be interpreted as the sine of the angle between β_0 and the subspace $\Lambda(\mathscr{V}_*)$. In other words, it measures how far the the GRR's subspace is from β_0 in squared-distance. This leads to the following definition.

Definition 5.2 *A GRR estimator is said to satisfy ideal variable selection if $\mathbb{D}(\Lambda; \beta_0) = 0$.*

Ideal variable selection is a type of oracle property. Achieving it requires that the GRR correctly estimates the zero coefficients and that its subspace contains the nonzero coefficients. Although we cannot expect to achieve this property in real problems, it is still interesting to consider whether this property holds theoretically. This analysis, in fact, reveals a shortcoming with GRR that will motivate a richer class of estimators with potentially better performance.

The following result shows that ideal variable selection is intimately tied to model sparsity. For the following, and throughout the remainder of this section, we assume that the first p_0 coefficients of β_0 are nonzero and that $p_0 \geq 1$. Let $\beta_{0,(p_0)}$ denote the first p_0 coefficients of β_0.

Theorem 5.4 *Consider a GRR estimator with ridge matrix of the form*

$$\Lambda = \sum_{k=1}^{p_0} \lambda_k \mathbb{J}_k \mathbb{J}_k^T + \infty \sum_{k=p_0+1}^{p} \mathbb{J}_k \mathbb{J}_k^T, \quad \text{where } 0 < \lambda_k < \infty, \text{ for } k = 1, \ldots, p_0.$$

Then, $\mathbb{D}(\Lambda; \beta_0) = 0$ if and only if $\beta_{0,(p_0)} \in \Lambda_{p_0}(\mathscr{V}_{*p_0})$ where $\mathscr{V}_{*p_0}$ is the span of the eigenvectors for $Q_{*p_0} = X_{*p_0}^T X_{*p_0}$, where $X_{*p_0} = X_{p_0} \Lambda_{p_0}^{-1/2}$, $X_{p_0} = (X_{(1)}, \ldots X_{(p_0)})$ and Λ_{p_0} is the upper $p_0 \times p_0$ submatrix of Λ. In particular, ideal variable selection holds if rank$(X_{p_0}) = p_0$.

The rank condition of Theorem 5.4 can be viewed as a sparsity condition. Because $\text{rank}(X_{p_0}) \leq n$, ideal variable selection is guaranteed only when the sparsity condition $p_0 \leq n$ is met. When $p_0 > n$, and sparsity does not hold, there is no guarantee that $\beta_{0,(p_0)} \in \Lambda(\mathscr{V}_{*p_0})$. These results are a direct consequence of Theorem 3 of [168] which has shown that the GRR must lie in low-dimensional subspace of dimension $d \leq n$.

Theorem 5.4 shows that finding a suitable orientation may be difficult for a single GRR estimator in non-sparse settings. To overcome this, one can instead use linear combinations of GRR estimators, or what we call weighted GRR (WGRR) estimation.

Our next result shows that weighted combinations of even elementary GRR estimators can produce both accurate variable selection and estimation.

Theorem 5.5 *Let $\hat{\beta}_{WG} = \sum_{k=1}^{p_0} w_k \hat{\beta}_G^k$, where $(w_k)_{k=1}^{p_0}$ are weights and $\hat{\beta}_G^k$ is the GRR estimator with ridge matrix*

$$\Lambda_k = \lambda_1 \mathbb{J}_k \mathbb{J}_k^T + \lambda_2 \sum_{j \neq k} \mathbb{J}_j \mathbb{J}_j^T.$$

Assume that $\sum_{i=1}^n y_i = 0$, $\sum_{i=1}^n x_{i,k} = 0$, and $\sum_{i=1}^n x_{i,k}^2 = 1$. Then, .

$$\lim_{\substack{\lambda_1 \to 0 \\ \lambda_2 \to \infty}} \hat{\beta}_{WG} = ||y||_2 \sum_{k=1}^{p_0} w_k \hat{\rho}_k \mathbb{J}_k = \sum_{k=1}^{p_0} w_k \Big(X_{(k)}^T \Theta_0 + \xi_k \Big) \mathbb{J}_k, \tag{5.9}$$

where $\Theta_0 = X\beta_0$, $(\xi_k)_{k=1}^{p_0}$ are dependent random variables such that $\mathbb{E}(\xi_k) = 0$ and $\text{Var}(\xi_k) = \sigma_0^2$, and $\hat{\rho}_k$ is the sample partial correlation of $X_{(k)}$ and y.

The second equality in (5.9) shows that the estimate for each nonzero coefficient depends upon two terms: one being an error term with mean zero and variance σ_0^2; and the other, the signal strength of the coefficient. The first equality shows that these two terms are the decomposition of the sample correlation between $X_{(k)}$ and y. Combined, this shows that if the coefficient signal is larger than the error in absolute size, or equivalently if the sample correlation is nonzero, then (5.9) correctly identifies the zero and nonzero coefficients. It is also apparent that by appropriately selecting weights, $(w_k)_{k=1}^{p_0}$, that $\hat{\beta}_{\text{WG}}$ can also accurately estimate the nonzero coefficients, thereby achieving both accurate prediction and variable selection. In practice, of course, selecting the weights for WGRR requires sophisticated methodology. We next describe a class of Bayesian models for this purpose that yields WGRR estimators that can be used effectively in practice.

5.5.3 Spike and slab regression

The term "spike and slab" was used first by Mitchell and Beauchamp who coined the expression to refer to the prior for β used in their model [255] (see also [216]). A modern prototype of this model appeared later in [106]. This differed by making use of a scale (variance) mixture of two normal distributions for the prior of β. The use of a normal distribution eliminated the degenerate spike at zero used in [255] and made it possible to efficiently calculate the posterior using Gibbs sampling. See [107, 58, 60, 209, 42, 163, 164, 327, 276] for related work on spike and slab models.

Models like those described in [106] were later characterized by [165] as being part of a broad class of models referred to as spike and slab models. This class was then extended to rescaled spike and slabs by rescaling the response. An example of a rescaled spike and slab model studied by [165], is described as follows:

$$\begin{aligned} (y^*|X, \beta) &\sim \mathrm{N}(X\beta, n\sigma^2 I_n), \quad y^* = n^{1/2}y \\ (\beta|\gamma) &\sim \mathrm{N}(0, \Gamma), \quad \Gamma = \mathrm{diag}\{\gamma_k\}_{k=1}^p \\ \gamma &\sim \pi(\cdot), \quad \gamma = (\gamma_1, \ldots, \gamma_p)^T \\ \sigma^2 &\sim \psi_{a,a}(\cdot), \quad 0 < a \ll 1. \end{aligned} \tag{5.10}$$

In the last line, $\psi_{a_1,a_2}(\cdot)$ denotes an inverse-gamma density with shape parameter $a_1 > 0$ and scale parameter $a_2 > 0$. In the second last line, π is the prior for the hypervariance γ.

Note that (5.10) makes use of the modified response y^* in place of y. Also note the rescaled variance appearing in the first level of the hierachy (5.10) (scaled by a factor of n). While these differences may appear cosmetic, the affects of rescaling are crucial to variable selection performance [165]. This is because rescaling functions as a penalty parameter. Without the right scaling (of size n), penalization vanishes asymptotically and the limiting distribution for the posterior mean equals that of the OLS. In contrast, rescaling ensures a different limit than the OLS. Furthermore, variable selection improves because the posterior mean acquires a selective shrinkage property. Selective shrinkage is a property where the posterior mean is shrunk towards zero for truly zero coefficients only. We adopt the following strong definition of selective shrinkage.

Definition 5.3 *Let* $\hat{\beta}_S^* = \mathbb{E}(\beta|y^*)$. *Then,* $\hat{\beta}_S^*$ *is said to possess the (strong) selective shrinkage property if* $n^{-1/2}\hat{\beta}_S^* \xrightarrow{\mathrm{P}} 0$ *if and only if* $\beta_{0,k} = 0$.

5.5.3.1 Selective shrinkage and the oracle property

Selective shrinkage is an important property that motivates rescaled spike and slab models. In this section we prove that selective shrinkage holds in general for these models. Currently, this property has only been shown to hold under orthogonal designs [165].

To establish this result we will prove the stronger assertion that the oracle property holds. An estimator has the Fan-Li oracle property ([92]) if it is sparse and asymptotically normal and possesses the same limiting distribution as the OLS constrained to the true nonzero coefficients.

Because this proof is difficult, we will make use of a modified rescaled spike and slab model for our arguments:

$$\begin{aligned}(\tilde{y}|X,\beta) &\stackrel{\text{ind}}{\sim} \text{N}(X\beta, nI_n), \quad \tilde{y} = \hat{\sigma}^{-1}n^{1/2}y \\ (\beta|\gamma) &\sim \text{N}(0,\Gamma).\end{aligned} \tag{5.11}$$

This model differs from (5.10) because we have replaced y^* by $\tilde{y}$, where $\tilde{y}$ is scaled by the additional factor $\hat{\sigma}^{-1}$ (here $\hat{\sigma}^2$ is an estimator for σ_0^2 satisfying certain properties; we say more about this shortly). Rescaling by $\hat{\sigma}^{-1}$ allows us to remove the prior for σ^2 which helps to simplify our arguments.

To complete the specifications for (5.11), we assume that γ_k has a *two-component prior*:

$$\begin{aligned}(\gamma_k|\varpi) &\stackrel{\text{ind}}{\sim} (1-\varpi)\,\delta_w(\cdot) + \varpi\,\delta_W(\cdot), \qquad k=1,\ldots,p \\ \varpi &\sim \text{Uniform}[0,1].\end{aligned} \tag{5.12}$$

The parameter ϖ appearing in (5.12) is a complexity parameter that controls overall model size. Thus, γ_k is either a small value $w > 0$ with probability $(1-\varpi)$ or a large value $W > w$ with probability ϖ. By allowing w and W to depend upon n we will show that the oracle property holds. Examples of this prior are shown in Figure 5.13 for $\varpi = 0.05$ and $\varpi = 0.95$. Interestingly, the height of the prior changes as a function of ϖ.

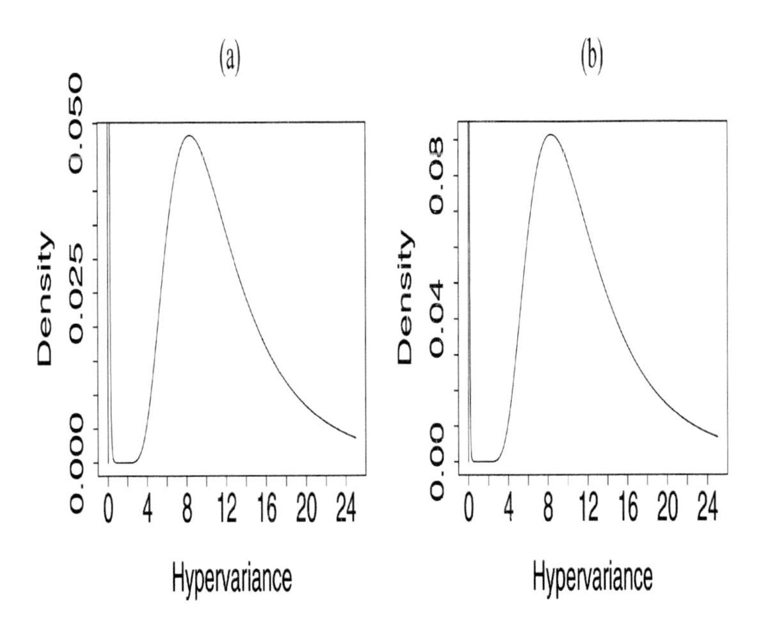

FIGURE 5.13: (Taken from Ishwaran and Rao (2005)[165]): Two component prior as a) $\varpi = 0.05$ and b) $\varpi = 0.95$.

We introduce the following notation. Map each γ to the model comprising those coefficients for which $\gamma_k = W$ (i.e., these are the promising variables not shrunk towards zero). Thus each γ is uniquely identified with a model comprising those regression coefficients with indices in some set $\alpha \subseteq \{1,\ldots,p\}$. One can think of α and the model corresponding to γ as being interchangeable.

Write α_0 for the true model. For our results, we make use of the following regularity conditions:

$$\sum_{i=1}^{n} y_i = 0, \sum_{i=1}^{n} x_{i,k} = 0, \text{ and } \sum_{i=1}^{n} x_{i,k}^2 = n\,, \text{ for } 1 \leq k \leq p. \tag{5.13}$$

$$\hat{\sigma}^2 \xrightarrow{\text{p}} s_0^2, \text{ where } 0 < s_0^2 < \infty. \tag{5.14}$$

$$\alpha_0 \neq \emptyset \text{ and } \alpha_0 \neq \{1,\ldots,p\}. \tag{5.15}$$

$$C_n = n^{-1}Q > 0 \text{ and } \lim_{n\to\infty} C_n = C > 0. \tag{5.16}$$

Assumption (5.13) requires that the data has been standardized. Condition (5.14) is mild and requires only that $\hat{\sigma}^2$ converges to a positive, finite value; a consistent estimator for σ_0^2 is not necessary. Condition (5.15) is purely a technical requirement: selective shrinkage is not well defined if all coefficients are zero, or if the true model is the full model. However, our results continue to hold even if (5.15) does not hold. Condition (5.16) assumes positive definiteness of C_n and is a standard assumption for the design matrix.

Let $\hat{\beta} = \hat{\sigma} n^{-1/2}\hat{\beta}_S$, where $\hat{\beta}_S$ is the posterior mean from (5.11)–(5.12). It is easily shown that

$$\hat{\beta} = n^{-1}\mathbb{E}(\Sigma|\tilde{y})X^T y, \tag{5.17}$$

where $\Sigma = (C_n + \Gamma^{-1})^{-1}$. This shows that the effects of shrinkage are captured exclusively by the posterior mean of the ridge matrix Σ. The following result establishes the frequentist properties of this quantity.

Lemma 2 *Assume that (5.2) is the true model and that regularity conditions (5.13)–(5.16) hold. Under the rescaled spike and slab model (5.11) with prior (5.12), if $W \to \infty$ and $w \to 0$ such that $W = O(n)$ and $w = O(n^{-1})$, then*

$$\mathbb{E}(\Sigma|\tilde{y}) \xrightarrow{\text{p}} C_{[\alpha_0]}^{-1},$$

where $C_{[\alpha_0]}^{-1}$ is the $p \times p$ symmetric matrix equal to zero everywhere except along the coordinates corresponding to α_0 where it equals $(C_{(\alpha_0)})^{-1}$, where the subscript (α) indicates a term including only those indices in α.

To understand how Lemma 2 implies the oracle property, it is instructive to consider the orthogonal setting, $C_n = I$. Under the asserted conditions, it follows that $\mathbb{E}(\Sigma|\tilde{y}) \xrightarrow{\text{p}} \sum_{k\in\alpha_0} \mathbb{J}_k \mathbb{J}_k^T$. Moreover, because $n^{-1/2}X^T y = n^{1/2}\beta_0 + O_p(1)$, this implies from (5.17) that

$$n^{1/2}\left(\hat{\beta} - (1 + o_p(1))\sum_{k\in\alpha_0} \beta_{0,k}\mathbb{J}_k\right) \overset{\text{d}}{\rightsquigarrow} \sigma_0 \left(\sum_{k\in\alpha_0} \mathbb{J}_k \mathbb{J}_k^T\right) Z,$$

for some random vector $Z \in \mathbb{R}^p$. Notice that the limiting covariance for $\hat{\beta}$ is zero if $\beta_{0,k} = 0$. Furthermore, by slightly tightening our assumptions regarding $(\varepsilon_i)_{i=1}^n$, we can assert asymptotic normality for Z, from which the oracle property follows.

Lemma 2 allows us to extend this argument to arbitrary X-designs. This leads to the following result.

Theorem 5.6 *Assume that the conditions of Lemma 2 hold and that $(\varepsilon_i)_{i=1}^n$ are i.i.d. and $n^{-1}\max_{i=1}^n ||x_i||_2^2 \to 0$, where x_i is the ith row of X. Then:*

(i) $\hat{\beta}_{(\alpha_0^c)} = o_p(1)$.

(ii) $n^{1/2}\left(\hat{\beta}_{(\alpha_0)} - (1 + o_p(1))\beta_{0,(\alpha_0)}\right) \overset{d}{\rightsquigarrow} N(0, \sigma_0^2(C_{(\alpha_0)})^{-1})$.

Thus, the rescaled posterior mean, $\hat{\beta}$, has the Fan-Li oracle property.

We make a few comments regarding Theorem 5.6:

1. Clearly (i) and (ii) imply that $n^{-1/2}\hat{\beta}_S$ shrinks to zero only for the truly zero coefficients. Thus the posterior mean, $\hat{\beta}_S$, has the strong selective shrinkage property.
2. The rate conditions for the prior can be considerably weakened in the orthogonal case. For W, any sequence satisfying $n - \log W \to \infty$ is permitted, whereas w can converge to zero at any rate. Interestingly, this shows that the growth rate for W and the shrinkage rate for w are considerably more stringent in correlated settings.
3. In the orthogonal case, the posterior has correct asymptotic complexity recovery. Under a Beta(a, a) prior for ϖ,

$$\mathbb{E}(\varpi|\tilde{y}) \overset{p}{\to} (p_0 + a)/(p + 2a).$$

If p is large this will be close to the true complexity p_0/p if a is chosen reasonably.

5.5.4 The elastic net (enet) and lasso

Consider the elastic net of [376]. Suppose that X and y have been standardized so that $\sum_{i=1}^n y_i = 0$, $\sum_{i=1}^n x_{i,k} = 0$, and $\sum_{i=1}^n x_{i,k}^2 = 1$ for $1 \le k \le p$. For a fixed $\lambda > 0$ (the ridge parameter) and a fixed $\lambda_0 > 0$ (the lasso parameter) the elastic net is defined as

$$\hat{\beta}_{\text{enet}} = (1 + \lambda) \operatorname*{arg\,min}_{\beta \in \mathbb{R}^p} \left\{ ||y - X\beta||_2^2 + \lambda||\beta||_2^2 + \lambda_0||\beta||_1 \right\},$$

where $||\cdot||_1$ is the ℓ_1-norm. Equivalently, by Lemma 1 of [376], $\hat{\beta}_{\text{enet}}$ can be written as a lasso-type optimization problem involving an augmented data matrix:

$$\hat{\beta}_{\text{enet}} = (1 + \lambda)^{1/2} \operatorname*{arg\,min}_{\beta \in \mathbb{R}^p} \left\{ ||y_A - X_A\beta||_2^2 + \lambda_0||\beta||_1 \right\}, \tag{5.18}$$

where

$$X_{\mathrm{A}} = (1+\lambda)^{-1/2} \begin{pmatrix} X \\ \lambda^{1/2} I_p \end{pmatrix}_{(n+p)\times p}, \qquad y_{\mathrm{A}} = \begin{pmatrix} y \\ 0 \end{pmatrix}_{(n+p)}.$$

This latter representation makes it possible to describe the geometry of the elastic net.

Theorem 5.7 *$\hat{\beta}_{enet}$ is the solution to the following optimization problem:*

$$\underset{\beta\in\mathbb{R}^p}{\text{minimize}}\ \mathbb{Q}_{\mathrm{A}}(\beta, \hat{\beta}_{\mathrm{SR}}) \quad \text{subject to} \quad ||\beta||_1 \leq L,$$

for some $L > 0$, where

$$\mathbb{Q}_A(\beta, \hat{\beta}_{SR}) = (\beta - \hat{\beta}_{SR})^T Q_A(\beta - \hat{\beta}_{SR}),$$

$\hat{\beta}_{SR} = (1+\lambda)\hat{\beta}_R$ and $Q_A = (1+\lambda)^{-1}(Q + \lambda I_p)$.

The geometry of the elastic net differs from the GRR in two important ways. First, the ellipsoid $\mathbb{Q}_{\mathrm{A}}(\cdot, \hat{\beta}_{\mathrm{SR}})$ in its optimation problem is centered at the rescaled ridge estimator $\hat{\beta}_{\mathrm{SR}}$. Here, $\hat{\beta}_{\mathrm{SR}}$ acts like the elastic net's OLS, in contrast to the modified MLS used by the GRR. Second, the orientation of the elastic net's ellipsoid depends upon the eigenvectors of Q_{A}, whose span is $\mathbb{R}^p$, and is unconstrained; whereas the GRR's orientation depends upon $\mathscr{V}_*$, and is focused along a low-dimensional subspace.

The above discussion also elucidates the geometry of the lasso shrinkage estimator which is simply the elastic net with $\lambda = 0$. The lasso stands for *least absolute selection and shrinkage operator* and was developed by [352] as a modification to the non-negative garrotte estimator ([36]). A quick peek into the citation history of the lasso quickly shows how impactful this estimator has been both in terms of spawning new paths for statistical methods development but also in a wide array of areas of application. The lasso ends up being a minimization problem like the enet, but now centered at the MLS solution $\hat{\beta}_{MLS}$. When X is full rank, the MLS solution reduces back down to the ordinary least squares (OLS) solution and more familiar lasso shrinkage plot is produced ([352]). Specifically, take the case when $p < n$ and $p = 2$ depicted in Figure 5.14. The plots both show the contours of the least squares objective function which are naturally centered at the least squares estimator (in this case plotted in the upper right hand quadrant). The shaded blue regions are the estimation constraint regions as imposed by ordinary ridge regression (right hand plot) and the lasso (left hand plot). The relative sizes of these regions are controlled by the shrinkage parameters. The first place the least square contours touch the constraint region is the shrinkage solution. The revelation of lasso was that the constraint regions contain corners sitting at the coordinate axes – resulting in possible zero solutions. This is what has been termed continuous variable selection. Notice also that all least square estimates are shrunk towards zero in both plots.

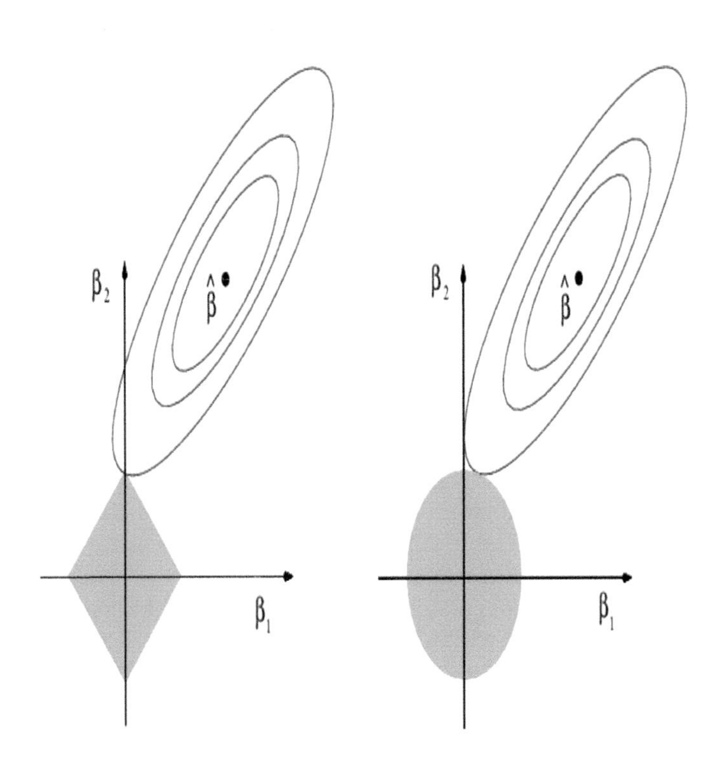

FIGURE 5.14: (Taken from Tibshirani (1996)[352]): Geometry of lasso shrinkage in two dimensions.

Example 5.5 Racial disparities in surgical interventions after lasso estimation of risk adjustment: Hammarlund (2020) [128] explored the observed finding that Black patients are less likely to receive certain surgical interventions than their white counterparts. To properly assess this apparent disparity, the fact that Black patients have increased health risk due to structural discrimination that appears in the form of poorer health upon arrival at a hospital needs to be taken into account ([332]). This is done by risk-adjusting surgery rates for clinically relevant factors that describe a patient's state of health ([52]). This is somewhat, in contrast, to directly trying to capture the effect of race which is not possible in observational studies ([359]). Instead, this direction of investigation asks whether the disparity in treatment rates remains after adjustment conditional on the many factors that are captured in the socially constructed variable we call race.

Hammarlund (2020) [128] focused on treatment disparity in the case of acute myocardial infarction (AMI) diagnosis and the subsequent decision to prescribe heart surgery or a non-invasive treatment regimen based on observed patient characteristics from which risk scores are estimated to determine the patient's health risk for surgery. Heart surgery encompassed both coronary artery bypass (CABG) or percutaneous coronary intervention (PCI) which can both relieve symptoms and delay death ([261, 291]). Data came from the Nationwide Inpatient Sample (NIS) and covered the years 2003 to 2011. The NIS is an annual, stratified sample of 20% of U.S. community hospitals (Healthcare Cost and Utilization Project 2017). Variables of interest were ICD-9 diagnosis codes, age, sex, year of admission, primary payer status and hospital identifier. The focus variable was race which was defined as the clinically derived version. That is, while self-reported race is the usual gold standard, each state and hospital employ different data collection standards making clinically recorded race an unknown combination of self-reported race and race as observed by others ([30]). The NIS sample size for AMI patients during the observed time period was 1,392,570 patients. Physician identifiers for a subset of physicians are also available in the NIS amounting to nearly 700,000 observations with such information. Patients were coded for their clinically defined race as White to indicate non-Black. The ICD-9 diagnosis fields described a wide variety of health conditions, some relevant to the heart surgery decision and some not. Hammarlund (2020) [128] created binary dummy variables for the presence of each unique ICD-9 code within the sample resulting in 2341 codes. He then built a logistic regression model with parameters estimated using the lasso with surgery (yes/no) as the outcome and ICD-9 codes as the potential set of risk adjustment covariates. He first removed ICD-9 codes that denoted outcomes of surgery or are otherwise determined after the surgery decision. This model was further adjusted for hospital location and year. The lasso identified 577 variables for surgery prediction from a candidate list of 1853 variables that met the candidate variable criteria. These were then taken forward as a risk adjustment set in a second logistic regression model that focused on the effect of race, specifically,

$$logit(p_{ithp}) = \beta_0 + \beta race_i + \gamma R_i + \delta_t + \nu_h + \phi_p,$$

where p_{ithp} is the probability of surgery for patient i in time period t evaluated at hospital h under physician p; R is the set of lasso-identified factors for risk adjustment, δ_t corresponds to time fixed effects, ν_h are hospital fixed effects and ϕ_p are physician fixed effects.

Hammarlund (2020) [128] found that raw disparity in surgical intervention rates was 8 percentage points with 29% of Black patients and 37% of Whites patients receiving invasive surgery for an AMI diagnosis. He found that the lasso-based risk adjustment could not explain the cardiac surgery disparity and that post-adjustments, Black patients are in fact 12.5% less likely to have surgery compared to White patients seen by the same physician. So in fact, the risk adjustments exacerbated the raw disparity estimate which can certainly happen depending on the directionality of the association of the risk factors to the probability of receiving surgery.

5.5.5 Model-assisted lasso for complex survey data

McConville *et al.* (2017) [240] derived a lasso estimator for complex survey data. Consider the typical complex survey setup. For element $j \in U$, define the inclusion probability as $\pi_i = P(i \in s) = \sum_{s:i\in s} p(s)$. Denote the superpopulation model that states, conditional on p-vector x,

$$y_i = f(x_i) + e_i,$$

where e_i are i.i.d. random errors with mean 0 and variance σ^2. McCoville *et al.* (2017) [240] utilized a design-based inference that assumes that the randomness stems only from the sampling design $p(s)$ and not the stochastic model. Thus all of their optimality properties are under this paradigm. Their rationale for this is to emphasize that the superpopulation model is considered a working model. Thus its focus is to aid in estimation and does not serve as a foundation for inference. As stated in Chapter 2, the working model can increase efficiency of survey estimators.

Under the specific case where $f(x_i) = x_i'\beta$, the least squares coefficients can be estimated by the Horvitz-Thompson "plug-in" estimator where population totals are each replaced by their Horvitz-Thompson estimator. Thus,

$$\hat{\beta}_s = (\sum_{i\in s} \frac{x_i x_i'}{\pi_i})^{-1} \sum_{i\in s} \frac{x_i y_i}{\pi_i} = (X_s' \varpi_s^{-1} X_s)^{-1} X_s' \varpi_s^{-1} y_s.$$

.

If β is potentially sparse in that only p_0 of its elements are non-zero where $p_0 < p$, then if the full model is fit, the design mean squared error of estimates for totals may be larger than that from a reduced (but correct) model. Thus [240] developed a survey-weighted model assisted estimator,

$$\hat{\beta}_s^{\text{lasso}} = argmin_\beta (y_s - X_s\beta)' \varpi_s^{-1} (y_s - X_s\beta) \quad \text{subject to} \quad ||\beta||_1 \leq L,$$

for some $L > 0$. As shown in Chapter 2, this one can use a simple transformation of the y_s and X_s to turn this into a usual lasso-constrained optimization which allows the use of efficient computing algorithms like coordinate descent search as implemented in the glmnet function in R.

Example 5.6 Age disparity in risk of Zika virus contraction on an isolated island Duffy *et al.* (2009) [83] conducted a household survey in order to better understand the risk factors and prevalence associated with contracting the Zika virus on the island of Yap in Micronesia. The island experienced an outbreak during the summer of 2007. The survey included demographic information, IgM antibody testing, and questions about each household member's activities during the time of the outbreak.

Yap residents older than 3 represented the finite population. The outcome variable was the presence or absence (0/1) of the IgM antibody in a blood test together with suspected disease symptoms during the outbreak period. Covariates included how many days an individual was crabbing during the outbreak period, if the perimeter of the house was free of vegetation, whether the house had air conditioning or not, and the age of the individual.

McConville (2011) [239] applied a survey-weighted lasso for GLMs because of the binary outcome to identify important covariates and specifically to identify if there were differences in risk of disease contraction for older individuals. The total number of households on the island was 1276 and the number sampled was 200. This yielded sampling design weights. McConville (2011) [239] went further and also defined what they termed stage II non-response rates which corresponded to members of an enrolled/sampled household who chose not to have their blood tested. The survey-weighted lasso shrinkage parameter was chosen by the AIC_c criterion (reference). Figure 5.15 shows the standard-

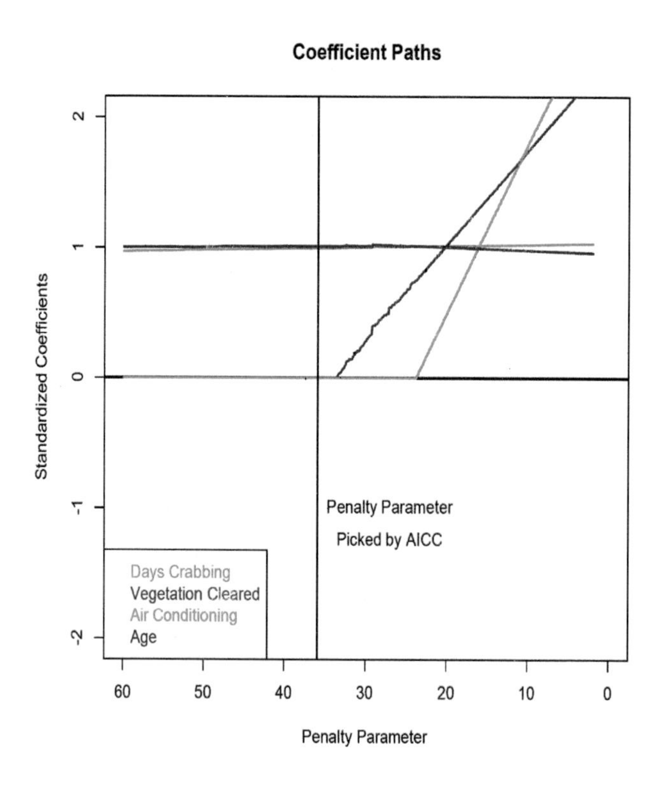

FIGURE 5.15: (Taken from McConville (2011) [239]): Standardized survey-weighted lasso trace plots for Zika risk from household survey.

ized lasso trace plots as a function of the penalty parameter. The vertical line shows the value of the penalty parameter chosen by AIC_c.

The analysis revealed that days crabbing and age were important predictors. For the age variable, the odds of contracting the disease was estimated to increase by 5.5% for every 10 years increase in age when the number of days crabbing was held constant. So clearly a disparity in Zika risk between elderly and younger individuals was detected.

5.6 Deep learning

Deep learning has become very popular in mainstream culture because it can potentially solve problems of automatic recognition of patterns in data often better than human beings can ([326]). It builds off of the older technology of artificial neural networks (ANNs) and allows a variety of different architectures and optimization protocols. While a revolution within the machine learning world, it is now starting to see a wider scope of application including in health disparity estimation (see, for example, [231]). In the review paper of [326], they give a nice primer on multilayer ANNs and deep learning but early pioneering work goes back to [243].

The overarching goal of ANNs is to mimic a connected neurons type structure within the human brain and by doing so, create a framework for learning from data much in the way that the human brain can learn through experience. An ANN consists of many interconnected simple functional units (neurons) that behave as parallel information processors to solve machine learning problems. They can be used for both classification or regression-type tasks and can also be used for unsupervised learning as well.

If the ANN is stacked into layers of connected neurons, then the network can receive information (input layers), pass information back and forth between layers (hidden layers) and output information (output layers). Within a hidden layer, each neuron is connected to outputs of the neuron in the previous layer with each multiplied by a *weight*. A neuron takes the sum of the products of its inputs and their corresponding weights. To allow non-linear predictions, each neuron can add a numerical *bias* to the result of its input sum of products and then pass this through a non-linear *activation function*.

Figure 5.16 shows a simple schematic of a single neuron learning model. The combined output of all neurons within a layer is either a linear classifier or a linear regression hyperplane (for the identity activation function). The hyperplane produces output points that are consistent with the original data in the sense of minimizing a chosen error function. Multiple layers whose output is the input of another are equivalent to having a complex single linear classifier or regression function ([326]). ANNs can learn because they can change the distribution of the weights to approximate functions that are

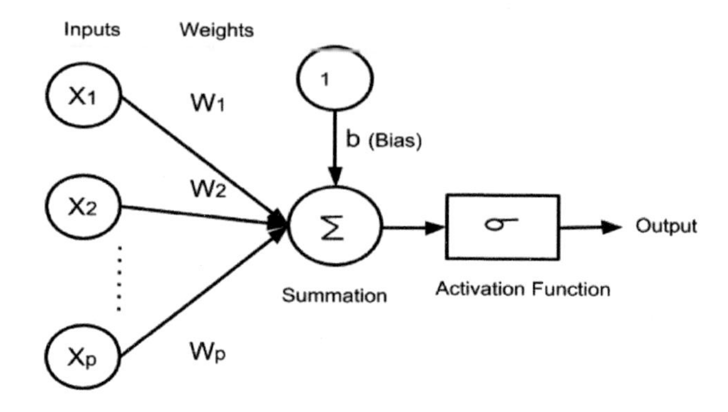

FIGURE 5.16: (Taken from Sengupta *et al.* (2020)[326]): Single neuron learning within an ANN.

representative of patterns in the inputs. The term *deep* is used to describe the fact that the ANN may consist of many hidden layers. The flexibility provided in the ANN architecture makes them very good adaptive learners, particularly with large training datasets and strong computing power like parallel computing platforms. In addition, better regularization techniques help avoid overfitting as the networks become more complex. Finally, improved optimization algorithms can produce near-optimal solutions. In such instances, complex ANNs can be learned which exhibit very good predictive performance. It is no wonder then that the number of application areas in which ANNs are being applied is growing by leaps and bounds and they have also caught the eye of health disparity researchers.

5.6.1 Deep architectures

There are a number of possible ways of arranging and connecting the hidden layers of an ANN. This is termed the deep architecture of the ANN. Different architectures have been shown to operate more effectively in different applications so no one architecture is always preferred. Very nice summaries of the most popular deep architectures are described in [326]. We will discuss only a few here.

Deep feed-forward ANNs impose the most basic architecture with the connections between the layers moving in a forward direction. Figure 5.17 shows a schematic of a deep feed-forward ANN. The multiple hidden layers help in modeling complex non-linear relationships more efficiently than can a shallow network architecture. Specifically, more complex functions can be modeled with less number of units compared to a shallow network due to the hierarchical learning associated with multiple levels of non-linearity.

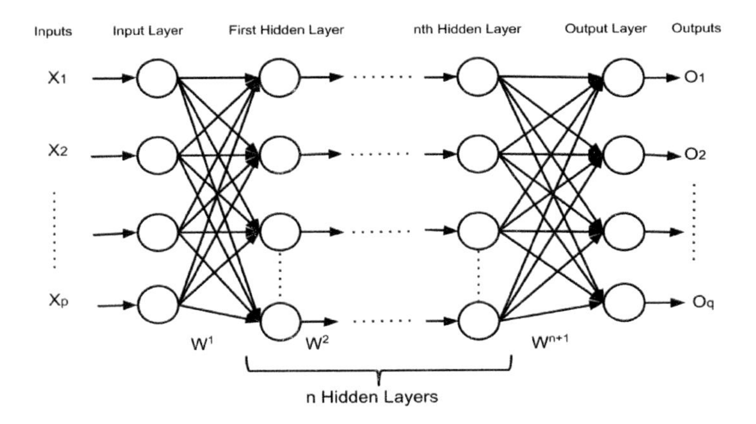

FIGURE 5.17: (Taken from Sengupta *et al.* (2020)[326]): A deep feed-forward ANN architecture.

Convolution neural networks (CNN) are another popular deep architecture that have proven to be particularly adept at image processing tasks. A CNN breaks down an image into simple properties like edges, contours, strokes, textures, orientation and color and learns them as representations in different layers. The idea traces back to [215]. The layers are known as convolution layers combined with pooling layers. The convolution layers retain spatial arrangements of pixels while the pooling layers allow summarization of pixel information. Figure 5.18 provides a schematic of a typical CNN.

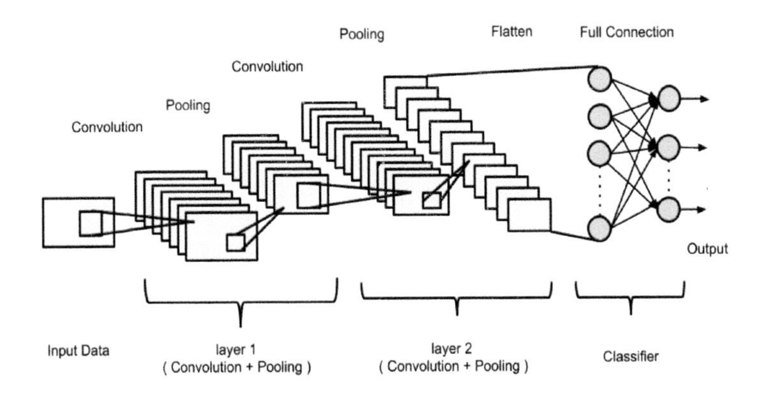

FIGURE 5.18: (Taken from Sengupta *et al.* (2020)[326]): Convolution neural network deep architecture.

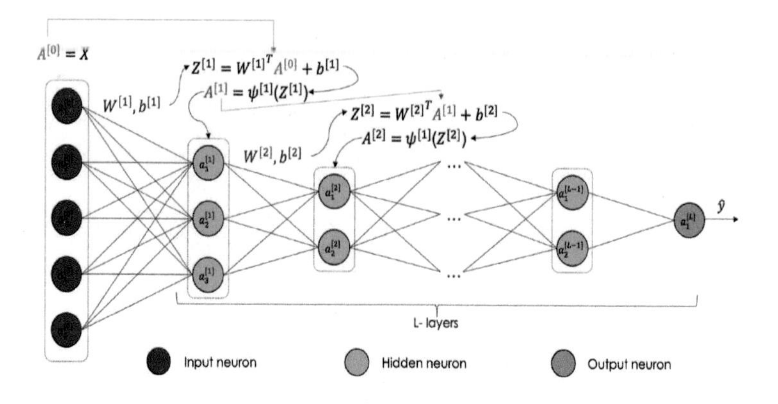

FIGURE 5.19: (Taken from Mebsout (2020)`https://www.ismailmebsout.com/deep-learning/`): Forward propagation parameter estimation.

5.6.2 Forward and backpropagation to train the ANN

The first step after defining the ANN architecture is to initialize the parameters. The parameters correspond to the weights W and the biases b across the entire network. The simplest form of initialization is to set $W = 0$ and $b = 0$. This forces all hidden layers to be symmetric. Other options include random initialization. Two examples include Xavier's and Glorot's method where initial values are drawn from specific normal distributions.

Learning for the network involves updating the parameters in order to minimize a loss function of interest. This involves two steps: forward propagation and backpropagation. In forward propagation, we pass the data through the network and calculate the loss function (e.g., sum of the errors based on output predictions). Figure 5.19 shows a schematic of the forward propagation process. Backpropagation then involves calculating gradients of the loss function with respect to the different parameters and applying a descent algorithm to update them. This process is repeated a number of times (known as epochs) until convergence of the parameter estimates is achieved.

This can be described in the following algorithm:

- Initialize model parameters $\theta = (W, b)$ for the network of a given architecture.

- For each epoch, compute $\hat{y}_i^{\theta}; i = i, \ldots, n$ where i indexes over the training data set.

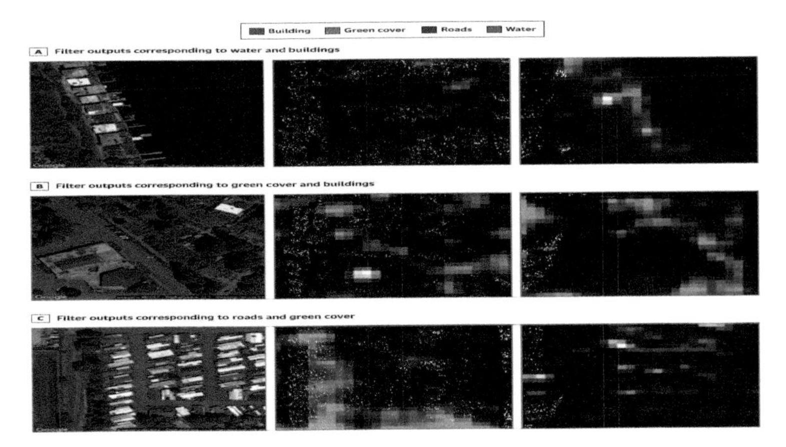

FIGURE 5.20: (Taken from Maharana and Nsoesie (2018)[231]): Deep learning identified features from a sample of 3 satellite images.

- Evaluate loss function $L(\theta) = \sum_i (y_i - \hat{y}_i^\theta)^2$.
- Apply a descent method to update the parameters: $\theta \to G(\theta)$.

Remark: Before optimizing the loss function, it's common to normalize (e.g., standardize) the inputs. This speeds up learning because $L(\theta)$ becomes more symmetric which helps the gradient descent find the minimum faster in fewer iterations. It is also typical to use convex and differentiable loss functions where any local minima will be a global one.
Remark: When training a ANN, it's also necessary to regularize parameter estimates to avoid overfitting. This can be done using $L1$ (lasso type) or $L2$ (ridge type) penalization to the parameter estimation steps.

Example 5.7 Using deep learning to assist in the understanding the association of the built environment with prevalence of neighborhood adult obesity [231] used deep learning via a convolution ANN to consistently measure features of the built environment (both natural and modified elements of the physical environment) extracted from high-resolution satellite images from Google Static Maps API. This analysis was done in Los Angeles, CA; Memphis, TN; San Antonio, TX; and Seattle, WA. These features were then fed into an elastic net regression model fit to data extracted on adult obesity prevalence from the Centers for Disease Control and Prevention's 500 Cities project. The regression models were used to quantify the association between the built environment features and obesity prevalence across U.S. census tracts.

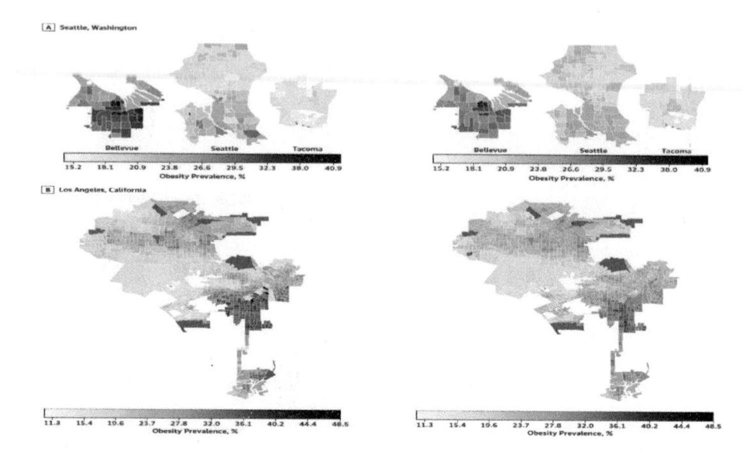

FIGURE 5.21: (Taken from Maharana and Nsoesie (2018)[231]): Elastic net cross-validated predictions (left) versus actual prevalence values (right) for two high prevalence regions.

5.7 Proofs

Proof of Lemma 1: We first show that $AA^+ = I_n$. Using $V^TV = I_n$, $Q = VD^2V^T$, and $V\Sigma_\lambda^{-1} = V(D^2 + \lambda I_n)^{-1}$, deduce that

$$\begin{aligned} AA^+ &= (D^2V^T + \lambda V^T)\Big[V(D^2 + \lambda I_n)^{-1}\Big] \\ &= (D^2 + \lambda I_n)(D^2 + \lambda I_n)^{-1} \\ &= I_n. \end{aligned}$$

From this it immediately follows that: (i) $AA^+A = A$; (ii) $A^+AA^+ = A^+$; and (iii) $(AA^+)^T = AA^+$. Furthermore,

$$A^+A = V(D^2 + \lambda I_n)^{-1}(D^2V^T + \lambda V^T) = VV^T.$$

Therefore: (iv) $(A^+A)^T = VV^T = A^+A$. Properties (i)-(iv) are the four criteria required for a Moore-Penrose generalized inverse.

Proof of Theorem 5.1: By (5.5), the GRR estimator can be expressed as a ridge estimator scaled by a diagonal matrix. Therefore, it suffices to prove that (5.7) holds and that the number of operations required to calculate (5.7) is of order $O(pn^2)$. Set $\Lambda = \lambda I_p$. Taking the derivative with respect to β in (5.3), setting this to zero, and multiplying right and left-hand sides by V^T, it follows that $\hat{\beta}_R$ must satisfy

$$A\hat{\beta}_R = V^TX^TY.$$

The solution must be $\hat{\beta}_{\mathrm{R}} = A^{+}V^{T}X^{T}Y$ because upon substituting this into the left-hand side we obtain

$$A\hat{\beta}_{\mathrm{R}} = AA^{+}V^{T}X^{T}Y = V^{T}X^{T}Y,$$

where we have used the fact that $AA^{+} = I_n$ from Lemma 1. Now substituting the right-hand side of (5.4) for A^{+}, yields

$$\hat{\beta}_{\mathrm{R}} = V\Sigma_{\lambda}^{-1}V^{T}X^{T}Y = V\Sigma_{\lambda}^{-1}\mathrm{R}^{T}Y.$$

To determine the number of operations required to compute $\hat{\beta}_{\mathrm{R}}$, note that the SVD for X requires $O(pn^2)$ operations. Once the SVD is obtained, inverting Σ_{λ}^{-1} requires $O(n)$ operations. Multiplying this (of size $n \times n$) by $V(p \times n)$ requires $O(pn^2)$ operations (note that because S_{λ}^{-1} is diagonal, this can be reduced further to $O(pn)$ operations, but this level of refinement is not essential). Multiplying by $\mathrm{R}^{T}Y$ requires a total of $O(pn)$ operations. The total number of operations equals

$$O(pn^2) + O(n) + O(pn^2) + O(pn) = O(pn^2).$$

Proof of Theorem 5.2: By (5.5), $\hat{\beta}_{\mathrm{G}} = \Lambda^{-1/2}\hat{\beta}_{\mathrm{R}}^{*}$ where $\hat{\beta}_{\mathrm{R}}^{*}$ is the ridge estimator under X_* with ridge parameter $\lambda = 1$. We show that $\Lambda^{-1/2}\hat{\beta}_{\mathrm{R}}^{*}$ is the solution to (5.8). As a Lagrangian problem, (5.8) can be written as

$$\underset{(\beta,\ell)\in\mathbb{R}^{p}\times\mathbb{R}_{+}}{\text{minimize}} \left\{\mathbb{Q}(\beta, \hat{\beta}_{\mathrm{MLS}}^{*}) + \ell(\beta^{T}\Lambda\beta - L)\right\},$$

where ℓ is the Lagrangian multiplier. Because L is arbitrary we can assume that $\ell = 1$ without loss of generality. Taking the derivative with respect to β, the solution is

$$2\Lambda\beta + 2\Lambda^{1/2}Q_*\Lambda^{1/2}(\beta - \hat{\beta}_{\mathrm{MLS}}^{*}) = 0.$$

Multiplying throughout by $\Lambda^{-1/2}$, β must satisfy

$$\begin{aligned}
(Q_* + I_p)\Lambda^{1/2}\beta &= Q_*\Lambda^{1/2}\hat{\beta}_{\mathrm{MLS}}^{*} \\
&= V_*D_*^2V_*^TV_*\Sigma_{*0}^{+}\mathrm{R}_*^TY \\
&= V_*D_*^2\Sigma_{*0}^{+}D_*U_*^TY \\
&= V_*D_*U_*^TY \\
&= X_*^TY.
\end{aligned}$$

Therefore, $\beta = \Lambda^{-1/2}\hat{\beta}_{\mathrm{R}}^{*}$; thus verifying that (5.8) is the optimization problem for $\hat{\beta}_{\mathrm{G}}$.

Proof of Theorem 5.3: Without loss of generality assume that the last $r \geq 1$ coordinates of Λ converge to ∞. Let $q = p - r$. It is easily seen that

$$X_\infty := \lim_{\substack{\lambda_k \to \infty \\ k \geq q+1}} X_* = X\Lambda_\infty^{-1/2} = X\Lambda_\infty^{-1/2}\left(I_p - \sum_{j=q+1}^{p} \mathbb{J}_j \mathbb{J}_j^T\right),$$

where $\Lambda_\infty^{-1/2}$ is the limit of $\Lambda^{-1/2}$. Express X_∞ as a SVD of the form $U_\infty D_\infty V_\infty^T$. If $k \geq q+1$,

$$U_* D_* V_*^T \mathbb{J}_k \to U_\infty D_\infty V_\infty^T \mathbb{J}_k = X\Lambda_\infty^{-1/2}\left(I_p - \sum_{j=q+1}^{p} \mathbb{J}_j \mathbb{J}_j^T\right)\mathbb{J}_k = 0.$$

Multiplying the left-hand side by U_∞^T, we have $D_\infty V_\infty^T \mathbb{J}_k \to 0$ for $1 \leq i \leq n$. Therefore, $\mathscr{V}_\infty \perp \mathbb{J}_k$.

To determine the limit of $\hat{\beta}_{\mathrm{G}}$, note that $X_\infty = (B, 0)$, where $B = X_q \Lambda_q^{-1/2}$ and X_q refers to X restricted to its first q columns and Λ_q is the upper $q \times q$ subdiagonal matrix of Λ_∞, which equals the upper $q \times q$ subdiagonal matrix of Λ. Therefore, by (5.5),

$$\begin{aligned}
\hat{\beta}_{\mathrm{G}} &\to \Lambda_\infty^{-1/2}(X_\infty^T X_\infty + I_p)^{-1} X_\infty^T y \\
&= \begin{bmatrix} \Lambda_q^{-1/2} & 0 \\ 0 & 0 \end{bmatrix} \begin{bmatrix} B^T B + I_q & 0 \\ 0 & I_r \end{bmatrix}^{-1} \begin{bmatrix} B^T y \\ 0 \end{bmatrix} \\
&= \begin{bmatrix} \Lambda_q^{-1/2}(B^T B + I_q)^{-1} B^T y \\ 0 \end{bmatrix} \\
&= \begin{bmatrix} (X_q^T X_q + \Lambda_q)^{-1} X_q^T y \\ 0 \end{bmatrix}. \qquad (5.19)
\end{aligned}$$

Therefore, only the first q coefficients are nonzero and these are determined from GRR under the design matrix X_q with ridge matrix Λ_q.

Proof of Theorem 5.4: The numerator of $\mathbb{D}(\Lambda; \beta_0)$ equals the squared-distance of the residual obtained from projecting β_0 onto $\Lambda(\mathscr{V}_*)$. Thus for $\mathbb{D}(\Lambda; \beta_0) = 0$, we must have $\beta_0 \in \Lambda(\mathscr{V}_*)$, or equivalently $\Lambda^{1/2}\beta_0 \in \mathscr{V}_*$. Thus, ideal variable selection holds if and only if

$$0 = \left\| \left(I_p - V_* D_* (V_* D_*)^+\right) \Lambda^{1/2} \beta_0 \right\|_2^2 = \left\| \left(I_p - V_* D_* D_*^+ V_*^T\right) \Lambda^{1/2} \beta_0 \right\|_2^2.$$

Applying Theorem 5.3 to each of the $n - p_0$ zero coefficients, we have $\mathscr{V}_* \perp \mathbb{J}_k$ for $k \geq p_0 + 1$. Thus, equivalently, ideal variable selection holds if and only if

$$\left\| \left(I_{p_0} - V_{*p_0} D_{*p_0} D_{*p_0}^+ V_{*p_0}^T\right) \Lambda_{p_0}^{1/2} \beta_{0,(p_0)} \right\|_2^2 = 0, \qquad (5.20)$$

where $U_{*p_0} D_{*p_0} V_{*p_0}^T$ is the SVD of X_{*p_0}. Therefore, for (5.20) to hold, we must have $\beta_{0,(p_0)} \in \Lambda_{p_0}(\mathscr{V}_{*p_0})$. Now if $\text{rank}(X_{p_0}) = p_0$, then $\Lambda_{p_0}(\mathscr{V}_{*p_0}) = \mathbb{R}^{p_0}$, and therefore $\beta_{0,(p_0)} \in \Lambda_{p_0}(\mathscr{V}_{*p_0})$.

Proof of Theorem 5.5: Using a similar argument as in (5.19), deduce that for each $1 \leq k \leq p_0$,

$$\begin{aligned} \lim_{\substack{\lambda_1 \to 0 \\ \lambda_2 \to \infty}} \hat{\beta}_{\mathrm{G}}^k &= \left[(X_{(k)}^T X_{(k)})^{-1} X_{(k)}^T y \right] \mathbb{J}_k \\ &= \left[X_{(k)}^T y \right] \mathbb{J}_k \\ &= \left[X_{(k)}^T \Theta_0 + X_{(k)}^T \varepsilon \right] \mathbb{J}_k. \end{aligned}$$

The first equality in (5.9) holds by the second line above. The last equality in (5.9) holds by the last equality above and by observing that $\xi_k = X_{(k)}^T \varepsilon$ has a mean of zero and a variance of σ_0^2.

Proof of Lemma 2: Throughout the proof we will use a subscript of α to indicate dependence upon γ whenever this distinction is necessary. For example, Σ_α will refer to $(C_n + \Gamma_\alpha^{-1})^{-1}$, where Γ_α is the diagonal matrix comprised of hypervariances defined by α. Subscripts of the form (α) will be used to indicate a term containing only those coordinates corresponding to α. Thus $X_{(\alpha)}$ is the X matrix constrained to those columns containing α. With a slight abuse of notation, $X_{(k)}$ will continue to denote the kth column of X.

One can show straightforwardly that the posterior density for γ and ϖ can be written as

$$d\pi(\gamma, \varpi | \tilde{y}) \propto \pi(\gamma | \varpi) \, |\Gamma \Sigma^{-1}|^{-1/2} \exp\left(\frac{1}{2\hat{\sigma}^2} Z_n^T \Sigma Z_n \right),$$

where $Z_n = n^{-1/2} X^T y$. Let $\Pr(\alpha) = \int_0^1 \varpi^{p_\alpha} (1 - \varpi)^{p - p_\alpha} d\varpi$ denote the prior probability for α, where $p_\alpha = |\alpha|$. Mapping each γ to its model α and integrating over ϖ, deduce that

$$\mathbb{E}(\Sigma | \tilde{y}) = \frac{\sum_\alpha \Pr(\alpha) \Sigma_\alpha |\Gamma_\alpha \Sigma_\alpha^{-1}|^{-1/2} \exp\left(\frac{1}{2\hat{\sigma}^2} Z_n^T \Sigma_\alpha Z_n \right)}{\sum_\alpha \Pr(\alpha) |\Gamma_\alpha \Sigma_\alpha^{-1}|^{-1/2} \exp\left(\frac{1}{2\hat{\sigma}^2} Z_n^T \Sigma_\alpha Z_n \right)}. \tag{5.21}$$

Let P_α be a $p \times p$ orthogonal matrix that rotates the coordinate axes so that the first p_α coordinates correspond to α. Partition $P_\alpha \Sigma_\alpha P_\alpha^T$ as follows:

$$P_\alpha \Sigma_\alpha P_\alpha^T = \left(P_\alpha C_n P_\alpha^T + P_\alpha \Gamma_\alpha^{-1} P_\alpha^T \right)^{-1} = \begin{pmatrix} A_{1,1} & A_{1,2} \\ A_{1,2}^T & w^{-1} A_{2,2} \end{pmatrix}^{-1},$$

where

$$\begin{aligned} A_{1,1} &= n^{-1}X_{(\alpha)}^T X_{(\alpha)} + W^{-1}I_{(\alpha)} \\ A_{1,2} &= n^{-1}X_{(\alpha)}^T X_{(\alpha^c)} \\ A_{2,2} &= n^{-1}wX_{(\alpha^c)}^T X_{(\alpha^c)} + I_{(\alpha^c)}. \end{aligned}$$

By standard matrix algebra,

$$P_\alpha \Sigma_\alpha P_\alpha^T = \begin{pmatrix} B_{1,1} & B_{1,2} \\ B_{1,2}^T & B_{2,2} \end{pmatrix}$$

where

$$\begin{aligned} B_{1,1} &= \left(A_{1,1} - wA_{1,2}A_{2,2}^{-1}A_{1,2}^T\right)^{-1} \\ B_{1,2} &= -A_{1,1}^{-1}A_{1,2}B_{2,2} \\ B_{2,2} &= w\left(A_{2,2} - wA_{1,2}^T A_{1,1}^{-1}A_{1,2}\right)^{-1}. \end{aligned}$$

By assumption (5.16), $A_{1,1}$, $A_{1,1}^{-1}$, $A_{2,2}$, $A_{2,2}^{-1}$, and $A_{1,2}$ are all well defined, and all have well defined limits. By the rates imposed on W and w, deduce that

$$\begin{aligned} \Sigma_\alpha &= P_\alpha^T \begin{pmatrix} (C_{n,(\alpha)})^{-1} & 0 \\ 0 & 0 \end{pmatrix} P_\alpha + O(n^{-1}) \\ &= C_{n,[\alpha]}^{-1} + O(n^{-1}). \end{aligned} \tag{5.22}$$

Now observe that $\Gamma_\alpha \Sigma_\alpha^{-1} = \Gamma_\alpha C_n + I$. Therefore,

$$P_\alpha \Gamma_\alpha \Sigma_\alpha^{-1} P_\alpha^T = \left(P_\alpha \Gamma_\alpha P_\alpha^T\right)\left(P_\alpha C_n P_\alpha^T\right) + I = \begin{pmatrix} WA_{1,1} & WA_{1,2} \\ wA_{1,2}^T & A_{2,2} \end{pmatrix}.$$

The determinant of the left-hand side equals $|\Gamma_\alpha \Sigma_\alpha^{-1}|$. Hence, using standard properties for determinants, we have

$$|\Gamma_\alpha \Sigma_\alpha^{-1}| = W^{p_\alpha}|A_{1,1}|\,|A_{2,2} - wA_{1,2}^T A_{1,1}^{-1}A_{1,2}|.$$

Observe that $A_{1,1} \to C_{(\alpha)}$, $A_{2,2} \to I_{(\alpha^c)}$, and $wA_{1,2}^T A_{1,1}^{-1}A_{1,2} \to 0$. Deduce that

$$W^{p_\alpha/2}|\Gamma_\alpha \Sigma_\alpha^{-1}|^{-1/2} \to |C_{(\alpha)}|^{-1/2}, \quad \text{as } n \to \infty. \tag{5.23}$$

Now multiply the numerator and denominator of (5.21) by the value

$$W^{p_0/2} \exp\left(-\frac{1}{2\hat{\sigma}^2} Z_n^T \Sigma_{\alpha_0} Z_n\right).$$

Using assumption (5.13) observe that $n^{-1/2}X^T\varepsilon = O_p(1)$, because

$$n^{-1}\mathbb{E}(X_{(k)}^T\varepsilon)^2 = \sigma_0^2 n^{-1}X_{(k)}X_{(k)}^T = \sigma_0^2, \quad 1 \le k \le p.$$

Hence, by (5.22),

$$\begin{aligned} &Z_n^T \Sigma_\alpha Z_n - Z_n^T \Sigma_{\alpha_0} Z_n \\ &\quad = Z_n^T \left(C_{n,[\alpha]}^{-1} - C_{n,[\alpha_0]}^{-1} \right) Z_n + O_p(1). \end{aligned} \tag{5.24}$$

The $O_p(1)$ term on the right-hand side of (5.24) holds because $Z_n^T Z_n = O_p(n)$ due to

$$Z_n = n^{-1/2} X^T X \beta_0 + n^{-1/2} X^T \varepsilon = n^{1/2} C_n \beta_0 + O_p(1).$$

By (5.23) and (5.24), the dominating term asymptotically for each term in the sum of the numerator (or the denominator) of (5.21) is

$$W^{(p_0 - p_\alpha)/2} \exp\left(\frac{1}{2\hat{\sigma}^2} \left[Z_n^T \left(C_{n,[\alpha]}^{-1} - C_{n,[\alpha_0]}^{-1} \right) Z_n + O_p(1) \right] \right). \tag{5.25}$$

Consider the exponent of (5.25). Let $\hat{\beta}_{\text{OLS},\alpha} = (X_{(\alpha)}^T X_{(\alpha)})^{-1} X_{(\alpha)}^T y$ denote the constrained OLS estimator for α. With rearrangement one can show

$$\begin{aligned} Z_n^T C_{n,[\alpha]}^{-1} Z_n &= n^{-1} y^T X_{(\alpha)} (C_{n,(\alpha)})^{-1} X_{(\alpha)}^T y \\ &= \left(X_{(\alpha)} \hat{\beta}_{\text{OLS},\alpha} \right)^T \left(X_{(\alpha)} \hat{\beta}_{\text{OLS},\alpha} \right). \end{aligned}$$

The right-hand side is the squared ℓ_2-length of the projection of y onto X_α.

For each α, let $\nu_1, \ldots, \nu_n$ be an orthonormal basis for $\mathbb{R}^n$ such that the first p_α vectors span the column space of X_α and the first p_{α_0} vectors span the column space of X_{α_0}. It is clear that such an orthonormal basis can always be constructed for α if either $\alpha \subseteq \alpha_0$ or $\alpha_0 \subset \alpha$. We assume that this is the case for now. Let $\theta_k = y^T \nu_k$. Then by the definition of the OLS, $X_{(\alpha)} \hat{\beta}_{\text{OLS},\alpha} = \sum_{k \le p_\alpha} \theta_k \nu_k$, and therefore

$$Z_n^T C_{n,[\alpha]}^{-1} Z_n = \sum_{k=1}^{p_\alpha} \theta_k^2.$$

Consequently if $\alpha \subseteq \alpha_0$,

$$Z_n^T \left(C_{n,[\alpha]}^{-1} - C_{n,[\alpha_0]}^{-1} \right) Z_n = - \sum_{k=p_\alpha+1}^{p_{\alpha_0}} \theta_k^2.$$

Because $\theta_k^2 = O_p(n)$ if $k \le p_{\alpha_0}$, the exponent in (5.25) converges to $-\infty$ in probability unless $\alpha = \alpha_0$ (when $\alpha = \alpha_0$ the exponent is exactly zero). On the other hand if $\alpha_0 \subset \alpha$, then $p_\alpha > p_0$ and $W^{(p_0 - p_\alpha)/2} \to 0$. Furthermore, $\theta_k^2 = O_p(1)$ for $k > p_{\alpha_0}$ (this follows from $y^T \nu_k = \varepsilon^T \nu_k$ and $\mathbb{E}(\varepsilon^T \nu_k)^2 = \sigma_0^2$, because $||\nu_k||_2^2 = 1$). Consequently, by the rate imposed on W, if α is a model such that either $\alpha \subseteq \alpha_0$ or $\alpha_0 \subset \alpha$, then the only such α with a nonzero limiting contribution to either the numerator or denominator of (5.21) is α_0.

Now we consider the scenario when $\alpha \subsetneq \alpha_0$ and $\alpha_0 \subsetneq \alpha$. In this case, we construct an orthonormal basis so that the first $P' = p_{\alpha'}$ vectors span the column space of $X_{\alpha'}$, the first $P'' = p_{\alpha'} + p_{\alpha''}$ vectors span the column space of $(X_{\alpha'}, X_{\alpha''})$, and the first $P''' = p_{\alpha'} + p_{\alpha''} + p_{\alpha'''}$ vectors span the column space of $(X_{\alpha'}, X_{\alpha''}, X_{\alpha'''})$, where $\alpha' = \alpha \cap \alpha_0^c$, $\alpha'' = \alpha \cap \alpha_0$, and $\alpha''' = \alpha^c \cap \alpha_0$. Because the squared-length of the projection of y onto $\{\nu_j\}_{j=P'+1}^{P'''}$ is less than the squared-length of the projection of y onto X_{α_0}, we have

$$Z_n^T \left(C_{n,[\alpha]}^{-1} - C_{n,[\alpha_0]}^{-1}\right) Z_n \leq \sum_{k=1}^{P''} \theta_k^2 - \sum_{k=P'+1}^{P'''} \theta_k^2 = \sum_{k=1}^{P'} \theta_k^2 - \sum_{k=P''+1}^{P'''} \theta_k^2.$$

On the right, the first sum is $O_p(1)$ while the second sum is $O_p(n)$. Thus, the right-hand side converges to $-\infty$ in probability. Because of this, even though p_α may be larger than p_{α_0}, the dominating term in (5.25) is the exponent and hence α has a vanishing contribution in (5.21).

Combining these results with (5.22) deduce that $\mathbb{E}(\Sigma|\tilde{y}) \xrightarrow{\text{p}} C_{[\alpha_0]}^{-1}$.

Proof of Theorem 5.6: Using Lemma 2, deduce that

$$\begin{aligned} n^{1/2}\hat{\beta} &= n^{-1/2}\mathbb{E}(\Sigma|\tilde{y})X^T y \\ &= n^{-1/2}\mathbb{E}(\Sigma|\tilde{y})X^T(X\beta_0 + \varepsilon) \\ &= n^{1/2}\mathbb{E}(\Sigma|\tilde{y})C_n\beta_0 + \left(C_{[\alpha_0]}^{-1} + o_p(1)\right) n^{-1/2}X^T\varepsilon. \end{aligned}$$

Invoking a standard triangular central limit theorem (Corollary B1, [340]) for $n^{-1/2}X^T\varepsilon$, deduce that

$$\left(C_{[\alpha_0]}^{-1} + o_p(1)\right) n^{-1/2}X^T\varepsilon \overset{\text{d}}{\rightsquigarrow} C_{[\alpha_0]}^{-1}N(0, \sigma_0^2 C).$$

Therefore,

$$n^{1/2}\left(\hat{\beta} - \left[C_{[\alpha_0]}^{-1} + o_p(1)\right] C_n\beta_0\right) \overset{\text{d}}{\rightsquigarrow} N(0, \sigma_0^2 C_{[\alpha_0]}^{-1}),$$

and (i) and (ii) now follow.

Proof of Theorem 5.7: Because the rank of X_{A} is p, the OLS exists and is well defined. Indeed, by direct calculation it is easily verified that $\hat{\beta}_{\text{OLS}}^{\text{A}} = (1+\lambda)^{-1/2}\hat{\beta}_{\text{SR}}$. By elementary properties of the OLS,

$$||y_{\text{A}} - X_{\text{A}}\beta||_2^2 = ||y_{\text{A}} - X_{\text{A}}\hat{\beta}_{\text{OLS}}^{\text{A}}||_2^2 + ||X_{\text{A}}\hat{\beta}_{\text{OLS}}^{\text{A}} - X_{\text{A}}\beta||_2^2.$$

Minimizing this with respect to β is equivalent to minimizing

$$||X_{\text{A}}\hat{\beta}_{\text{OLS}}^{\text{A}} - X_{\text{A}}\beta||_2^2 = (\beta - \hat{\beta}_{\text{OLS}}^{\text{A}})^T Q_{\text{A}}(\beta - \hat{\beta}_{\text{OLS}}^{\text{A}}).$$

Substitute $(1+\lambda)^{-1/2}\hat{\beta}_{\text{SR}}$ for $\hat{\beta}^{\text{A}}_{\text{OLS}}$, use the representation (5.18), and reparameterizing β by $\tilde{\beta} = (1+\lambda)^{-1/2}\beta$. The optimization problem for $\hat{\beta}_{\text{enet}}$ is

$$\underset{\tilde{\beta}\in\mathbb{R}^p}{\text{minimize}}\ \mathbb{Q}_{\text{A}}(\tilde{\beta}, \hat{\beta}_{\text{SR}})/(1+\lambda) \quad \text{subject to} \quad ||\beta||_1 \leq (1+\lambda)^{1/2}L.$$

Now absorb the scaling factor $(1+\lambda)^{1/2}$ into a new generic constant L.

6

Health Disparity Estimation under a Precision Medicine Paradigm

6.1 What is precision medicine?

"Precision medicine refers to the tailoring of medical treatment to the individual characteristics of each patient. It does not literally mean the creation of drugs or medical devices that are unique to a patient, but rather the ability to *classify individuals into subpopulations* that differ in their susceptibility to a particular disease, in the biology and/or prognosis of those diseases they may develop, or in their response to a specific treatment. Preventive or therapeutic interventions can then be concentrated on those who will benefit, sparing expense and side effects for those who will not.".

While often seen as focusing on the individual, " Precision in the context of public health has been described as improving the ability to prevent disease, promote health, and reduce health disparities in populations by (1) applying emerging methods and technologies for measuring disease, pathogens, exposures, behaviors, and susceptibility in populations; and (2) developing policies and targeted implementation programs to improve health." So there is still a focus on targeted implementations to improve health.

In the context of health disparities, where population or group differences are the focus, this amounts to targeting specific subpopulations with varying levels of group differences. So in other words, precision medicine in the context of health disparities would imply heterogeneity in differences in health outcomes across subpopulations. The focus of this chapter is to develop different statistical frameworks to identify such subpopulations as well as new methods for modeling and prediction in the presence of such heterogeneity.

6.1.1 The role of genomic data

Precision medicine-based research involves the study of multi-level determinants to understand how disease differentially affects different groups ([21]). So while precision medicine is often associated with molecular determinants of disease and other factors that currently reside in medical health systems, a complete study will involve factors involving lifestyle, nutrition, environment, and access to care. Current research in the area of wearables and mobile health

DOI: 10.1201/9781003119449-6

devices aims to improve tracking of these behavioral, environmental, and social determinants of health. In fact, it is estimated that these make up about 60% of the overall determinants of health while genes account for about 30% and medical history about 10% ([193]). So while the field initially focused on developing a new classification of human disease based on molecular biology, it has evolved to recognize that there are complex interactions at play between our genes and these other important determinants ([193]).

6.2 Disparity subtype identification using tree-based methods

We first consider methods for the data-based identification of disparity subgroups within a tree-based modeling paradigm. This methodology will also facilitate the identification of interactions between covariates, some of which may be across levels within a multi-level design (so-called hierarchical interactions). In order to fit hierarchical interactions between individual-level variables and contextual ones, we first introduce a generalized surface varying coefficient model. The focus of the presentation will be on a survival outcome but similar ideas can be used to model continuous or class-valued outcomes.

First, let T be the logarithm of the failure time and $x = (x_1, \ldots, x_p)'$ be a p-dimensional covariate vector of focus-level variables and z a K-dimensional vector of individual-level potential moderator variables. In most applications for health disparity estimation, x will be a scalar but we continue in full generality here for the discussion.

Since T is subject to right censoring, we observe (y, δ, x, z) with $y = min(T, C)$, where C is the logarithm of the censoring time and $\delta = 1\{T \leq C\}$ is the censoring indicator. Since we will also want to incorporate contextual level moderators, we will assume that we have drawn a random sample $\{y_{im}, \delta_{im}, x_{i,m}, z_{im}\}; i = 1, \ldots, n_m, m = 1, \ldots, M$ where M represents the total number of areas and n_m the number of observations in area m from the parent distribution. Here area is meant to imply contextual domain which could be more general than a geographical area. We will first assume the relationship between y and x and z follows the model,

$$y = x'\beta(z) + e, \tag{6.1}$$

where $\beta(z)' = (\beta_1(z), \ldots, \beta_p(z))$. The e are errors with an unknown distribution. Here the individual level moderator variables z are seen to be moderating the effect of x on y. The true underlying form for $\beta_j(z); j = 1, \ldots, p$ is an unknown complex p-dimensional hypersurface which modulates the effect of each x_j. This is a multivariable analog of the varying coefficient models introduced by [134].

6.2.1 PRISM approximation

Estimating the model above directly proves challenging in higher dimensions due to the curse of dimensionality, and thus [305] developed a structured approximation that takes the form for each $\beta_j(z)$ as,

$$\beta_j(z) = \sum_{l=1}^{L} \theta_{jl} I(z \in A_l), \tag{6.2}$$

where A_l is a partition of the predictor space determined by z. All A_l are assumed mutually exclusive. We will designate this model as *Partially Recursively Induced Structured Moderation (PRISM)* regression approximation to 6.1 and formally define it as,

$$y = \sum_{j=1}^{p} x_j \sum_{l=1}^{L} \theta_{jl} I(z \in A_l) + e. \tag{6.3}$$

So this approximation fits separate linear models with focus variables x to observations in each A_l whose membership in which are determined by individual-level moderator variables. This is done using a weighted least squares approach to account for censoring. For each A_l, let $\hat{F}_{nl}$ be the Kaplan-Meier estimator of the distribution function F of T for observations in A_l. Following [343, 344], we can write $\hat{F}_{nl} = \sum_{i \in A_l} d_{ni}(y_{(i)} \leq y)$ where the d_{ni} are the Kaplan-Meier weights representing the jump points in the Kaplan-Meier estimator. Specifically, $d_{n1} = \delta_{(1)}/n$ and $d_{ni} = \delta_{(i)}/(n-i+1) \prod_{j=1}^{i-1}((n-j)/(n-j+1))^{\delta_{(j)}}; i \in A_l$.

Contextual level variables w (say a q-vector) can be further incorporated into the structured moderation model as $\beta_j(z(w))$. This allows for multilevel moderation of the effect of x on y by now both z and w and we term this model hierarchical PRISM or HPRISM. We use a tree-structured regression approach to fit the model [38]. As is well known, there are many advantages of this approach over traditional multilevel models based on linear (mixed) models. These tree-based models are generally good predictors for complex data. They are non-linear, non-parametric, resistant to outliers and missing values and because of their piecewise structure, provide ease of interpretation. In addition, they naturally find complex interactions which may not be known apriori.

In order to fit HPRISM models using our sample $\{y_{i,m}, \delta_{im}, \mathbf{x}_{im}, \mathbf{z}_{im}, \mathbf{w}_m\}$; $i = 1, \ldots, n_m, m = 1, \ldots, M$ where M, we use a recursive partitioning approach as follows: For ease of discussion, take for example, $p = 1, x = race, z_1, \ldots, z_K$ and a single contextual level variable $w = percentpov$ and $n = \sum_{m=1}^{M} n_m m$ observations. Consider z_k and all observed values $z_{k1}, \ldots, z_{kn}$. Index the root node as τ that pools all of the observations.

That is, (x_i, y_i, w_i), $i = 1, \ldots, \sum_{m=1}^{M} n_m m$, and with some abuse of notation, $w' = \{(w_1)_{n_1}, \ldots, (w_M)_{n_M}\}$. Consider a split $z_{ki} < s$ that generates daughter nodes τ_L and τ_R. Then define the change in residual sum of squares (RSS) for this split as,

$$\Delta RSS(s) = \sum_{i \in \tau} \hat{r_i}^2 - \{\sum_{i \in \tau_L} \hat{r_i}^2 + \sum_{i \in \tau_R} \hat{r_i}^2\},$$

where $\hat{r_i} = \Delta_i r_i + (1 - \Delta_i) E(e|e > r_i)$ with Δ_i being the censoring indicator and $r_i = y_i - \theta_0 - \theta_1 x_i - \theta_2 x_i * w_i$ and $E(e|e > r_i)$ is estimated as the mean value of all residuals of uncensored observations greater than r_i [268].

Then choose the split value among all z_k's that maximizes the $\Delta RSS(s)$. *Recurse* till a stopping rule is satisfied. This can be visualized as a *binary tree* consisting of a set of terminal nodes whose corresponding branches are the recursively applied splitting rule from the root node onwards.

6.2.2 Level set estimation (LSE) for disparity subtypes

Level sets correspond to regions of the input space where functions of interest exceed fixed thresholds. There are a number of interesting papers which describe methods to identify such sets. This includes formalizing the task as a classification problem with sequential measurements and modeling the unknown function as a sample from a Gaussian process ([118]), or using tree-based approaches to partition the input space and then collapsing partitions by optimizing a penalized goodness-of-fit criterion ([366]), or using piecewise polynomial estimators which maximize local empirical excess masses ([49]).

A level set ([212]) $\{l : \theta_{0L} \leq \theta_l(\mathbf{w}) \leq \theta_{0R}\}$ will consist of a union of those regions A_l for which $\theta_l(\mathbf{w})$ are close enough to each other as defined by $[\theta_{0L}, \theta_{0R}]$. In order to estimate level sets, the terminal node parameter estimates can be clustered together indicating similar group effects. This can be done using any reasonable clustering algorithm (e.g., kmeans clustering).

In order to determine the appropriate number of clusters, we can employ a measure like the gap statistic ([294]) to determine $\tilde{m}$ – the number of disparity subtypes. Specifically, for a candidate number of clusters k, we define the sum of the pairwise distances for all points in a particular cluster r and from this, derive the pooled within-cluster sum of squares W_k around the k cluster means. We then compare (the log) of this value with its expectation under a null reference distribution of the data (e..g a permutation distribution). The optimal $\tilde{m}$ is the value for which W_k is the farthest away from its null counterpart. Additionally, it's straightforward to assign each observation to a subtype based on the terminal node in the tree to which it fell.

Example 6.1 PRISM modeling to identify disparities in survival for ovarian cancer patients as a function of DNA methylation profiles:

We will now illustrate our disparity subtyping methods using The Cancer Genome Atlas (TCGA), specifically focusing on ovarian cancer. A detailed integrated genomic analysis of this data was done by The Cancer Genome Atlas Research Network ([348]) and found that most tumors (96%) at the time of analysis had *TP53* mutations, and low but important prevalence of somatic mutations in 9 additional genes including *NF1, BRCA1, BRCA2, RB1 and CDK12*. Additionally, a number of significant DNA copy number aberrations were detected and significant differentially methylated regions (as compared to matched normal tissue). Four transcriptional subtypes were discovered, three miRNA subtypes as well as four methylation subtypes.

As background, ovarian cancer is the fifth leading cause of cancer death among women in the U.S. Mortality is associated heavily with patients presenting with advanced stage, high-grade serous ovarian cancer. Standard of care is surgery followed by platinum therapy. The majority of ovarian cancers occur in women older than 65 years of age. Age-specific analyses show that incidence and mortality rates continuously increase in the elderly population ([282]). More advanced stage at diagnosis is one of the determinants of the poorer prognosis in elderly patients but treatment guidelines are still vague for these women because of the feasibility of chemotherapy or reduction in remaining years of quality of life due to treatment side effects. Hence if more refined disparity subtypes (beyond just the advanced stage at diagnosis) as a function of age exist, it might shed additional light on which elderly patients should receive more aggressive therapy.

As of August 31, 2018, The TCGA repository had 575 clinically annotated stage II-IV high-grade serous ovarian cancer cases. After removing cases with missing survival outcome information and age information, this number was reduced to 549 cases. Clinical data included age at diagnosis, race, tumor grade and stage, and surgical outcome although much missingness exists on many of these clinical variables for the ovarian cancer type. The median overall survival of this cohort was 1013 days and 40.1% were still alive at the time of the last follow-up. Median follow-time time was 828 days. We will classify those patients ≥ 65 years of age as elderly and everyone else in the younger age category and apply both level set identification and peeling to try and identify and then validate disparity subtypes. For validation purposes, we will randomly split the dataset up into a training set (50%) and a test or validation set (50%) using stratified (by age category) random sampling without replacement. This splitting proportion helps to reduce some of the instability inherent in subgroup discovery studies due to sampling and sample size effects. While it's also known that racial/ethnic disparities exist in ovarian cancer survival with African American women experiencing poorer survival as compared to other race/ethnic groups ([16]), TCGA does not contain enough racial diversity for this cohort to do a meaningful analysis ([337]).

We were interested in studying whether epigenetic determinants as embodied by DNA methylation could be used to identify age group-related disparity subtypes. There is a growing recognition that while it's likely that social, environmental, and genetic factors are at play, epigenetic changes might act as a liaison between the three ([341]). In addition, epigenetic changes that might explain disparate susceptibilities to age-related disease have been discovered ([315]). While we would have liked to incorporate clinical information (particularly stage at diagnosis), a large amount of missingness in these variables prevented us from doing so. Still, if DNA methylation markers alone could identify disparity subtypes and then these subtypes could be statistically validated, the finding would still indicate that these subtypes likely exist and could be further refined by incorporating complete clinical information. TCGA provides two methylation profiles – the 27K chip and the 450K chip. For the ovarian cancer dataset, the 27K chip had many more samples available and so we focused on that. This is older data than that of the 450K chip but represents methylation profiling done using the Infinium HumanMethylation27 BeadChip 27K array where 27,578 probes of CpG sites were included. Details on how these profiles were generated can be found in [228]. There are no contextual variables so we are fitting PRISM models only.

We first split the dataset into 50% training data and 50% test/validation data set. We next screened methylation markers by fitting univariate Cox regression models in the training data to overall survival using the methylation marker-age group variable interaction as the only covariate. Those methylation markers that resulted in p-values less than 10^{-6} were kept for further analysis. This is a similar threshold to what's used for genome-wide control of SNP testing in GWAS studies. Post-filtering, 47 methylation sites remained.

Figure 6.1 shows the level sets identified by the fitted PRISM model (blue, green and pink terminal nodes, respectively). The determination of three-level sets was made by use of the gap statistic whose graphical summary is presented in Figure 6.2. These level sets were then labeled as disparity subtypes and the Kaplan-Meier survival curves for each subtype between younger and elder patients are presented for the training set in Figure 6.3 and the test set in Figure 6.4 which demonstrates some degree of validation of the subtyping.

We next wanted to study the nature of these subtypes a little more deeply. Figure 6.5 shows heatmaps of the three subtypes found by LSE as defined by their methylation markers. The columns represent the TCGA samples in a subtype, and the rows, the defining methylation values. Further, samples have colored bars above them to indicate if they were part of the older age group or younger group of women. Hypermethylation was coded in blue and hypomethylation in red with white representing intermediate values. This proved not all that satisfying because the subtype-specfiic group differences in DNA methylation were not clearly obvious. Further work to determine an appropriate cut point scheme for the methlylation coloring would be required.

Figure 6.6 provides an alternative view of the result (as opposed to a heat map) of the description of the disparity subtypes as a function of the 47 methylation markers that survived univariate filtering. From top to bottom are colored parallel coordinate plots (red are the younger aged women, blue the older aged women) for each subtype 1, 2, and 3, respectively. Each line

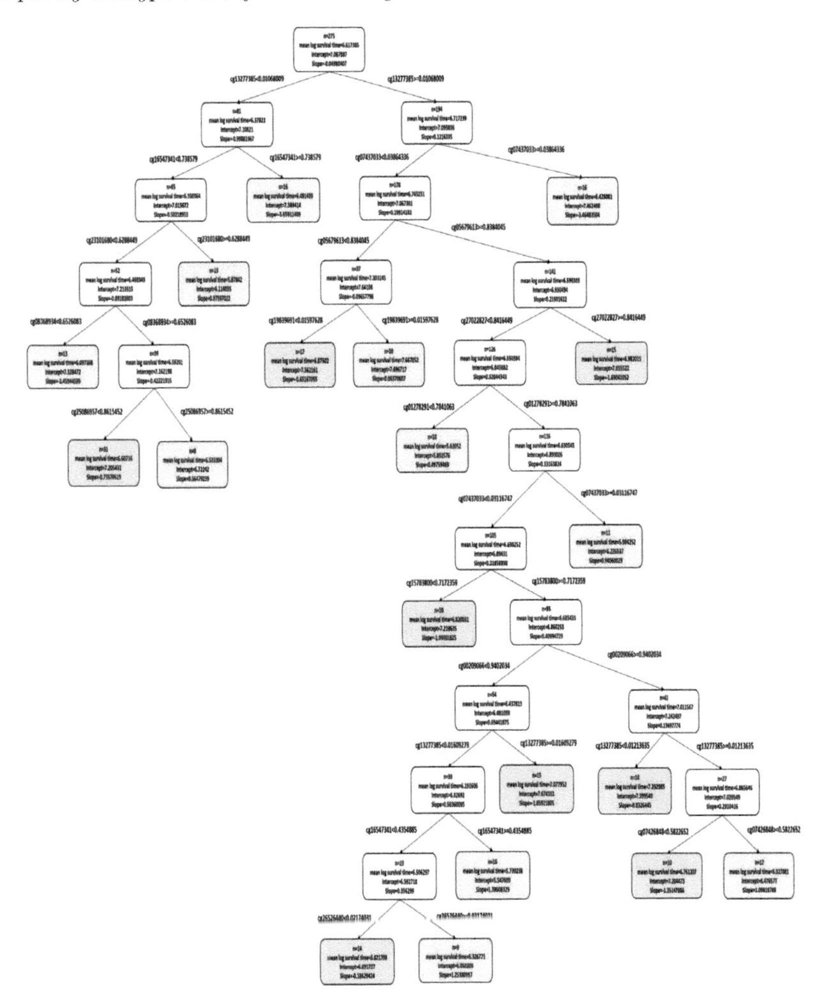

FIGURE 6.1: Level sets identified in the ovarian cancer training data.

represents standardized methylation values for a particular woman across the 47 methylation sites of focus. While as in the previous heat map, complex interactions are difficult to see, some useful conclusions are still immediate. First, subtype 3 which had no survival difference between the age groups shows no obvious difference in methylation profile lines (in fact the two groups are quite homogeneous). Next, subtype 1 and 2 do indeed show some subtype-specific differences in profiles for a number of women between age groups.

Instead, we turned to a very different exploration of the methylation patterns between young and older women in each disparity subtype. For ease of presentation, we will focus only on the subtypes found by LSE. We generated predicted epigenetic ages based on Horvath's epigenetic clock ([148]) for each

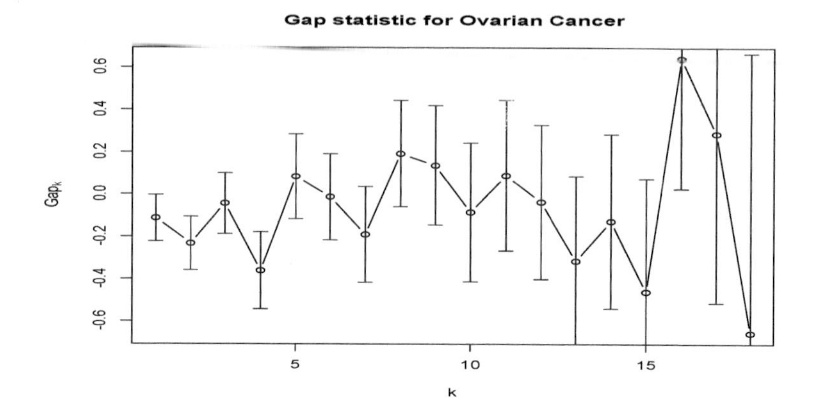

FIGURE 6.2: Gap plot for ovarian cancer training data

sample in each subtype. Horvath's clock was designed as a regression-based prediction of chronological age using DNA methylation markers from either the 27K Illumina methylation chip or the 450K version. Specifically, approximately 353 CpG locations were identified and then an elastic net regression model was estimated. Among the quantities that can be predicted is chrono-

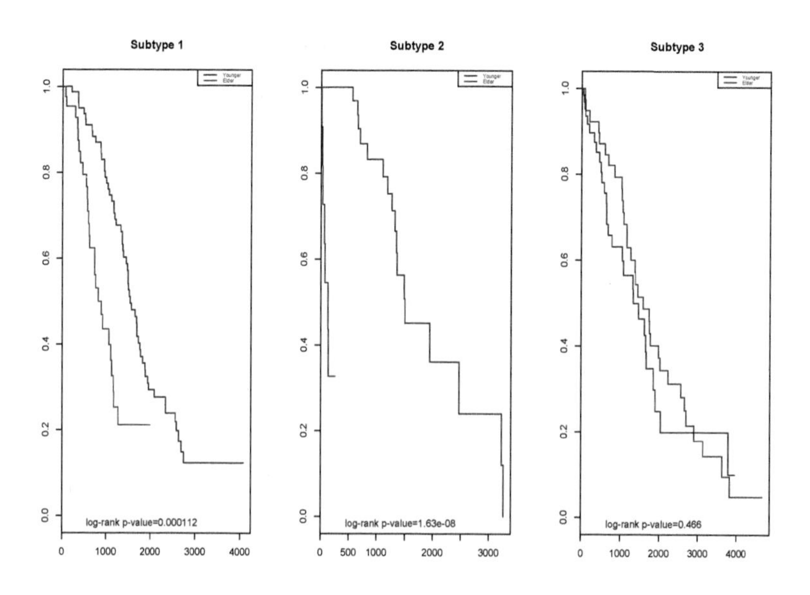

FIGURE 6.3: Level set disparity subtype (clusters 1, 2, 3) survival curves found in ovarian cancer TCGA training dataset.

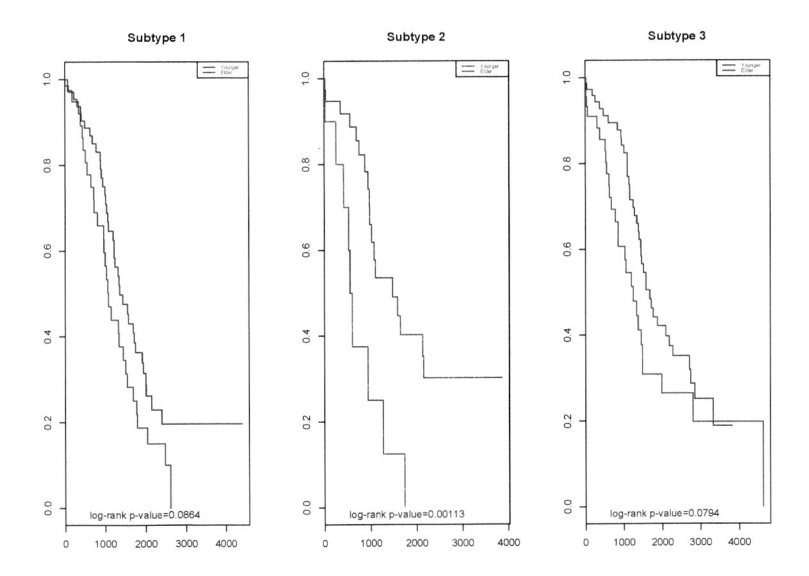

FIGURE 6.4: Test dataset predicted disparity subtypes (clusters 1, 2, 3) survival curves for the ovarian cancer TCGA dataset. Clear evidence of disparity subtype validation is evident.

logical age (the predicted values are termed epigenetic ages because they are based on the methylation markers). Interestingly, Horvath found that these predictions were quite accurate and seemed to be tissue-independent. Software to generate such predictions is readily available at dnamage.genetics.ucla.edu.

Figure 6.7 shows our findings of this analysis. Each plot corresponds to a particular disparity subtype. The x-axis is predicted epigenetic age, the y-axis is chronological age-at-diagnosis. The line of identity is included in all plots. Blue circles are the younger women and red triangles are the older women. Additionally, horizontal dashed lines in blue and red represent median chronological age values for each age group within a subtype, and vertical dashed lines the median predicted epigenetic age value for each age group within a subtype.

An immediate observation is that in this set of data, epigenetic age is in fact significantly underestimating chronological age systematically. Interestingly, this phenomenon was also noticed by [91]. But other more interesting conclusions emerge. The difference in chronological age medians is about constant across subtypes. *However*, the difference in predicted epigenetic age medians grows with growing survival disparity across the subtypes with subtype 1 showing no difference in predicted epigenetic age and subtype 2 showing the largest difference. This is both extremely interesting and reassuring because the LSE has simply not identified the largest survival disparity subtype as

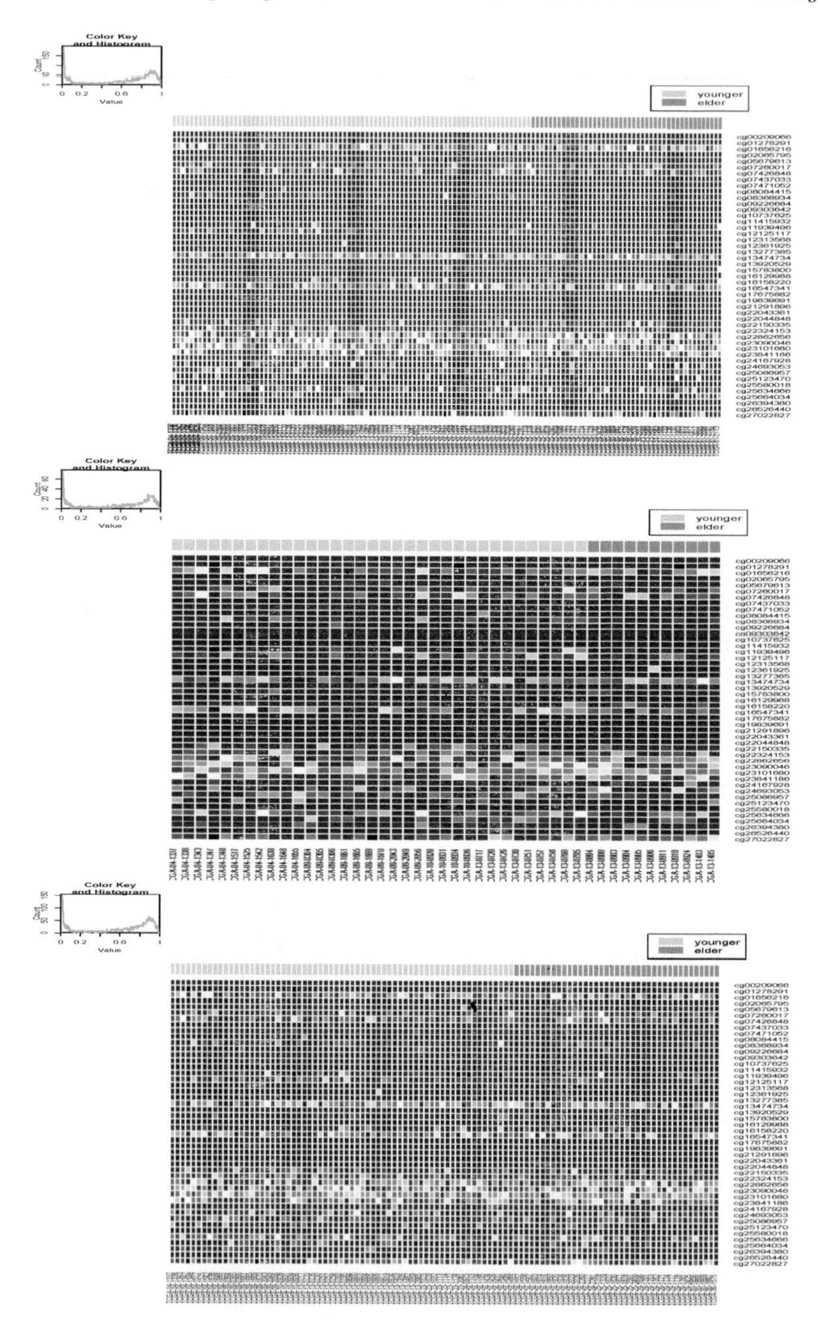

FIGURE 6.5: Heat map of defining methylation markers of level set disparity subtypes. Shown are (from the top then down), subtype 1, subtype 2 and subtype 3. Columns represent the TCGA ovarian cancer samples and rows the particular methylation markers.

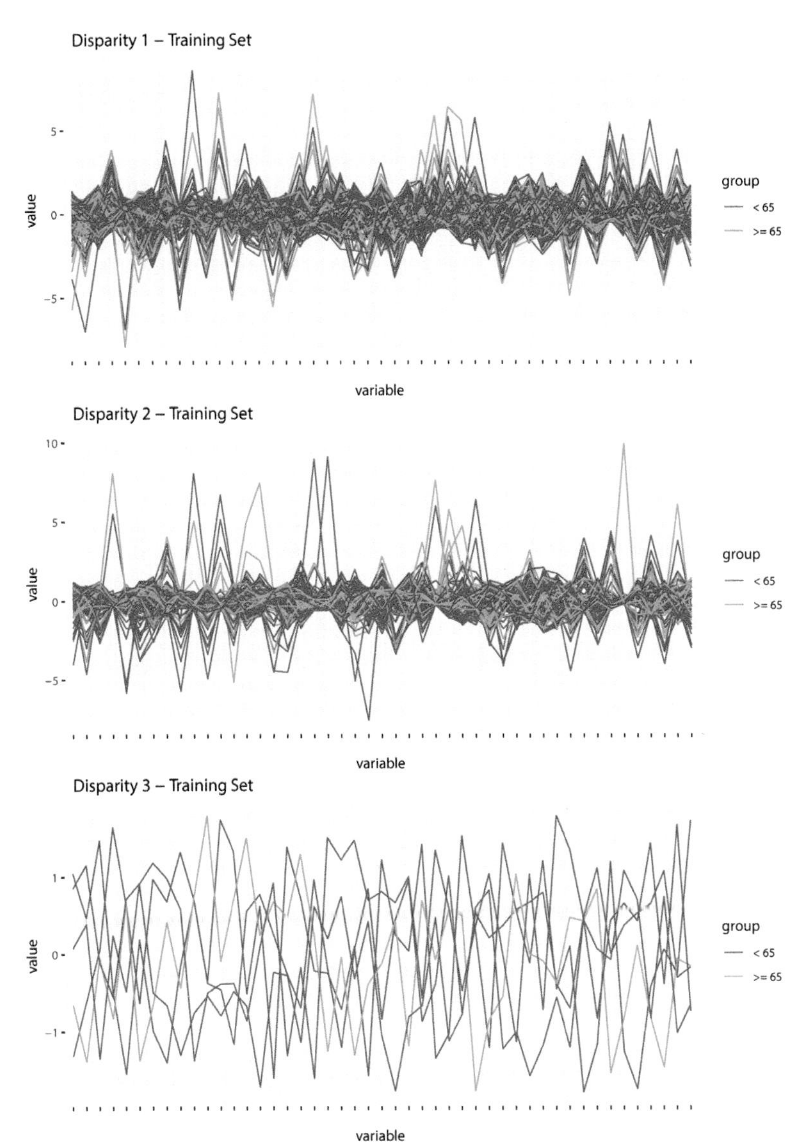

FIGURE 6.6: Training set Parallel Coordinate Plots of methylation profiles for the "inbox" observations in age group $' \leq 65'$ vs. $' > 65'$, for the real ovarian cancer dataset. Top: First estimated disparity; Middle: Second estimated disparity; Bottom: Third (leftover) disparity. Each curve represents a methylation profile of one patient, that is, the methylation value (y-axis) for each covariate gene (x-axis) and each patient. The red and cyan curves represent the observations in age group $' \leq 65'$ and $' > 65'$, respectively. The methylation signal is univariately standardized.

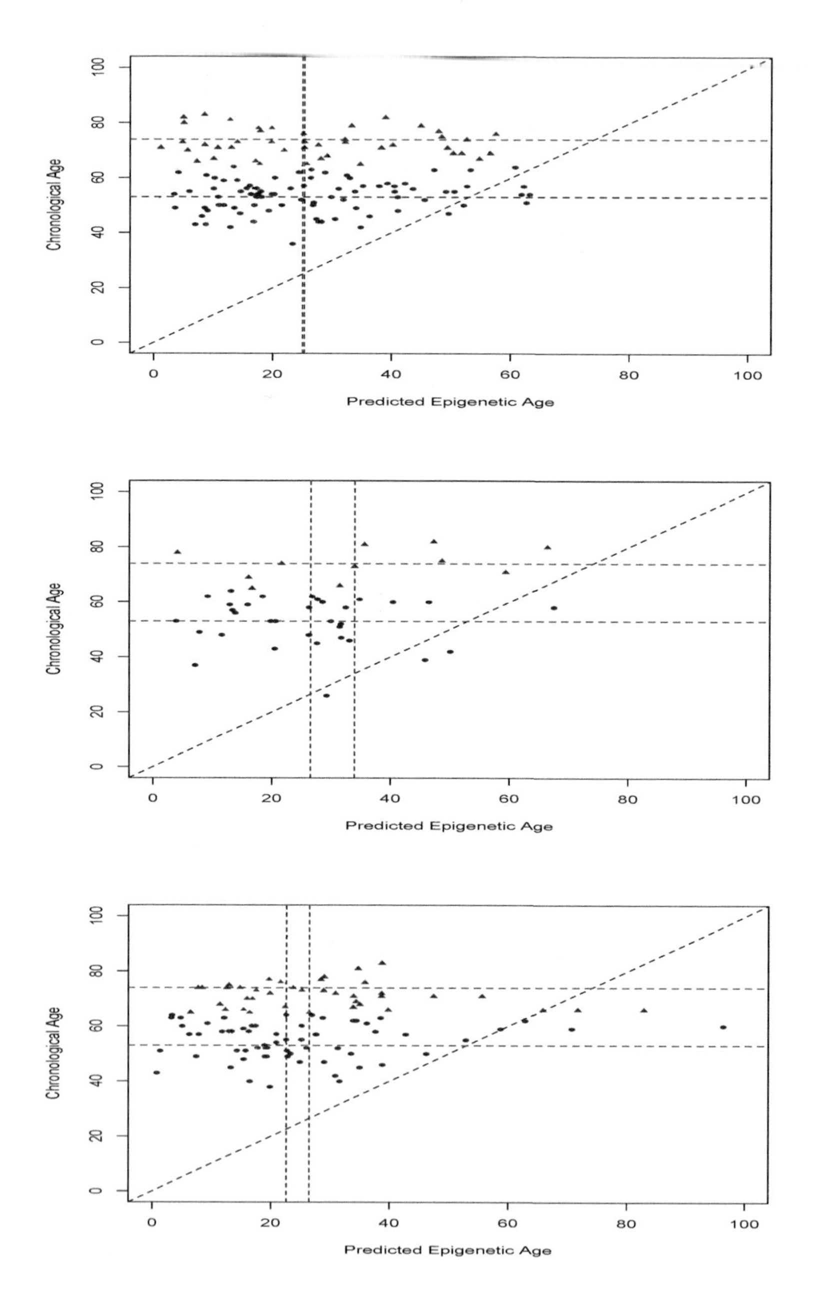

FIGURE 6.7: Epigenetic age (x-axis) versus chronological age (y-axis) for disparity subtype 1, 2 and 3 (from top to bottom). Blue circles represent younger age women, and red triangles are older age women. Also plotted are the median chronological ages by age group (horizontal lines) and median epigenetic ages by age group (vertical lines).

consisting of the chronologically oldest and youngest women because subtypes are discovered via the moderation of the age-group effect by the methylation markers. So the disparity subtypes are in fact picking up epigenetic structure that at least in part can be explained through predicted epigenetic ages.

Example 6.2 HPRISM and PRISM modeling to identify racial differences in endometrial cancer survival as a function of clinical covariates and social determinants of health:

Rao *et al.* (2022)[305] utilized a cohort of data from the Florida Cancer Data System (FCDS) consisting of female Non-Hispanic White (NHW) and Non-Hispanic Black (NHB) endometrial cancer cases in FCDS from 2005 to 2014. The primary outcome of interest was overall survival measured in days from the date of diagnosis. They included the following individual-level characteristics in these analyses based on data in the FCDS: (a)race; (b)marital status; (c)insurance type; (d)age at diagnosis; (e)histologic type; (f)grade; (g)stage; and (h)course of treatment.

Race was operationalized as an indicator variable corresponding to identifying as non-Hispanic Black (NHB) or not (binary). Other covariates included marital status, insurance type, age at diagnosis, histological type, tumor grade, and treatment (radiation, chemotherapy, and surgery). Explicit details of how these variables were defined can be found in [305].

Patients were geo-coded (see Chapter 7) to their census tracts which enabled the characterization of neighborhoods by key social determinants. Rao *et al.* (2022)[305] considered the following census-tract-level variables that were extracted from American Community Survey (ACS) based on their potential for mediating, moderating, driving, and/or confounding racial disparities in cancer: (a) median household income, (b) GINI coefficient (a measure of income inequality), (c) percent of individuals living below the poverty line, (d) percent of individuals 16+ in the civilian labor force who are unemployed, (e) percent of adults 25+ with less than a high school education, (f) percent of housing units with more than 1 resident per room, (g) percent of housing units with no access to a vehicle, and (h) percent of housing units that are renter-occupied.

PRISM and HPRISM models were fit to the data and were evaluated for their predictive performance. The FCDS cohort was stratified by censoring status and then split by strata into an 80% training set and a 20% test set. Models were built on the training set and then test observations were fed down each tree based on their x and w values, and a predicted value of the log survival time was estimated from the terminal nodes that each test observation fell into. This process was repeated 100 times and the mean empirical test set Harrell's c statistic [132] and standard error (SE) was reported. Harrell's c statistic is a widely accepted measure of predictive performance based on validation data that may be subject to right censoring. The c statistics are routinely used in the medical literature to quantify the capacity of an estimated risk score in discriminating among subjects with different event times. It provides a global assessment of a fitted survival model rather than focusing on the prediction for a fixed time.

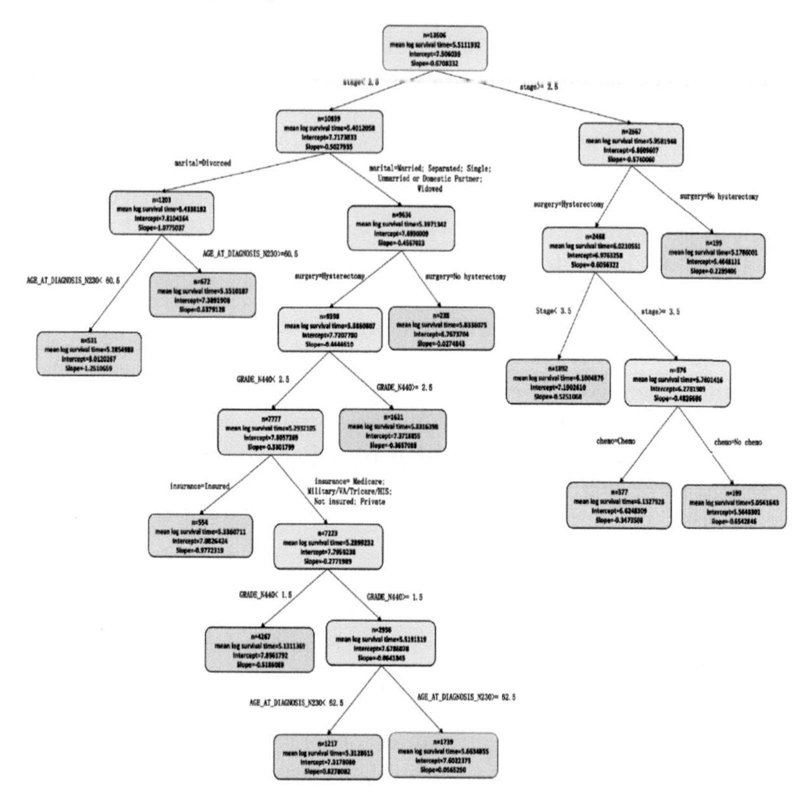

FIGURE 6.8: (Taken from Rao *et al.* (2022)[305]): PRISM tree. Inside each terminal node of the PRISM tree is printed sample size, mean log survival time, the intercept and slope effect for race.

Understanding how disparity is distributed and (hierarchically) moderated within a geographical area at the tract level is of great interest. Direct estimation at the tract level is not possible because all individuals in a tract share the same value of the social determinant. However, the HPRISM model allows such an estimate to be reverse-engineered. Notice that within each terminal node, we have estimated $\theta_l' = (\theta_{0l}, \theta_{1l}, \theta_{2l})$ locally and each terminal node consists of a mixture of observations from different census tracts (areas). Thus, for $x = 0$ if White and $x = 1$ if Black, the predicted mean log survival difference (i.e., disparity) for observations in a terminal node is $\hat{d}_l = (\hat{y}|x = 1) - (\hat{y}|x = 0) = (\hat{\theta}_{0l} + \hat{\theta}_{1l} + \hat{\theta}_{2l} * w_l) - \hat{\theta}_{0l}$.

To go back to the tract level itself, they gathered all of the observations from tract m from each terminal node and form the weighted average $\hat{d}_m = \sum_l \eta_{lm} d_{lm}$. The weights η_{lm} can be made flexible but typically correspond to the relative proportions of individuals from a given tract in a terminal node. We call this the *specific area-level disparity estimate or SPADE.*

Figures 6.8 and 6.9 show the PRISM and HPRISM median income fits, respectively (as depicted by tree-like topological graphs), to the FCDS cohort.

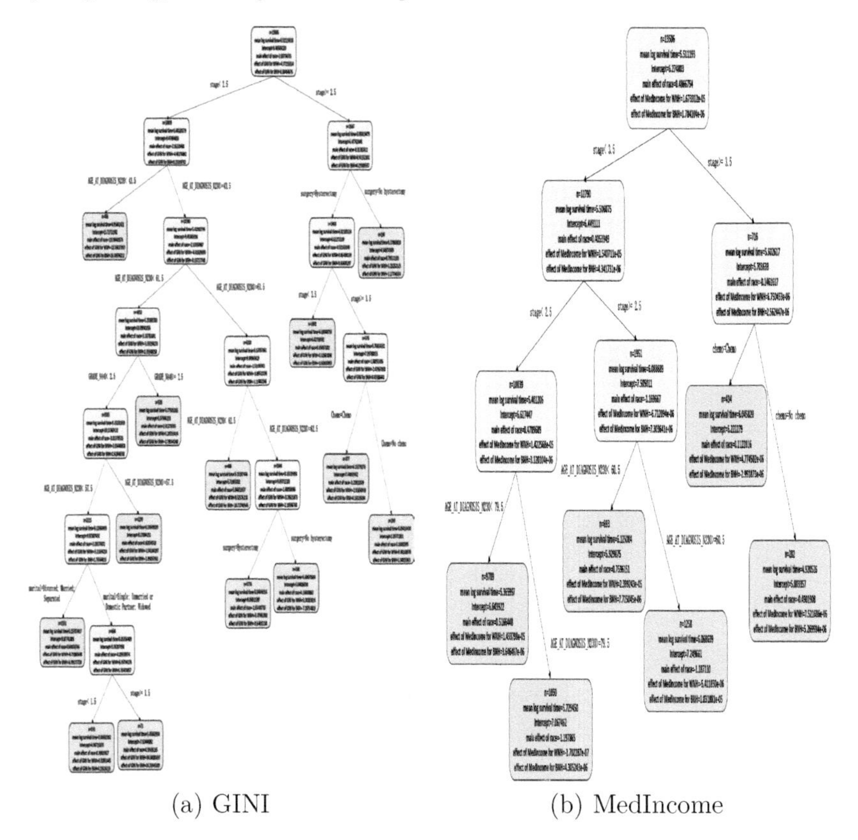

(a) GINI (b) MedIncome

FIGURE 6.9: (Taken from Rao *et al.* (2022)[305]): HPRISM tree for GINI and MedIncome. Inside each node, the HPRISM tree additionally adds the GINI or MedIncome slopes by racial group to each node.

Each node is split at a value of one of the individual level variables and observations are sent to the left or right resulting daughter nodes (colored blue) according to whether they affirmatively obey the split rule or not and this process is recursively repeated until the stopping rule is invoked, at which point an observation reaches a terminal node (colored pink). Within each node is printed the mean log survival time, the intercept, race effect, and additionally the interaction of race with tract median income (for the HPRISM tree). Each terminal node represents a discovered subgroup where the racial effect on survival is moderated significantly differently from the root node. In this analysis, we are treating each terminal node as its own level set.

Test set predictive accuracy was done via Harrell's c statistic. Table 6.1 shows Harrell c comparisons of the PRISM model versus the various HPRISM models along with accompanying standard error estimates. Increases in empirical test set Harrell c statistic were seen for all HPRISM models over the

TABLE 6.1: (Taken from Rao *et al.* (2022)[305]): Test set prediction performance of the various models

Model	Harrell C Statistic (SE)
PRISM	0.538 (0.012)
HPRISM with GINI	0.531 (0.018)
HPRISM with MedIncome	0.576 (0.021)
HPRISM with PercentCrowd	0.533 (0.016)
HPRISM with PercentNoVeh	0.544 (0.021)
HPRISM with PercentRent	0.552 (0.016)
HPRISM with PercentUnEmp	0.544 (0.019)

PRISM model. This provides unbiased validation of the fact that multilevel determinants at the individual and contextual level are indeed important in explaining racial disparity in endometrial cancer survival in the FCDS cohort.

Rao *et al.* (2022) [305] then dug deeper with an examination of the HPRISM tree topologies. Each branch path to a terminal node for an HPRISM tree explicitly details a discovered hierarchical interaction. Figure 6.10 shows another way to display such interactions. For illustration, plotted are the differences in log survival time between White non-Hispanic Black and Black non-Hispanics groups versus GINI and MedIncome, respectively. Each dotted line represents a different terminal node from the HPRISM tree. Conditioning on a particular value of the social determinant variable, we see that the data points on the line do not coincide. This indicates the first layer of interaction (i.e., the interaction of individual-level variables defining the terminal nodes with race). The fact the lines are not parallel across different values of GINI is indicative of the hierarchical interaction of race with the individual level variables that define the terminal nodes with the social determinant. It is interesting that for MedIncome, the lines are nearly parallel indicating a much weaker hierarchical moderation effect.

Figure 6.11 plots Andrews curves [11] for the PRISM and HPRISM GINI and MedIncome trees to visualize how different or similar the terminal nodes are with respect to racial disparity. Each line represents a unique observation and all observations of the same color are within the same terminal node. This is a technique to visualize multivariate distributions using connections to Fourier series. Notice how the PRISM tree is less able to find distinct subgroups than either of the HPRISM trees. In particular, the MedIncome HPRISM tree found wider differences across terminal nodes (i.e., different disparity subgroups) than the GINI tree did.

Figure 6.12 (right-hand plot) puts everything together in a composite heat map showing the combined effect of all social determinants using the approximation described above. As a comparison, we show the direct Kaplan-Meier estimate in the left-hand plot of Figure 6. For the direct estimate, there are many tracts where the Kaplan-Meier curves do not drop to 50% survival and so a difference between median survivals between racial groups could not be estimated.

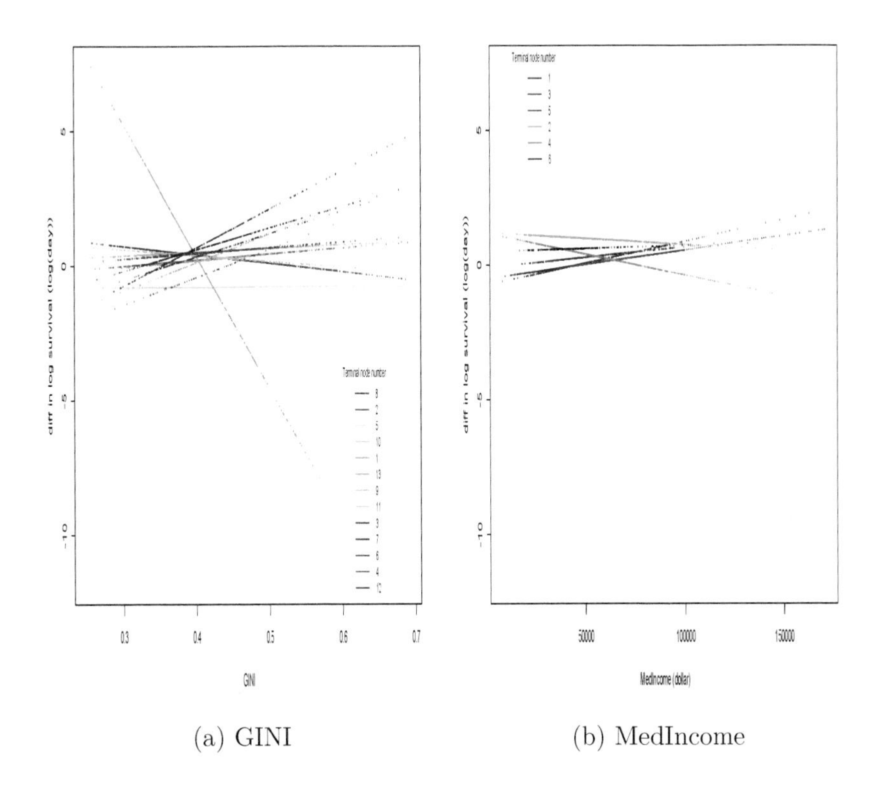

(a) GINI (b) MedIncome

FIGURE 6.10: (Taken from Rao *et al.* (2022)[305]): HPRISM hierarchical moderation plots for GINI and MedIncome. Each color represents a different terminal node (defined by the individual level variables) in the HPRISM tree. The y-axis plots mean the difference in log survival between Whites and Blacks at given values of the social determinant. Hierarchical moderation is visible as follows: at the level of individual variables because the y-axis values do not overlap at fixed x-values; at the level of the social determinant, when the lines are not parallel. Notice though for MedIncome, the lines are nearly parallel.

6.3 Classified mixed model prediction

We now turn our attention to the problem of prediction associated with data with a subgrouping structure. Our focus will be on improving predictions within a mixed model context. The idea here is that such predictions can be made for new observations whether yet seen or not. In particular, we will discuss a method that makes effective use of the random effect structure in the

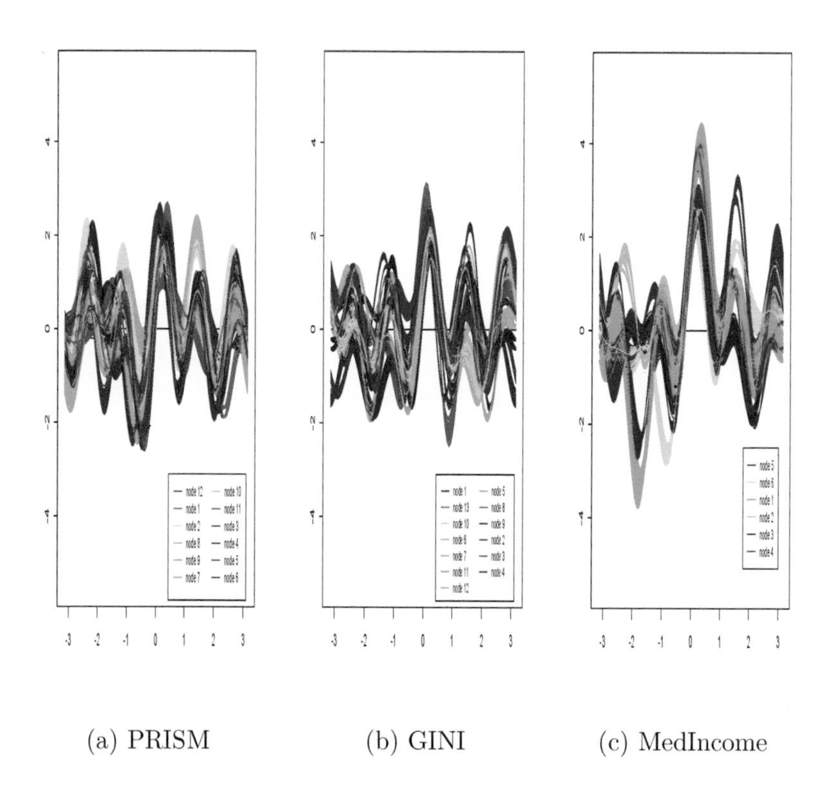

(a) PRISM (b) GINI (c) MedIncome

FIGURE 6.11: (Taken from Rao *et al.* (2022)[305]): Andrews curves for PRISM and HPRISM models for GINI and MedIncome, respectively.

mixed model thereby keeping the predictions focused at the subject level. As noted in [173] (sec. 2.3), there are two types of prediction problems associated with the mixed effects models. The first type, which is encountered more often in practice, is the prediction of mixed effects; the second type is the prediction of new responses.

For the first problem, we will start out assuming that there is a match between the group to which the new subject belongs and a group within the training data set, and then relax this assumption. We will then focus our attention on the second problem of predicting new responses. A more detailed description of the ideas can be found in [178].

6.3.1 Prediction of mixed effects associated with new observations

Suppose that we have a set of grouped training data, $y_{ij}, i = 1, \ldots, m, j = 1, \ldots, n_i$ in the sense that their *classifications* are known, that is, one knows which group, i, that y_{ij} belongs to. The structured linear mixed model (LMM)

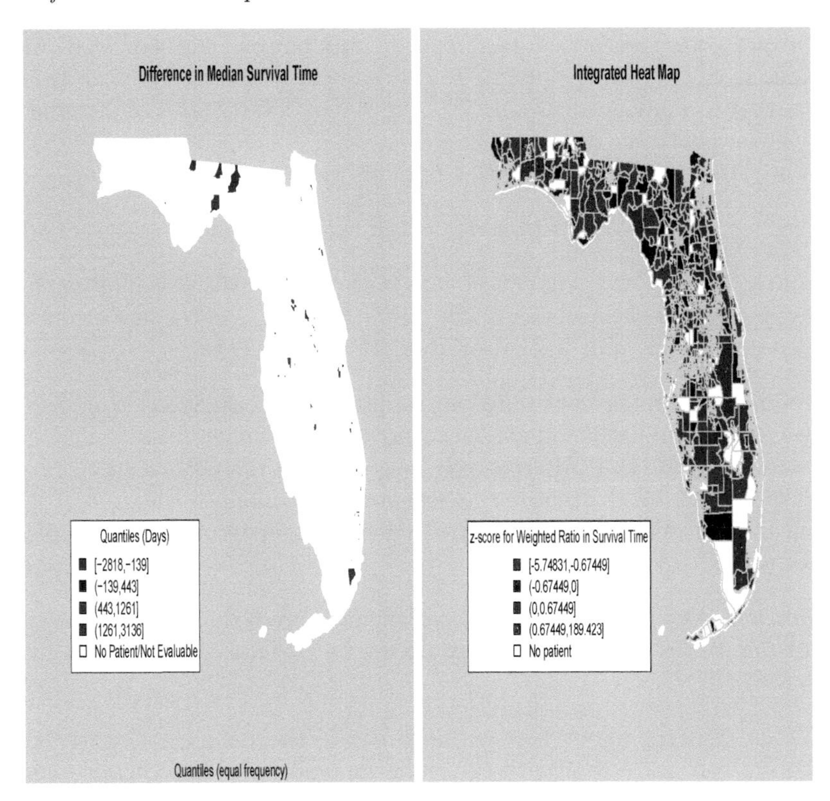

FIGURE 6.12: (Taken from Rao *et al.* (2022)[305]): Direct estimate of tract-specific median differences in survival (left). Integrated composite SPADE heat map (right).

assumed for the training data is

$$y_i = X_i\beta + Z_i\alpha_i + \epsilon_i, \tag{6.4}$$

where $y_i = (y_{ij})_{1\le j\le n_i}$, $X_i = (x'_{ij})_{1\le j\le n_i}$ is a matrix of known covariates, β is a vector of unknown regression coefficients (the fixed effects), Z_i is a known $n_i \times q$ matrix, α_i is a $q \times 1$ vector of group-specific random effects, and ϵ_i is an $n_i \times 1$ vector of errors. It is assumed that the α_i's and ϵ_i's are independent, with $\alpha_i \sim N(0, G)$ and $\epsilon_i \sim N(0, R_i)$, where the covariance matrices G and R_i depend on a vector ψ of variance components.

The first type of prediction problem of interest is to make a classified prediction for a mixed effect associated with a set of new observations, $y_{\mathrm{n},j}$, $1 \le j \le n_{\mathrm{new}}$ (the subscript n refers to "new"). Suppose that

$$y_{\mathrm{n},j} = x'_{\mathrm{n}}\beta + z'_{\mathrm{n}}\alpha_{\mathrm{I}} + \epsilon_{\mathrm{n},j}, \quad 1 \le j \le n_{\mathrm{new}}, \tag{6.5}$$

where $x_{\rm n}, z_{\rm n}$ are known vectors, $I \in \{1, \ldots, m\}$ but one does not know which element i, $1 \leq i \leq m$, is equal to I. Furthermore, $\epsilon_{{\rm n},j}, 1 \leq j \leq n_{\rm new}$ are new errors that are independent with $\mathrm{E}(\epsilon_{{\rm n},j}) = 0$ and $\mathrm{var}(\epsilon_{{\rm n},j}) = R_{\rm new}$, and are independent with the α_is and ϵ_is.

The mixed effect that we wish to predict is

$$\theta = \mathrm{E}(y_{{\rm n},j}|\alpha_I) = x_{\rm n}'\beta + z_{\rm n}'\alpha_{\rm I}. \tag{6.6}$$

Remark 2 Two important caveats are that the normality assumption is not always needed for the new errors and the variance $R_{\rm new}$ of the new errors does not have to be the same as the variance of ϵ_{ij} (see [178]).

From the training data, one can estimate the parameters, β and ψ using say maximum likelihood (ML) or restricted maximum likelihood (REML) estimators (e.g., [173]). Alternatively, one may use the OBP method (Jiang, Nguyen & Rao 2011) discussed in Chapter 3 to obtain estimators of β, ψ, which is more robust to model misspecifications in terms of the predictive performance.

Remark 3 As a point of comparison standard predictor would be based on *regression prediction* (RP) which would use only the fixed effects $x_{\rm n}$ and the estimate of β.

When thinking about how to make use of the random effect structure in 6.4, we can ask how accurately could we predict the new mixed effect if the new observations were classified to each of the training data groups, and then choose that group with the highest accuracy. To do so, suppose that $I = i$. Then, we know that the vectors $y_1, \ldots, y_{i-1}, (y_i', \theta)', y_{i+1}, \ldots, y_m$ are independent. Thus, we have $\mathrm{E}(\theta|y_1, \ldots, y_m) = \mathrm{E}(\theta|y_i)$. Using normal theory, we can write

$$\mathrm{E}(\theta|y_i) = x_{\rm n}'\beta + z_{\rm n}'GZ_i'(R_i + Z_iGZ_i')^{-1}(y_i - X_i\beta). \tag{6.7}$$

The right side of (6.7) is the BP under the assumed LMM, if the true parameters, β and ψ, are known. Because the latter is unknown, we replace them by $\hat{\beta}$ and $\hat{\psi}$, respectively. The result is what we call empirical best predictor (EBP), denoted by $\tilde{\theta}_{(i)}$.

In practice since I is unknown and treated as a parameter which we want to optimize. In order to identify an optimal I, we consider the mean squared prediction error (MSPE) of θ by the BP when I is classified as i, which we can write out as $\mathrm{MSPE}_i = \mathrm{E}\{\tilde{\theta}_{(i)} - \theta\}^2 = \mathrm{E}\{\tilde{\theta}_{(i)}^2\} - 2\mathrm{E}\{\tilde{\theta}_{(i)}\theta\} + \mathrm{E}(\theta^2)$. Using the expression $\theta = \bar{y}_{\rm n} - \bar{\epsilon}_{\rm n}$, where $\bar{y}_{\rm n} = n_{\rm new}^{-1}\sum_{j=1}^{n_{\rm new}} y_{{\rm n},j}$ and $\bar{\epsilon}_{\rm n}$ is defined similarly, we have $\mathrm{E}\{\tilde{\theta}_{(i)}\theta\} = \mathrm{E}\{\tilde{\theta}_{(i)}\bar{y}_{\rm n}\} - \mathrm{E}\{\tilde{\theta}_{(i)}\bar{\epsilon}_{\rm n}\} = \mathrm{E}\{\tilde{\theta}_{(i)}\bar{y}_{\rm n}\}$. Thus, we have the expression:

$$\mathrm{MSPE}_i = \mathrm{E}\{\tilde{\theta}_{(i)}^2 - 2\tilde{\theta}_{(i)}\bar{y}_{\rm n} + \theta^2\}. \tag{6.8}$$

Using similar ideas to the OBP in Chapter 3, the observed MSPE corresponding to (6.8) is the expression inside the expectation. Therefore, a natural idea is to identify I as the index i that minimizes the observed MSPE. Because θ^2 does not depend on i, the minimizer is given by

$$\hat{I} \quad = \quad \text{argmin}_i \left\{ \tilde{\theta}_{(i)}^2 - 2\tilde{\theta}_{(i)}\bar{y}_{\mathrm{n}} \right\}. \tag{6.9}$$

The classified mixed-effect predictor (CMEP) of θ is then given by $\hat{\theta} = \tilde{\theta}_{(\hat{I})}$. Jiang *et al.* (2018) [178]| were then able to prove the following consistency result about the CMEP.

Theorem 6.1 (Consistency of CMMP). *Suppose that A1–A5 in the Appendix hold. Then, we have* $\hat{\theta} - \theta \xrightarrow{\mathrm{P}} 0$, *that is, the CMEP is consistent.*

Remark. It should be noted that the result can be generalized to not require normality of the random effects and errors, either for the training data or for the new observations. In fact, the normal distribution can be replaced by any distribution that maintains the up-to-second-moment properties (i.e., mean zero and constant variance) of the normal distribution however, in such cases, the BP would become the best linear predictor instead (Jiang *et. al* 2018).

6.3.2 CMMP without matching assumption

Let us now drop the assumption regarding the new observations matching one of the training data groups. A direct extension of the CMMP is to continue to use (6.9) to identify I, regardless of whether there is an actual match.

Jiang *et al.* (2018)[178] described a modified procedure. According to the earlier results, if $I \in \{1, \dots, m\}$, we have (6.8), where $\theta_{(i)}$ is the BP with the unknown parameters, β and ψ, replaced by their, say, REML estimators based on the training data, denoted by $\hat{\beta}$ and $\hat{\psi}$. On the other hand, if $I \notin \{1, \dots, m\}$, (θ, e_{n}) is independent with the training data. Therefore, the BP of θ is given by

$$\mathrm{E}(\theta|y_1, \dots, y_m) = \mathrm{E}(\theta) = x_{\mathrm{n}}'\beta, \tag{6.10}$$

where β is the same β as appeared in (6.4). Once again, we replace the β by the same $\hat{\beta}$, and denote the corresponding EBP by $\tilde{\theta} = x_{\mathrm{n}}'\hat{\beta}$. By the same argument, it can be shown that

$$\mathrm{E}(\tilde{\theta} - \theta)^2 \quad = \quad \mathrm{E}(\tilde{\theta}^2 - 2\tilde{\theta}\bar{y}_{\mathrm{n}} + \theta^2). \tag{6.11}$$

Comparing (6.11) with (6.8), it is clear that the only difference is that $\tilde{\theta}_{(i)}$ is replaced by $\tilde{\theta}$. From this we can derive the following extension to the CMMP: Let $\hat{I}$ be given by (6.9). Compare $\tilde{\theta}_{(\hat{I})}^2 - 2\tilde{\theta}_{(\hat{I})}\bar{y}_{\mathrm{n}}$ with $\tilde{\theta}^2 - 2\tilde{\theta}\bar{y}_{\mathrm{n}}$. If the former is smaller, the CMEP of θ is $\tilde{\theta}_{(\hat{I})}$; otherwise, the CMEP of θ is $\tilde{\theta}$.

Jiang *et al.* (2018)[178] also proved consistency of the non-matched version of the CMMP as stated in the following theorem. They also showed that the CMMP has lower MSPE than the standard regression prediction (RP) estimator.

Theorem 6.2 *Under suitable regularity conditions as described in [178], and* $\text{var}(\alpha_{\text{new}}) > 0$. *Then, we have*

$$\text{E}\{(\hat{\theta}_{\text{n}} - \theta_{\text{n}})^2\} \to 0 \text{ and } \liminf \left\{\text{E}(\hat{\theta}_{\text{n,r}} - \theta_{\text{n}})^2\right\} \geq \delta$$

for some constant $\delta > 0$. *It follows that the CMEP,* $\hat{\theta}_{\text{n}}$, *is consistent and, asymptotically, has smaller MSPE than the RP,* $\hat{\theta}_{\text{n,r}}$.

To provide some more intuition about this result, we note that the way one identifies I is to find the index i whose corresponding EBP for the mixed effect, θ, is closest to the "observed" θ, which is $\bar{y}_{\text{n}}$. So, even if the class membership is estimated wrong, the corresponding EBP is still the closest to θ, in a certain sense, which is the most important consideration for our prediction problem.

Remark 4 Jiang *et al.* (2018)[178] highlighted the fact that consistency here is not about estimating the class membership, I. In fact, as m, the number of classes increases, the probability of identifying the true index I decreases, even in the matched case; thus, there is no consistency in terms of estimating I, even in the matched case. In the unmatched case, of course, there is also no consistency. More recent work by [227] using a pseudo-Bayesian procedure showed that they can indeed choose group membership consistently. The price paid however is additional complexity in specifying the model (in particular model priors) and in computational burden.

6.3.3 Prediction of responses of future observations

We now turn our attention to the problem of predicting the responses themselves for future observations which we will call y_{f}, that belongs to an unknown group that matches one of the existing groups. It should be noted that it is impossible, in general, to do better with CMMP, if one does not have any other observations that are known to be from the same group as y_{f}. For example, take a look at the simplest case when there is no covariates, that is, $X_i\beta = (\mu, \ldots, \mu)'$, $Z_i\alpha_i = (\alpha_i, \ldots, \alpha_i)'$ in (6.4), and $x_{\text{f}}'\beta = \mu, z_{\text{f}}'\alpha_I = \alpha_I$ in (6.5). In this case, one knows nothing about y_{f} and without additional information we do not know which group the new observation y_{f} belongs to. Therefore, to circumvent this issue one needs to assume that one has some *intermediate* observation(s) that are known to be from the same group (but this group is unknown) as y_{f}, in addition to the training data.

Let $y_{\text{n},j}, 1 \leq j \leq n_{\text{new}}$ be the additional intermediate observations. Suppose that y_{f} satisfies (6.5), that is, $y_{\text{f}} = x_{\text{f}}'\beta + z_{\text{f}}'\alpha_I + \epsilon_{\text{f}}$, where ϵ_{f} is the new error that is independent with the training data. It follows that

$$\text{E}(y_{\text{f}}|y_1, \ldots, y_m) = \text{E}(\theta|y_1, \ldots, y_m) + \text{E}(\epsilon_{\text{f}}|y_1, \ldots, y_m) = \text{E}(\theta|y_1, \ldots, y_m) \quad (6.12)$$

with $\theta = x_f'\beta + z_f'\alpha_I$. Equation (6.12) shows that the BP for y_f is the same as the BP for θ, which is the right side of (6.7), that is, $\theta_{(i)}$ with x_n, z_n replaced by x_f, z_f, respectively, when $I = i$. Suppose that the additional observations satisfy $y_{n,j} = x_{n,j}'\beta + z_{n,j}'\alpha_I + \epsilon_{n,j}, 1 \leq j \leq n_{new}$. If $x_{n,j}, z_{n,j}$ do not depend on j (which includes the special case of $n_{new} = 1$), we can treat $y_{n,j}, 1 \leq j \leq n_{new}$ the same way as the new observations before, and identify the classification number, $\hat{I}$, by (6.9). The CMMP of y_f is then given by the right side of (6.7) with $i = \hat{I}$, β, ψ replaced by $\hat{\beta}, \hat{\psi}$, and x_n, z_n replaced by x_f, z_f, respectively.

Remark 5 Following the same line of logic that we described earlier, we can also extend the above idea to prediction of a future observation without assuming a match group in the training data. For example consider the following simple modified procedure, where we data-adaptively determine if there is a match among the existing random effects by comparing the observed MSPEs between matched and unmatched predictions, as described earlier. If the data think that there is a match, the result is a CMMP predictor; otherwise, it is a regression predictor.

6.3.4 Some simulations

Jiang *et al.* (2018)[178] considered a situation where there may or may not be matches between the group of the new observation(s) and one of the groups in the training data. They then estimated empirical prediction errors for the two scenarios with some interesting results. The simulation used the following model:

$$y_{ij} = 1 + 2x_{1,ij} + 3x_{2,ij} + \alpha_i + \epsilon_{ij}, \tag{6.13}$$

$i = 1, \ldots, m$, $j = 1, \ldots, n$, with $n = 5$, $\alpha_i \sim N(0, C)$, $\epsilon_{ij} \sim N(0, 1)$, and α_i's, ϵ_{ij}'s are independent. The $x_{k,ij}, k = 1, 2$ were generated from the $N(0, 1)$ distribution, then fixed throughout the simulation. There are $K = 10$ new observations, generated under two scenarios. Scenario I: The new observations have the same α_i as the first K groups in the training data ($K \leq m$), but independent ϵ's; that is, they have "matches". Scenario II: The new observations have independent α's and ϵ's; that is, they are "unmatched".

Table 6.2 reports the average of the simulated MSPEs, obtained based on $T = 1000$ simulation runs. Two different numbers of training data groups were considered, namely $m = 10$ and $m = 50$. What is very interesting is that whether the new observations actually have matches or not, CMMP matches them anyway to a training data group. However, there is some sort of matching that is still present in the simulation design. There is at least a "match" in terms of the random effects distribution, that is, the new random effect is generated from the same distribution that has generated the training-data random effects.; therefore, it is not surprising that one can find one among the latter that is close to the new random effect. This provides some empirical evidence to the result derived in Theorem 6.2.

TABLE 6.2: (Taken from Jiang *et al.* (2018)[178]) : Average MSPE for Prediction of Mixed Effects for CMMP simulation study. %MATCH = % of times that the new observations were matched to some of the groups in the training data.

	Scenario	σ_α^2	0.1	1	2	3
$m = 10$	I	RP	0.157	1.002	1.940	2.878
	I	CMMP	0.206	0.653	0.774	0.836
	I	%MATCH	91.5	94.6	93.6	93.2
	II	RP	0.176	1.189	2.314	3.439
	II	CMMP	0.225	0.765	0.992	1.147
	II	%MATCH	91.2	94.1	92.6	92.5
$m = 50$	I	RP	0.112	1.013	2.014	3.016
	I	CMMP	0.193	0.799	0.897	0.930
	I	%MATCH	98.7	98.5	98.6	98.2
	II	RP	0.113	1.025	2.038	3.050
	II	CMMP	0.195	0.800	0.909	0.954
	II	%MATCH	98.8	98.7	98.4	98.4

Example 6.3 Predicting DNA methylation in cervical cancer from genetic data using shared classified random effects Epigenetics describes factors beyond the genetic code that are typically modifications to DNA which regulate whether genes turn on or off. These "marks" are attached to the DNA and do not change the actual sequence itself. Two common types of epigenetic modifications includes DNA methylation (DNAm) and histone modifications.

As illustrated in our previous example on ovarian cancer, there is growing interest in epigenetic markers not only for a better mechanistic understanding of cancer, but since these marks are potentially modifiable, this opens the door to new epigenetic therapies for cancer. Therefore understanding epigenetic profiles is potentially very useful. Additionally, African Americans have a higher incidence of many cancers and often worse survival but little is known about their differential methylation patterns since public repositories of genomic data are known to lack racial and ethnic diversity.

Also, while the amount of epigenetic data is increasing all the time, it's still not as ubiquitously found as other genomic profiles. So it would be very useful to predict methylation values using the mountains of cancer-related genetic data that does exist today in the form of genotyping data. Rao *et al.* (2021)[297] used CMMP methodology to help *capture the unmeasured* sources of variation in DNAm not captured by the genetic and clinical data alone. Additionally, they employed a clustering step of the DNAm profiles executed prior to fitting the mixed models producing clusters of observations with racial diversity that allowed for borrowing strength across races to improve race-specific predictions.

The data used by [297] can from the TCGA cervical and endocervical cancers (CESC) raw data which contained information on 305 patients. The data was comprised of 482421 methylation features (450K platform) and 22618 gene features with somatic copy number alterations (sCNA). The CESC methylation data and sCNA data along with clinical data which includes demographic and staging information were downloaded using TCGA2STAT R package [361].

Patients with race other than White or Black were excluded, which reduced sample size to 230, among which 23 (12.2%) were Black and 202 (87.8%) were White. Methylation based on raw Beta values were filtered to the top 0.01-percentile in terms of empirical variance, resulting in 38 features selected. Two further methylation variables were removed due to missingness resulting in 36 methylation responses used in the analyses. The sCNAs were filtered to only including the top 0.5-percentile in terms of variance, which resulted in 114 features selected. Due to the existence of high correlation among some of the genes which would cause model singularity, one gene in any pair with a correlation greater than 0.7 were removed. The final number of sCNAs included in the analyses was 61.

Clinical variables included in the analysis were *age*; *gender*; *race*; and *Stage*. The *Stage* variable was manually created as described in [297].

Clustering using the pam algorithm was performed using the 36 methylation values per individual in a training dataset which came from an 70% random split of the full training data the optimal cluster number was calculated based on elbow Gap statistic[294] using R package cluster. Three clusters were selected and the groupid variable, indicating cluster membership, was created. The distribution of individuals by race across clusters is shown in Figure 6.13.

Methylation values were transformed using either the M value transformation [82] or RAU transformation [328] as below. This was done to better satisfy normality model assumptions for the mixed model framework.

$$M_i = \log_2(\frac{Beta_i}{1 - Beta_i})$$

$$RAU_i = 2(146/\pi)\text{arcsin}(Beta_i^{0.5}) - 23$$

Rao *et al.* (2021)[297] compared a number of different methods (CMMP, regression prediction and elastic net) in terms of test set prediction accuracy based on empirical mean square prediction error (MSPE) averaging over 100 training/test splits. For the elastic net they also entertained the possibility of sCNA by race interactions. If any of these were found to be important, they would also be entered into the CMMP and linear models. Figure 6.14 shows the results in a violin plot for all 36 methylation responses with empirical standard deviations overlayed (horizontal lines). It is quite clear that CMMP only marginally improves over the linear model (lm) both overall and by racial

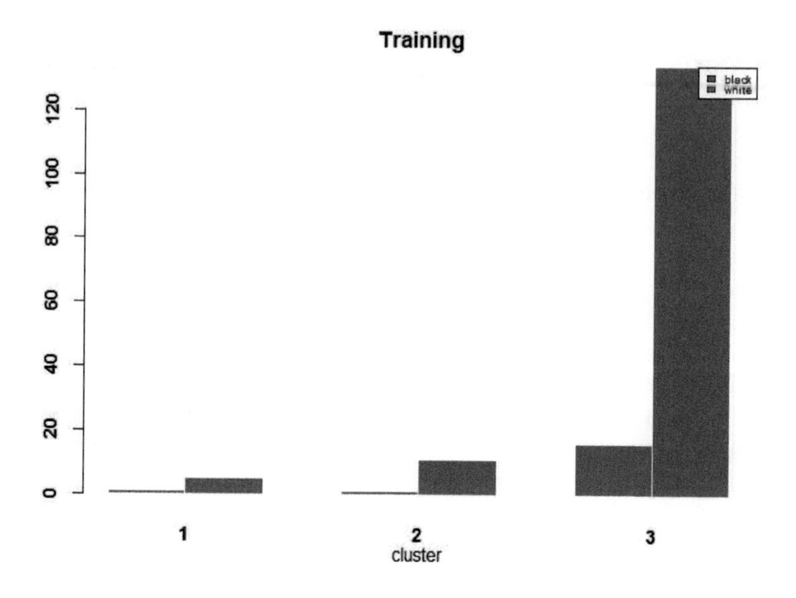

FIGURE 6.13: (Taken from Rao *et al.* (2021)[297]): Clustering of CESC samples for one training set.

group. The elastic net models provide significantly lower MSPE values compared to the other methods and that adding CMMP on top of elastic net does not further improve things.

Rao *et al.* (2021)[297] then further enhanced their mixed model by including additional cancers into the analysis and then including a fixed effect covariate for cancer type in the model. This allowed for potential borrowing strength across cancer types. To conduct the clustering, they used a hybrid goodness of fit measure.

The first measure is the Gini statistic calculation from [112]:

$$\text{Gini}_{\max} = \max_{i \in k} \sum_{j=1}^{C} \frac{n_{ij}}{n_i}\{1 - \frac{n_{ij}}{n_i}\},$$

where k is the number of clusters, C is the number of cancer types included, n_i is the total number of observations in cluster i, $n_i j$ is the number of observations in cancer type j in cluster i.

The second measure is the Gap statistic from [294]:

$$\text{Gap}(k) = \mathbb{E}_n^*\{log(W_k))\} - log(W_k).$$

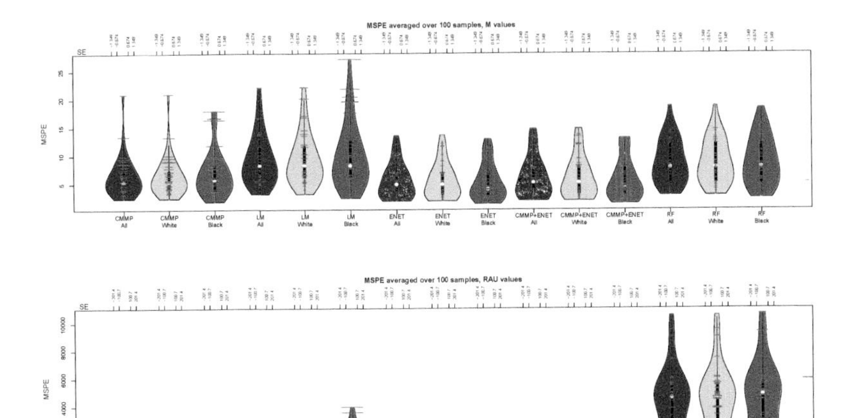

FIGURE 6.14: (Taken from Rao *et al.* (2021)[297]): Average empirical test set MSPE Violin plots with individual methylation response empirical standard deviation bars overlayed. Only CESC training samples used. Top plot is the M transformation and bottom plot is the RAU transformation.

The number of clusters k is then selected used the maxSE method in [294]:

$$k_{\text{optimal}} = \max k \in K \text{ s.t } \text{Gap}(k_{\max}) - \text{Gap}(k) < \text{Gap\_SE}(k_{\max})$$

where k is the number of clusters, K is the maximal number of clusters tested, $\mathbb{E}_n^*$ is the expected value taking a sample size of n, and W_k is the within-cluster sum of squares pooled between all clusters, Gap_SE(k) is the standard error of the bootstrap Gap values calculated, and $k_{\max}$ is the k value that gives the global maximal Gap statistic.

Combining the two measures together allows the identification of the optimal number of clusters with sufficient cancer type diversity:

$$\text{Gap+Gini} = \text{Gini}_{\max} + \text{Gap}(k_{\text{optimal}})$$

Figure 6.15 plots this convolution measure against different combinations of cancers from TCGA (each downloaded separately and then merged with other cancers). The plot indicates that combining CESC with lung adenocarcinoma (LUAD) results in an increase in the Gap+Gini. Adding additional cancers does not improve fit much more.

The TCGA Lung adenocarcinoma (LUAD) raw data contained 569 patients and removing all patients who were not Black or White further reduces the sample size to 401. Once all merging was complete, there were 631 patients available of which 230 had CESC (36.5%) and 401 had LUAD (63.5%)

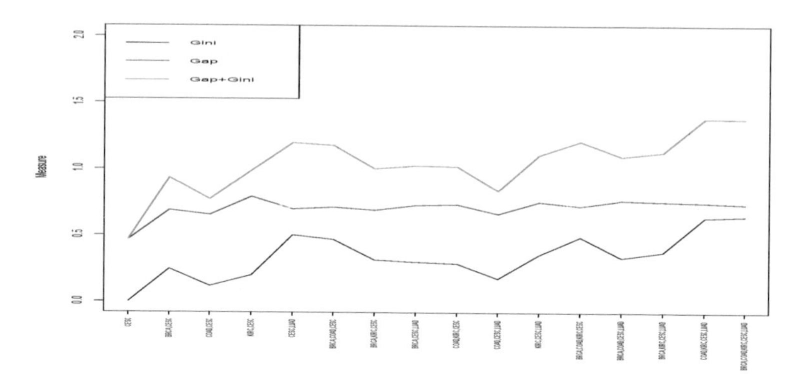

FIGURE 6.15: (Taken from Rao *et al.* (2021)[297]): Combining cancer types goodness of fit measure

and 78 were Black or African American (12.4%), and 553 were white (87.6%). Figure 6.16 summarizes the 5 clusters that were found (by the Gap statistic) and gives the racial composition of each. This is important since our goal is the borrowing of information between races; therefore, it is imperative that we have a mixture of representations of each race in our clusters.

Once again, the dataset was repeatedly randomly split (100 times) into training and test partitions of 70% and 30%, respectively. Covariates included were CSNAs and clinical variables with an additional variable indicating cancer type. The analysis procedure was similar to what was described earlier except that they also entertained the possibility of cancer type-by-stage interactions. Empirical mean MSPEs *for CESC samples only* reported together with their empirical standard deviations (SD) are graphically depicted in Figure 6.17 which shows MSPE performance across all methods by race and combined across racial groups. Now, MSPE values are systematically lower (by race and overall) for CMMP, and the distribution of values is much more skewed towards small values as compared to the other methods. Thus borrowing strength across cancer types has greatly improved CMMP performance.

To demonstrate the borrowing strength effect across races (within the same clusters) using CMMP, [297] plotted the classified random effects for test observations. One training-test split plot using the methylation response cg01315092 is shown in Figure 6.18. The y-axis plots the cluster-specific intercept (i.e., random effect) and the x-axis identifies a test patient ID. Red circles are Black individuals and black circles are White individuals. Fully 6 out of the 7 Black individuals in the test set were assigned a non-zero classified (group-specific) random effect shared also with White individuals in the same cluster. Only one test set Black individual was given a value of zero which indicates that because we used the no-match version of CMMP, this test observation was not classified to any of the training set clusters, and usual regression prediction was done.

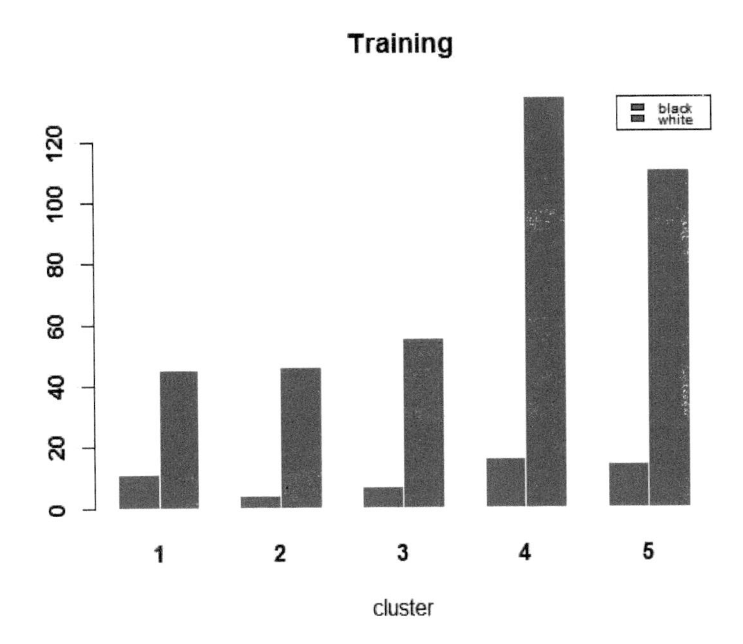

FIGURE 6.16: (Taken from Rao *et al.* (2021)[297]): Clustering for combined CESC and LUAD samples for one training set.

6.4 Assessing the uncertainty in classified mixed model predictions

An important issue is producing a measure of uncertainty of classified mixed model predictions. A measure of uncertainty in mixed model prediction (MMP), especially in terms of the mean squared prediction error (MSPE), has been well studied, in the context of small area estimation (SAE; e.g., [300]). However, CMMP is more complicated than MMP in that there is a matching procedure prior to the prediction. In a way, it retains some of the issues around post-model selection (PMS) inference. Jiang & Torabi (2020)[190] proposed a new method for MSPE estimation that applies to PMS prediction problems called "Sumca" which stands for "simple, unified, Monte-Carlo assisted" and [266] developed this for CMMP.

6.4.1 Overview of Sumca

Let θ denote a mixed effect of interest, and $\hat{\theta}$ a predictor of θ. Then, the MSPE is defined as $\text{MSPE}(\hat{\theta}) = \text{E}(\hat{\theta} - \theta)^2$. A standard method for

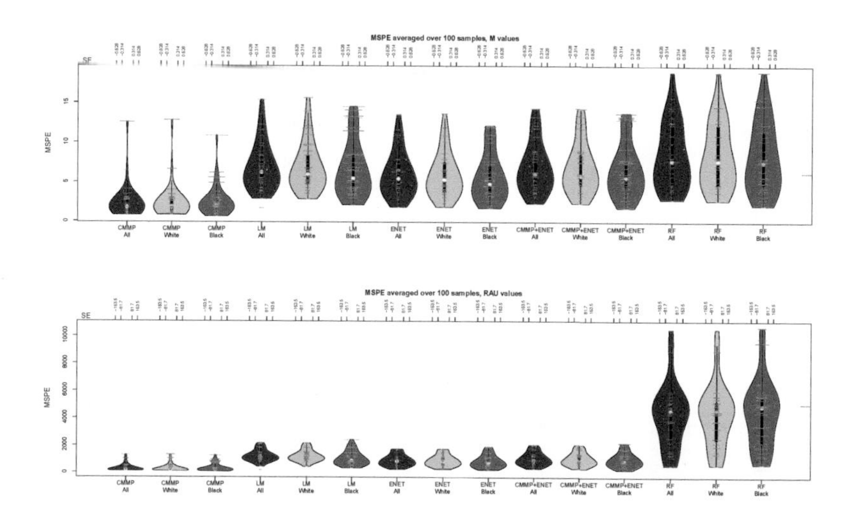

FIGURE 6.17: (Taken from Rao *et al.* (2021)[297]): Average empirical test set MSPE Violin plot with individual methylation response empirical standard deviation bars overlayed for M and RAU transformations.

obtaining a second-order unbiased MSPE estimator, in the sense that $E(\widehat{MSPE}) = MSPE + o(m^{-1})$, is the Prasad-Rao linearization method (PR; [287]), however, PR method requires differentiability in order to use the Taylor series expansion for approximation. In the case of CMMP, the procedure

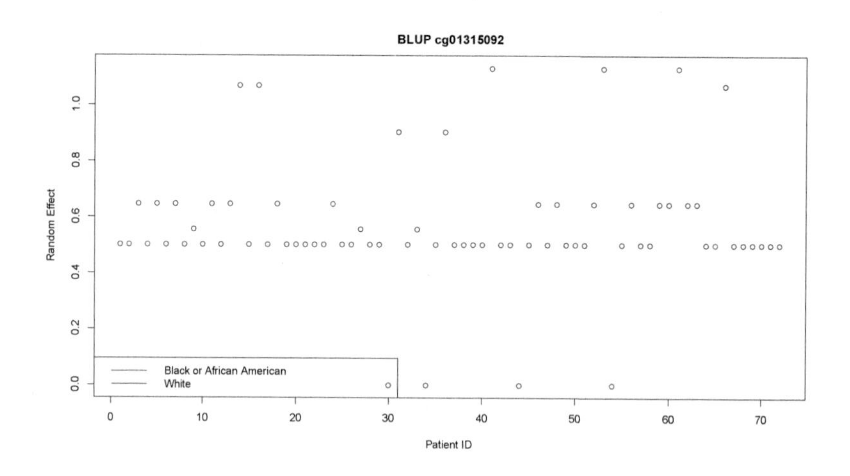

FIGURE 6.18: (Taken from Rao *et al.* (2021)[297]): Classified random effects for test data points for a particular split of full dataset

involves a non-differentiable process, that is, the selection of i over a discrete space, $i \in \{1, \dots, m\}$; as a result, the PR method may not apply.

The choice of the class index for the new observations may actually be viewed as a model selection problem so that the selected model connects the training data and new data in a specified way. We can write the MSPE of $\hat{\theta}_{\rm n}$ as

$$\text{MSPE} = \text{E}(\hat{\theta} - \theta)^2 = \text{E}\left[\text{E}\{(\hat{\theta} - \theta)^2 | Y\}\right], \tag{6.14}$$

where $Y = (y, y_{\rm n})$, y denotes the training data, and $y_{\rm n}$ the new observations. The conditional expectation inside the outer expectation on the right side of (6.14) is a function of Y and ψ, a vector of unknown parameters associated with the distribution of Y, that is,

$$\begin{aligned} a(Y, \psi) &= \text{E}\{(\hat{\theta} - \theta)^2 | Y\} \\ &= \hat{\theta}^2 - 2\hat{\theta}\text{E}(\theta | Y) + \text{E}(\theta^2 | Y) \\ &= \hat{\theta}^2 - 2\hat{\theta} a_1(Y, \psi) + a_2(Y, \psi), \end{aligned} \tag{6.15}$$

where $a_s(Y, \psi) = \text{E}(\theta^j | Y), s = 1, 2$. Note that $\hat{\theta}$ does not depend on ψ. If we replace the ψ in (6.15) by $\hat{\psi}$, a consistent estimator, the result is a first-order unbiased estimator, that is,

$$\text{E}\{a(Y, \hat{\psi}) - a(Y, \psi)\} = O(m^{-1}). \tag{6.16}$$

On the other hand, both MSPE $= \text{E}\{a(Y, \psi)\}$ [by (6.14), (6.15)] and $\text{E}\{a(Y, \hat{\psi})\}$ are functions of ψ. Let $b(\psi) = \text{E}\{a(Y, \psi)\}$, $c(\psi) = \text{E}\{a(Y, \hat{\psi})\}$, and $d(\psi) = b(\psi) - c(\psi)$. Then, (6.16) implies that $d(\psi) = O(m^{-1})$; thus, if we replace, again, ψ by $\hat{\psi}$ in $d(\psi)$, the difference is a lower-order term, that is $d(\hat{\psi}) - d(\psi) = o(m^{-1})$. Now consider the following estimator:

$$\widehat{\text{MSPE}} = a(Y, \hat{\psi}) + b(\hat{\psi}) - c(\hat{\psi}). \tag{6.17}$$

We have, by combining the above arguments, that $\text{E}(\widehat{\text{MSPE}}) = \text{E}\{a(Y, \psi)\} + \text{E}\{a(Y, \hat{\psi}) - a(Y, \psi)\} + \text{E}\{d(\hat{\psi})\} = \text{MSPE} + \text{E}\{d(\hat{\psi}) - d(\psi)\} = \text{MSPE} + o(m^{-1})$.

One can re-express $a(Y, \psi)$ in a different way:

$$a(Y, \psi) = \{\hat{\theta} - \text{E}_\psi(\theta | Y)\}^2 + \text{var}_\psi(\theta | Y). \tag{6.18}$$

Note that, in (6.17), $a(Y, \hat{\psi})$ is the leading term which is typically $O(1)$; the remaining term, $d(\hat{\psi}) = b(\hat{\psi}) - c(\hat{\psi})$ is typically $O(m^{-1})$. However, the remaining term is usually much more difficult to evaluate than the leading term. Jiang and Torabi (2020)[190] propose to evaluate this term via a Monte-Carlo method. Let P_ψ denote the distribution of Y with ψ being the true parameter vector. Given ψ, one can generate Y under P_ψ. Let $Y_{[b]}$ denote Y generated under the bth Monte-Carlo sample, $b = 1, \dots, B$. Then, we have

$$b(\psi) - c(\psi) \approx \frac{1}{B} \sum_{b=1}^{B} \left\{ a(Y_{[b]}, \psi) - a(Y_{[b]}, \hat{\psi}_{[b]}) \right\}, \tag{6.19}$$

where $\hat{\psi}_{[b]}$ denotes $\hat{\psi}$ based on $Y_{[b]}$. Jiang and Torabi argued that a reasonable choice for the Monte-Carlo sample size, B, is $B = m$. Thus, we can replace the term $b(\hat{\psi}) - c(\hat{\psi})$ in (6.17) by the right side of (6.19) with ψ replaced by $\hat{\psi}$, leading to the Sumca MSPE estimator:

$$\widehat{\text{MSPE}}_B = a(Y, \hat{\psi}) + \frac{1}{B}\sum_{b=1}^{B}\left\{a(Y_{[b]}, \hat{\psi}) - a(Y_{[b]}, \hat{\psi}_{[b]})\right\}, \quad (6.20)$$

where $Y_{[b]}, b = 1, \ldots, B$ are generated as described above (6.19), with $\psi = \hat{\psi}$, and $\hat{\psi}_{[b]}$ is the estimator of ψ based on $Y_{[b]}$.

6.4.2 Implementation of Sumca to CMMP

Following [178], [266] assumed that the training data satisfy the following nested-error regression (NER; [24]) model:

$$y_{ij} = x_{ij}'\beta + \alpha_i + \epsilon_{ij}, \quad (6.21)$$

$i = 1, \ldots, m$, $j = 1, \ldots, k_i$, where i represents the group index corresponding to the training data, k_i is the group size for group i; y_{ij} is the outcome of interest, x_{ij} is a vector of associated covariates, β is an unknown vector of regression coefficients (the fixed effects), α_i is a group-specific random effect, and ϵ_{ij} is an error. It is assumed that the random effects and errors are independent with $\alpha_i \sim N(0, G)$ and $\epsilon_{ij} \sim N(0, R)$, where $G > 0, R > 0$ are unknown variances. Furthermore, suppose that the outcomes of interest corresponding to a new subject, $y_{\text{n}j}, 1 \leq j \leq k_{\text{n}}$, satisfy

$$y_{\text{n}j} = x_{\text{n}j}'\beta + \alpha_I + \epsilon_{\text{n}j}, \quad (6.22)$$

$1 \leq j \leq k_{\text{n}}$, where $x_{\text{n}j}$ is the corresponding vector of covariates; I is an unknown group index that is thought to be one of the $1, \ldots, m$ corresponding to the training data groups, although, in reality, this may or may not be true; and $\epsilon_{\text{n}j}$s are the new errors that are independent and distributed as $N(0, R)$, and are independent with the α_is and ϵ_{ij}s.

To apply the Sumca method, note that, here, $\psi = (\beta', G, R, I)'$, where I is the true group index treated as another unknown parameter, and $\theta = x_{\text{n}}'\beta + \alpha_I$ is the mixed effect of interest that one wishes to predict. By the normal theory, it can be derived that

$$\text{E}_\psi(\theta|Y) = x_{\text{n}}'\beta + \frac{(k_I + k_{\text{n}})G}{R + (k_I + k_{\text{n}})G}(\bar{y}_{I\cup\text{n}\cdot} - \bar{x}_{I\cup\text{n}\cdot}'\beta), \quad (6.23)$$

$$\text{var}_\psi(\theta|Y) = \frac{GR}{R + (k_I + k_{\text{n}})G}, \quad (6.24)$$

where $\bar{y}_{I\cup\text{n}\cdot} = (k_I + k_{\text{n}})^{-1}(\sum_{j=1}^{k_I} y_{Ij} + \sum_{j=1}^{k_{\text{n}}} y_{\text{n}j})$ and $\bar{x}_{I\cup\text{n}\cdot}$ is defined similarly. Note the similarity, and difference, between (6.24) and the empirical best predictor (EBP) based on the training data (only), which is used in CMMP ([178]):

$$\hat{\theta}_{(i)} = x_{\rm n}'\hat{\beta} + \frac{k_i\hat{G}}{\hat{R} + k_i\hat{G}}(\bar{y}_{i\cdot} - \bar{x}_{i\cdot}'\beta), \tag{6.25}$$

where $\bar{y}_{i\cdot} = k_i^{-1}\sum_{j=1}^{k_i} y_{ij}$, $\bar{x}_{i\cdot} = k_i^{-1}\sum_{j=1}^{k_i} x_{ij}$, and $\hat{\beta}, \hat{G}, \hat{R}$ are also based on the training data. The Sumca estimator of the MSPE of $\hat{\theta}$ is then obtained by (6.20) with $a(Y, \psi)$ given by (6.18), (6.24), (6.25) and $\hat{\psi} = (\hat{\beta}', \hat{G}, \hat{R}, \hat{I})'$, where $\hat{\beta}, \hat{G}, \hat{R}$ are the (consistent) estimators mentioned, and $\hat{I}$ is obtained from CMMP by minimizing the distance between $\hat{\theta}_{(i)}$ and $\bar{y}_{\rm n} = k_{\rm n}^{-1}\sum_{j=1}^{k_{\rm n}} y_{{\rm n}j}$ ([178], p. 278). Specifically, we have

$$\begin{aligned} a(Y, \hat{\psi}) &= \{\hat{\theta} - {\rm E}_{\hat{\psi}}(\theta|Y)\}^2 + {\rm var}_{\hat{\psi}}(\theta|Y) \\ &= \left\{\frac{k_{\hat{I}}\hat{G}}{\hat{R} + k_{\hat{I}}\hat{G}}(\bar{y}_{\hat{I}\cdot} - \bar{x}_{\hat{I}\cdot}'\hat{\beta}) - \frac{(k_{\hat{I}} + k_{\rm n})\hat{G}}{\hat{R} + (k_{\hat{I}} + k_{\rm n})\hat{G}}(\bar{y}_{\hat{I}\cup{\rm n}\cdot} - \bar{x}_{\hat{I}\cup{\rm n}\cdot}'\hat{\beta})\right\}^2 \\ &\quad + \frac{\hat{G}\hat{R}}{\hat{R} + (k_{\hat{I}} + k_{\rm n})\hat{G}}; \end{aligned} \tag{6.26}$$

$$\begin{aligned} a(Y_{[b]}, \hat{\psi}) &= \{\hat{\theta}_{[b]} - {\rm E}_{\hat{\psi}}(\theta_{[b]}|Y_{[b]})\}^2 + {\rm var}_{\hat{\psi}}(\theta_{[b]}|Y_{[b]}) \\ &= \left\{x_{\rm n}'(\hat{\beta}_{[b]} - \hat{\beta}) + \frac{k_{\hat{I}_{[b]}}\hat{G}_{[b]}}{\hat{R}_{[b]} + k_{\hat{I}_{[b]}}\hat{G}_{[b]}}(y_{[b]\hat{I}_{[b]}\cdot} - x_{[b]\hat{I}_{[b]}\cdot}'\hat{\beta}_{[b]})\right. \\ &\quad \left. - \frac{(k_{\hat{I}} + k_{\rm n})\hat{G}}{\hat{R} + (k_{\hat{I}} + k_{\rm n})\hat{G}}(\bar{y}_{[b]\hat{I}\cup{\rm n}\cdot} - \bar{x}_{[b]I\cup{\rm n}\cdot}'\hat{\beta})\right\}^2 \\ &\quad + \frac{\hat{G}\hat{R}}{\hat{R} + (k_{\hat{I}} + k_{\rm n})\hat{G}}; \end{aligned} \tag{6.27}$$

$$\begin{aligned} a(Y_{[b]}, \hat{\psi}_{[b]}) &= \{\hat{\theta}_{[b]} - {\rm E}_{\hat{\psi}_{[b]}}(\theta_{[b]}|Y_{[b]})\}^2 + {\rm var}_{\hat{\psi}_{[b]}}(\theta_{[b]}|Y_{[b]}) \\ &= \left\{\frac{k_{\hat{I}_{[b]}}\hat{G}_{[b]}}{\hat{R}_{[b]} + k_{\hat{I}_{[b]}}\hat{G}_{[b]}}(\bar{y}_{[b]\hat{I}_{[b]}\cdot} - \bar{x}_{[b]\hat{I}_{[b]}\cdot}'\hat{\beta}_{[b]})\right. \\ &\quad \left. - \frac{(k_{\hat{I}_{[b]}} + k_{\rm n})\hat{G}_{[b]}}{\hat{R}_{[b]} + (k_{\hat{I}_{[b]}} + k_{\rm n})\hat{G}_{[b]}}(\bar{y}_{[b]\hat{I}_{[b]}\cup{\rm n}\cdot} - \bar{x}_{[b]\hat{I}_{[b]}\cup{\rm n}\cdot}'\hat{\beta}_{[b]})\right\}^2 \\ &\quad + \frac{\hat{G}_{[b]}\hat{R}_{[b]}}{\hat{R}_{[b]} + (k_{\hat{I}_{[b]}} + k_{\rm n})\hat{G}_{[b]}}. \end{aligned} \tag{6.28}$$

6.4.3 A simulation study of Sumca

Nguyen, Jiang and Rao (2022)[266] considered the same simulation setting in Jiang *et al.* (2018) where the underlying model can be expressed as

$$y_{ij} \quad = \quad 1 + 2x_{ij,1} + 3x_{ij,2} + \alpha_i + \epsilon_{ij}, \tag{6.29}$$

$i = 1, \ldots, m$, $j = 1, \ldots, k$. The new observations satisfy (6.29) with $\theta_{\rm n} = 1 + 2x_{{\rm n},1} + 3x_{{\rm n},2} + \alpha_I$, where $\alpha_i, \epsilon_{ij}, \alpha_I, \epsilon_{{\rm n},j}$ are the same as in the previous subsection, with G varies among $0.25, 1.0, 2.0$ and R fixed at 1.0. Three combinations of sample sizes are considered: $m = 50, k = 5$; $m = 50, k = 25$, and $m = 100, k = 25$; $k_{\rm n} = 10$ in all cases. Both the matched and unmatched scenarios were considered.

In addition to the Sumca estimator, they considered three alternative methods of MSPE estimation. The first is a brute-force (parametric) bootstrap (Boots) where one treats β, G, R and I, the unknown group index for the new observations, as unknown parameters. Then, from CMMP, one obtains estimates of β, G, R (e.g., REML), say, $\hat{\beta}, \hat{G}, \hat{R}$, respectively, and $\hat{I}$, the matched group index. One then treats $\hat{\beta}, \hat{G}, \hat{R}, \hat{I}$ as the true parameters to regenerate both the training data and the new data. The number of bootstrap replicates, B, is chosen as the same as the B for Sumca, which is 100. The second alternative is to simply use the leading term in (6.18) or (6.20), that is, $a(Y, \hat{\psi})$. This is called the naive estimator (Naive). The third alternative is the PR estimator at matched index (Prami). Note that, given the group index i, the PR MSPE estimator, with REML estimator of the variance components, can be computed as

$$\widehat{\rm MSPE}_{{\rm PR},i} \quad = \quad g_{1i}(\hat{\sigma}^2) + g_{2i}(\hat{\sigma}^2) + 2g_{3i}(\hat{\sigma}^2), \tag{6.30}$$

where $\hat{\sigma}^2 = (\hat{G}, \hat{R})'$ is the REML estimator of $\sigma^2 = (G, R)'$. Datta & Lahiri (2000) gave more specific expressions of the terms on the right side of (6.30). The Prami estimator is given by (19) with $i = \hat{I}$, the matched index by CMMP.

A total of $L = 500$ simulation runs were performed that compared the four methodsin terms of percent relative bias (%RB). The results are presented in Table 2. It is seen that both Sumca and Boots significantly outperform Naive and Prami in terms of %RB. There also seems to be no obvious patterns between different scenarios, matched or unmatched. The %RBs of Naive are consistently negative, while those of Prami are consistently positive when k is smaller, and consistently negative when k is larger. The picture is less clear, however, regarding the comparison between Sumca and Boots. It appears that Sumca performs slightly better than Boots in terms of the number of double-digit %RB cases (3 vs 5) and in terms of the maximum absolute value of %RB (14.72 vs 18.60).

Remark 6 Sumca is known to be second-order unbiased ([190]), while bootstrap without double-bootstrap bias correction is typically first-order unbiased

TABLE 6.3: (Taken from Nguyen, Jiang and Rao (2022)[266]): Simulated %RB of Sumca, Boots, Naive and Prami Estimators: M–Matched; UM–Unmatched

			Matched				Unmatched			
m	k	G	Sumca	Boots	Naive	Prami	Sumca	Boots	Naive	Prami
50	5	0.25	1.53	6.51	−34.98	37.22	−2.88	−10.89	−37.48	30.44
50	5	1.0	−5.23	−1.94	−36.30	69.19	−9.80	−9.74	−37.73	47.53
50	5	2.0	−10.20	−4.11	−40.03	57.70	−1.68	−18.60	−30.08	62.45
50	25	0.25	−0.80	0.75	−71.00	−58.67	−1.06	−1.66	−70.97	−60.88
50	25	1.0	6.98	0.83	−69.19	−57.58	−3.24	−2.58	−72.13	−58.84
50	25	2.0	5.39	1.16	−69.95	−56.68	−14.72	−9.57	−74.65	−67.01
100	25	0.25	−3.22	−13.83	−72.96	−63.69	−0.45	−1.67	−72.15	−62.68
100	25	1.0	−9.04	−11.74	−74.34	−62.80	−11.55	−5.70	−74.21	−65.52
100	25	2.0	4.05	−12.26	−70.52	−58.77	0.32	−7.80	−71.44	−59.56

(e.g., Hall & Maiti 2006; however, the double-bootstrap method is computationally too intensive). On the other hand, Boots has some advantages of its own. First, it is guaranteed positive; second, Boots is relatively simpler to program than Sumca.

6.5 Proofs

Proof of Theorem 6.1

Assumptions: Let $N = (m, n_i, 1 \le i \le m, n_{\text{new}})$ denote the vector of all of the sample sizes involved. Let Ψ denote the parameter space for ψ. The parameter space for β is assumed to be R^p, the p-dimensional Euclidean space. The norm of a matrix, A, is defined as $\|A\| = \sqrt{\lambda_{\max}(A'A)}$. Let $\theta_{(0i')}$ denote the right side of (4) with i replaced by i' and β, ψ being the true parameter vectors; when β, ψ are replaced by $\hat{\beta}, \hat{\psi}$, the corresponding notation is $\tilde{\theta}_{(i')}$, as in (6).

A1. Conditioning on $I = i$, model (1) holds with all the i replaced by i', and model (2) holds with I replaced by i.

A2. The true ψ is in the interior of Ψ.

A3. $x_{ijk}, 1 \le i \le m, 1 \le j \le n_i$ are bound, where x_{ijk} is the kth component of x_{ij}.

A4. $\|B_i X_i\|$, $g_{N,i}\|\partial B_i/\partial\psi_k\|$, $\|(\partial B_i/\partial\psi_k)X_i\|, 1 \le k \le q$ are bounded in a neighborhood $S = \{\psi : |\psi - \psi_0| \le \delta\}$, where ψ_0 is true ψ, δ is some positive number, and $g_{N,i}$ are positive constants such that $\max_{1 \le i \le m}(|y_i|/g_{N,i}) = O_{\text{P}}(1)$.

A5. $m \to \infty, \min_{1\le i\le m} n_i \to \infty, n_{\rm new} \to \infty$ so that $\hat{\beta} - \beta_0 = O_{\rm P}(a_N)$, $\hat{\psi} - \psi_0 = O_{\rm P}(b_N)$, $\max_{1\le i\le m} |\alpha_i| = O_{\rm P}(c_N)$, $\max_{1\le i\le m} \|B_i Z_i - I_q\| = O(d_N)$, $\max_{1\le i\le m} |B_i\epsilon_i|) = O_{\rm P}(f_N)$ when $\psi = \psi_0$, where a_N, b_N, etc. are sequences of positive constants such that $c_N(a_N + f_N) \to 0$ and $c_N^2(b_N + d_N) \to 0$, assuming $c_N \ge 1$ without loss of generality.

Consider the case $I = i$. Let $B_{0i'}$ denote $B_{i'}$ with $\beta = \beta_0$ and $\psi = \psi_0$. First note that we can write $\theta_{(0i')} = x_{\rm n}'\beta_0 + z_{\rm n}'B_{0i'}(y_{i'} - X_{i'}\beta_0) = x_{\rm n}'\beta_0 + z_{\rm n}'B_{0i'}(Z_{i'}\alpha_{i'} + \epsilon_{i'})$, and $\theta = x_{\rm n}'\beta_0 + z_{\rm n}'\alpha_i$. Thus, we have

$$\theta_{(0i')} - \theta = z_{\rm n}'(\alpha_{i'} - \alpha_i) + z_{\rm n}'(B_{0i'}Z_{i'} - I_q)\alpha_{i'} + z_{\rm n}'B_{0i'}\epsilon_{i'}. \quad (A.1)$$

On the other hand, by Taylor series expansion, we have

$$\tilde{\theta}_{(i')} - \theta_{(0i')} = \frac{\partial\tilde{\theta}_{(i)}}{\partial\beta'}(\hat{\beta} - \beta_0) + \frac{\partial\tilde{\theta}_{(i)}}{\partial\psi'}(\hat{\psi} - \psi_0), \quad (A.2)$$

where $\partial\tilde{\theta}_{(i)}/\partial\beta'$ denotes $\partial\theta_{(i)}/\partial\beta$ evaluated at a point $(\tilde{\beta}', \tilde{\psi}')'$ that lies between $(\beta_0', \psi_0')'$ and $(\hat{\beta}', \hat{\psi}')'$, etc. By (A.1), (A.2), and the fact that $y_{{\rm n},j} = \theta + \epsilon_{{\rm n},j}$, it can be shown that $\tilde{\theta}_{(i')} - y_{{\rm n},j} = z_{\rm n}'(\alpha_{i'} - \alpha_i) - \epsilon_{{\rm n},j} + \cdots$ with

$$|\cdots| \le O_{\rm P}(a_N) + O_{\rm P}\{(c_N + 1)b_N\} + O_{\rm P}(c_N d_N) + O_{\rm P}(f_N). \quad (A.3)$$

Note that the $O_{\rm P}$'s on the right side of (A.3) do not depend on i', or i, neither do they depend on the new observation $y_{{\rm n},j}$. It follows that

$$\tilde{\theta}_{(i')} - \bar{y}_{\rm n} = z_{\rm n}'(\alpha_{i'} - \alpha_I) - \bar{\epsilon}_{\rm n} + \cdots, \quad 1 \le i' \le m, \quad (A.4)$$

where the $\cdots$ satisfies (A.3) uniformly for $1 \le i' \le m$. On the other hand, it is easy to see that $\hat{I}$ minimizes $\{\tilde{\theta}_{(i')} - \bar{y}_{\rm n}\}^2$ over $1 \le i' \le m$. Thus, at least, we have

$$\{\tilde{\theta}_{(\hat{I})} - \bar{y}_{\rm n}\}^2 \le \{\tilde{\theta}_{(I)} - \bar{y}_{\rm n}\}^2. \quad (A.5)$$

Let $\xi_{\hat{I}}$ and ξ_I denote the $\cdots$ corresponding to $\hat{I}$ and I, respectively. Also denote the right side of (A.3) by s_N. Then, by (A.4), we have

$$\begin{aligned}\{\tilde{\theta}_{(\hat{I})} - \bar{y}_{\rm n}\}^2 &= \{z_{\rm n}'(\alpha_{\hat{I}} - \alpha_I) - \bar{\epsilon}_{\rm n} + \xi_{\hat{I}}\}^2 \\ &= \{z_{\rm n}'(\alpha_{\hat{I}} - \alpha_I) - \bar{\epsilon}_{\rm n}\}^2 + 2\{z_{\rm n}'(\alpha_{\hat{I}} - \alpha_I) - \bar{\epsilon}_{\rm n}\}\xi_{\hat{I}} + \xi_{\hat{I}}^2 \\ &\ge \{z_{\rm n}'(\alpha_{\hat{I}} - \alpha_I) - \bar{\epsilon}_{\rm n}\}^2 - O_{\rm P}(c_N)s_N - 2\xi_{\hat{I}}\bar{\epsilon}_{\rm n}. \quad (A.6)\end{aligned}$$

On the other hand, again by (A.4), we have

$$\begin{aligned}\{\tilde{\theta}_{(I)} - y_{\rm n}\}^2 &= \{-\bar{\epsilon}_{\rm n} + \xi_I\}^2 \\ &= \bar{\epsilon}_{\rm n}^2 - 2\bar{\epsilon}_{\rm n}\xi_I + \xi_I^2 \\ &\le \bar{\epsilon}_{\rm n}^2 - 2\xi_I\bar{\epsilon}_{\rm n} + s_N^2. \quad (A.7)\end{aligned}$$

Combining (A.5)–(A.7), we have $\{z_{\rm n}'(\alpha_{\hat{I}} - \alpha_I)\}^2 - 2\{z_{\rm n}'(\alpha_{\hat{I}} - \alpha_I) + \xi_{\hat{I}}\}\bar{\epsilon}_{\rm n} + \bar{\epsilon}_{\rm n}^2 - O_{\rm P}(c_N)s_N \le \bar{\epsilon}_{\rm n}^2 - 2\xi_I\bar{\epsilon}_{\rm n} + s_N^2$, leading to the inequality

$$\{z_{\rm n}'(\alpha_{\hat{I}} - \alpha_I)\}^2 \le 2\{z_{\rm n}'(\alpha_{\hat{I}} - \alpha_I) + \xi_{\hat{I}} - \xi_I\}\bar{\epsilon}_{\rm n} + O_{\rm P}(c_N)s_N + s_N^2. \quad (A.8)$$

Now observe that $\hat{\theta} - \theta = \tilde{\theta}_{(\hat{I})} - \bar{y}_{\rm n} + \bar{y}_{\rm n} - \theta = z_{\rm n}'(\alpha_{\hat{I}} - \alpha_I) - \bar{\epsilon}_{\rm n} + \xi_{\hat{I}} + \bar{\epsilon}_{\rm n} = z_{\rm n}'(\alpha_{\hat{I}} - \alpha_I) + \xi_{\hat{I}}$, using (A.4). Thus, combined with (A.8), we have

$$\begin{aligned} (\hat{\theta} - \theta)^2 &= \{z_{\rm n}(\alpha_{\hat{I}} - \alpha_I)\}^2 + 2\{z_{\rm n}(\alpha_{\hat{I}} - \alpha_I)\}\xi_{\hat{I}} + \xi_{\hat{I}}^2 \\ &\le 2\{z_{\rm n}'(\alpha_{\hat{I}} - \alpha_I) + \xi_{\hat{I}} - \xi_I\}\bar{\epsilon}_{\rm n} + O_{\rm P}(c_N)s_N + 2s_N^2. \qquad (A.9) \end{aligned}$$

To complete the proof, write $\hat{\eta} = \xi_{\hat{I}} - \bar{\epsilon}_{\rm n}$ and $\eta_1 = \xi_1 - \bar{\epsilon}_{\rm n}$, where ξ_1 is the $\cdots$ in (A.4) with $i' = 1$. Then, we have $|\hat{\eta}| \vee |\eta_1| \le s_N + |\epsilon_{\rm n}| = o_{\rm P}(1)$. On the set $\mathcal{A} = \{|z_{\rm n}'(\alpha_{\hat{I}} - \alpha_I)| \ge 1, |\hat{\eta}| \le 1/4\}$, we have, by (A.4), that, on the one hand, $\{\tilde{\theta}_{(\hat{I})} - \bar{y}_{\rm n}\}^2 = \{z_{\rm n}'(\alpha_{\hat{I}} - \alpha_I) + \hat{\eta}\}^2 \ge (1/2)\{z_{\rm n}'(\alpha_{\hat{I}} - \alpha_I)\}^2$, and, on the other hand, $\{\tilde{\theta}_{(1)} - \bar{y}_{\rm n}\}^2 = \{z_{\rm n}'(\alpha_1 - \alpha_I) + \eta_1\}^2 \le 2[\{z_{\rm n}'(\alpha_1 - \alpha_I)\}^2 + \eta_1^2]$. Note that, similar to (A.5), we have $\{\tilde{\theta}_{(\hat{I})} - \bar{y}_{\rm n}\}^2 \le \{\tilde{\theta}_{(1)} - \bar{y}_{\rm n}\}^2$. Thus, by combining the inequalities, we have, $|z_{\rm n}'(\alpha_{\hat{I}} - \alpha_I)| \le 2\sqrt{\{z_{\rm n}'(\alpha_1 - \alpha_I)\}^2 + \eta_1^2}$ if $|z_{\rm n}'(\alpha_{\hat{I}} - \alpha_I)| \ge 1$ and $|\hat{\eta}| \le 1/4$. It follows that $|z_{\rm n}'(\alpha_{\hat{I}} - \alpha_I)| \le 1 \vee [2\sqrt{\{z_{\rm n}'(\alpha_1 - \alpha_I)\}^2 + \eta_1^2}] = O_{\rm P}(1)$, if $|\hat{\eta}| \le 1/4$, hence $z_{\rm n}'(\alpha_{\hat{I}} - \alpha_I) = O_{\rm P}(1)$. Then, by (A.9), we have $(\hat{\theta} - \theta)^2 \le 2\{O_{\rm P}(1) + o_{\rm P}(1)\}o_{\rm P}(1) + O_{\rm P}(c_N)s_N + s_N^2 = o_{\rm P}(1)$.

Proof of Theorem 6.2

Let $\tilde{I} = \text{argmin}_{1 \le i \le m}(\alpha_i - \alpha_{\rm new})^2$. Note that $\theta_{\rm n} = \bar{y}_{\rm n} - \bar{\epsilon}_{\rm n}$. Thus, we have

$$\begin{aligned} {\rm E}(\hat{\theta}_{\rm n} - \theta_{\rm n})^2 &= {\rm E}(\hat{\theta}_{{\rm n},\hat{I}}^2 - 2\hat{\theta}_{{\rm n},\hat{I}}\theta_{\rm n} + \theta_{\rm n}^2) \\ &= {\rm E}(\hat{\theta}_{{\rm n},\hat{I}}^2 - 2\hat{\theta}_{{\rm n},\hat{I}}\bar{y}_{\rm n} + \theta_{\rm n}^2) - 2{\rm E}(\hat{\theta}_{{\rm n},\hat{I}}\bar{\epsilon}_{\rm n}) \\ &\le {\rm E}(\hat{\theta}_{{\rm n},\tilde{I}}^2 - 2\hat{\theta}_{{\rm n},\tilde{I}}\bar{y}_{\rm n} + \theta_{\rm n}^2) - 2{\rm E}(\hat{\theta}_{{\rm n},\hat{I}}\bar{\epsilon}_{\rm n}). \qquad (A.10) \end{aligned}$$

The last inequality is by the definition of $\hat{I}$. Note that $\bar{\epsilon}_{\rm n}$ is not independent with $\hat{I}$; otherwise, the last term would vanish. However, we have $|{\rm E}(\hat{\theta}_{{\rm n},\hat{I}}\bar{\epsilon}_{\rm n})| \le |{\rm E}\{(\hat{\theta}_{{\rm n},\hat{I}} - \bar{y}_{\rm n})\bar{\epsilon}_{\rm n}\}| + {\rm E}(\bar{\epsilon}_{\rm n}^2) \le \{{\rm E}(\hat{\theta}_{{\rm n},\hat{I}} - \bar{y}_{\rm n})^2\}^{1/2}\{{\rm E}(\bar{\epsilon}_{\rm n}^2)\}^{1/2} + {\rm E}(\bar{\epsilon}_{\rm n}^2) \le \{{\rm E}(\hat{\theta}_{{\rm n},\tilde{I}} - \bar{y}_{\rm n})^2\}^{1/2}\{{\rm E}(\bar{\epsilon}_{\rm n}^2)\}^{1/2} + {\rm E}(\bar{\epsilon}_{\rm n}^2)$. The last inequality is due to the fact that $\hat{\theta}_{{\rm n},i}^2 - 2\hat{\theta}_{{\rm n},i}\bar{y}_{\rm n} = (\hat{\theta}_{{\rm n},i} - \bar{y}_{\rm n})^2 - \bar{y}_{\rm n}^2$ for any i; therefore, $\hat{\theta}_{{\rm n},\hat{I}}$ mininizes $(\hat{\theta}_{{\rm n},i} - \bar{y}_{\rm n})^2$ over $1 \le i \le m$. Furthermore, we have ${\rm E}(\hat{\theta}_{{\rm n},\tilde{I}} - \bar{y}_{\rm n})^2 = {\rm E}(\hat{\theta}_{{\rm n},\tilde{I}} - \theta_{\rm n})^2 - 2{\rm E}\{(\hat{\theta}_{{\rm n},\tilde{I}} - \theta_{\rm n})\bar{\epsilon}_{\rm n}\} + {\rm E}(\bar{\epsilon}_{\rm n}^2) = {\rm E}(\hat{\theta}_{{\rm n},\tilde{I}} - \theta_{\rm n})^2 + {\rm E}(\bar{\epsilon}_{\rm n}^2)$ due to the fact that $\bar{\epsilon}_{\rm n}$ is independent with $\hat{\theta}_{{\rm n},i}, 1 \le i \le m, \tilde{I}, \theta_{\rm n}$, by *B1*, hence ${\rm E}\{(\hat{\theta}_{{\rm n},\tilde{I}} - \theta_{\rm n})\bar{\epsilon}_{\rm n}\} = {\rm E}(\hat{\theta}_{{\rm n},\tilde{I}} - \theta_{\rm n}){\rm E}(\bar{\epsilon}_{\rm n}) = 0$. It follows that $\{{\rm E}\{(\hat{\theta}_{{\rm n},\tilde{I}} - \bar{y}_{\rm n})^2\}^{1/2} \le \{{\rm E}(\hat{\theta}_{{\rm n},\tilde{I}} - \theta_{\rm n})^2\}^{1/2} + \{{\rm E}(\bar{\epsilon}_{\rm n}^2)\}^{1/2}$ by the inequality $\sqrt{a+b} \le \sqrt{a} + \sqrt{b}$ for $a, b > 0$. Thus, by combining the result, we obtain the inequality:

$$|{\rm E}(\hat{\theta}_{{\rm n},\hat{I}}\bar{\epsilon}_{\rm n})| \le \sqrt{{\rm E}(\hat{\theta}_{{\rm n},\tilde{I}} - \theta_{\rm n})^2{\rm E}(\bar{\epsilon}_{\rm n}^2)} + 2{\rm E}(\bar{\epsilon}_{\rm n}^2) \le \frac{1}{2}{\rm E}(\hat{\theta}_{{\rm n},\tilde{I}} - \theta_{\rm n})^2 + \frac{5}{2}{\rm E}(\bar{\epsilon}_{\rm n}^2). \qquad (A.11)$$

Thus, continuing from (A.10), we have

$$\begin{aligned}
\mathrm{E}(\hat{\theta}_{\mathrm{n}} - \theta_{\mathrm{n}})^2 &\leq \mathrm{E}(\hat{\theta}^2_{\mathrm{n},\tilde{I}} - 2\hat{\theta}_{\mathrm{n},\tilde{I}}\theta_{\mathrm{n}} + \theta^2_{\mathrm{n}}) - 2\mathrm{E}(\hat{\theta}_{\mathrm{n},\tilde{I}}\bar{\epsilon}_{\mathrm{n}}) \quad 2\mathrm{E}(\hat{\theta}_{\mathrm{n},\tilde{I}}\bar{\epsilon}_{\mathrm{n}}) \\
&= \mathrm{E}(\hat{\theta}_{\mathrm{n},\tilde{I}} - \theta_{\mathrm{n}})^2 - 2\mathrm{E}(\hat{\theta}_{\mathrm{n},\tilde{I}}\bar{\epsilon}_{\mathrm{n}}) \\
&\leq 2\mathrm{E}(\hat{\theta}_{\mathrm{n},\tilde{I}} - \theta_{\mathrm{n}})^2 + 5\mathrm{E}(\bar{\epsilon}^2_{\mathrm{n}}), \qquad (\mathrm{A.12})
\end{aligned}$$

again using the independence of $\bar{\epsilon}_{\mathrm{n}}$ and $\hat{\theta}_{\mathrm{n},\tilde{I}}$.

Next, it is easy to derive the following expression:

$$\hat{\theta}_{\mathrm{n},\tilde{I}} - \theta_{\mathrm{n}} = \left(x_{\mathrm{n}} - \frac{n_{\tilde{I}}\hat{G}}{\hat{R} + n_{\tilde{I}}\hat{G}}\bar{x}_{\tilde{I}\cdot}\right)'(\hat{\beta} - \beta) + \frac{n_{\tilde{I}}\hat{G}}{\hat{R} + n_{\tilde{I}}\hat{G}}(\alpha_{\tilde{I}} - \alpha_{\mathrm{new}} + \bar{\epsilon}_{\tilde{I}\cdot}) - \frac{\hat{R}\alpha_{\mathrm{new}}}{\hat{R} + n_{\tilde{I}}\hat{G}},$$

where $\bar{x}_{i\cdot} = n_i^{-1}\sum_{j=1}^{n_i} x_{ij}$ and $\bar{\epsilon}_{i\cdot}$ is defined similarly, $1 \leq i \leq m$. It follows that there is a constant $c > 0$ such that

$$\begin{aligned}
\mathrm{E}(\hat{\theta}_{\mathrm{n},\tilde{I}} - \theta_{\mathrm{n}})^2 &\leq c\left[\mathrm{E}(|\hat{\beta} - \beta|^2) + \mathrm{E}(\alpha_{\tilde{I}} - \alpha_{\mathrm{new}})^2 + \mathrm{E}(\bar{\epsilon}^2_{\tilde{I}\cdot}) + \left\{\frac{(\log m)^{2\nu}}{n_{\min}}\right\}^2 R_{\mathrm{new}}\right] \\
&= c\{\mathrm{E}(\alpha_{\tilde{I}} - \alpha_{\mathrm{new}})^2 + \mathrm{E}(\bar{\epsilon}^2_{\tilde{I}\cdot})\} + o(1), \qquad (\mathrm{A.13})
\end{aligned}$$

by *B2*–*B4*, where $R_{\mathrm{new}} = \mathrm{var}(\alpha_{\mathrm{new}})$. Also, we have $\mathrm{E}(\bar{\epsilon}^2_{\tilde{I}\cdot}) = \sum_{i=1}^m \mathrm{E}\{\bar{\epsilon}^2_{i\cdot}1_{(\tilde{I}=i)}\} = \sum_{i=1}^m \mathrm{E}(\bar{\epsilon}^2_{i\cdot})\mathrm{P}(\tilde{I} = i) = R\sum_{i=1}^m n_i^{-1}\mathrm{P}(\tilde{I} = i) \leq R/n_{\min} = o(1)$, using the fact that $\tilde{I}$ depends only on the α's, and *B1*, *B4*.

If case (b), then, by definition, we must have $\alpha_{\tilde{I}} = \alpha_{\mathrm{new}}$. Thus, by (A.13), we have $\mathrm{E}(\hat{\theta}_{\mathrm{n},\tilde{I}} - \theta_{\mathrm{n}})^2 = o(1)$, hence $\mathrm{E}(\hat{\theta}_{\mathrm{n}} - \theta_{\mathrm{n}})^2 = o(1)$ by (A.12), and *B4*. Now suppose that case (a) holds. We have, for any $x > 0$,

$$\mathrm{P}\left\{\min_{1\leq i\leq m}(\alpha_i - \alpha_{\mathrm{new}})^2 > x\right\} = \mathrm{E}\left[\mathrm{P}\left\{(\alpha_i - \alpha_{\mathrm{new}}))^2 > x, 1 \leq i \leq m \middle| \alpha_{\mathrm{new}}\right\}\right].$$

For any fixed $u \in R$, we have, by independence, and i.i.d. of $\alpha_i, 1 \leq i \leq m$,

$$\begin{aligned}
\mathrm{P}\left\{(\alpha_i - \alpha_{\mathrm{new}}))^2 > x, 1 \leq i \leq m \middle| \alpha_{\mathrm{new}} = u\right\} &= \mathrm{P}\{(\alpha_i - u)^2 > x, 1 \leq i \leq m\} \\
&= [\mathrm{P}\{(\alpha_1 - u)^2 > x\}]^m.
\end{aligned}$$

Furthermore, it is easy to show that

$$\mathrm{P}\{(\alpha_1 - u)^2 > x\} = 1 - \Phi\left(\frac{u + \sqrt{x}}{\sqrt{G}}\right) + \Phi\left(\frac{u - \sqrt{x}}{\sqrt{G}}\right),$$

where $\Phi(\cdot)$ is the cdf of $N(0, 1)$. Thus, we have

$$\begin{aligned}
\mathrm{E}\{(\alpha_{\tilde{I}} - \alpha_{\mathrm{new}})^2\} &= \mathrm{E}\left\{\min_{1\leq i\leq m}(\alpha_i - \alpha_{\mathrm{new}})^2\right\} \\
&= \int_0^\infty \mathrm{P}\left\{\min_{1\leq i\leq m}(\alpha_i - \alpha_{\mathrm{new}})^2 > x\right\}dx \\
&= \int_0^\infty \mathrm{E}\left[\left\{1 - \Phi\left(\frac{\alpha_{\mathrm{new}} + \sqrt{x}}{\sqrt{G}}\right) + \Phi\left(\frac{\alpha_{\mathrm{new}} - \sqrt{x}}{\sqrt{G}}\right)\right\}^m\right]dx.
\end{aligned}$$

The expression inside the E in the last expression is bounded by 1 (because it is a probability), and goes to 0 as $m \to \infty$. Therefore, by the dominated convergence theorem, we have $\mathrm{E}\{(\alpha_{\tilde{I}} - \alpha_{\mathrm{new}})^2\} \to 0$, hence, by (A.12), (A.13) and earlier results, $\mathrm{E}(\hat{\theta}_{\mathrm{n}} - \theta_{\mathrm{n}})^2 = o(1)$.

Finally, denoting the LS estimator of β by $\tilde{\beta} = (X'X)^{-1}X'y$, we have $\mathrm{E}(\hat{\theta}_{\mathrm{n,r}} - \theta_{\mathrm{n}})^2 = \mathrm{E}\{x_{\mathrm{n}}'(\tilde{\beta} - \beta) - \alpha_{\mathrm{new}}\}^2 = x_{\mathrm{n}}'\mathrm{Var}(\tilde{\beta})x_{\mathrm{n}} + R_{\mathrm{new}} \geq R_{\mathrm{new}} > 0$, by *B1*.

7

Extended topics

In this chapter, we will discuss some miscellaneous topics with implications for health disparity research. First, we will examine the impact of biased sampling on estimated population disease prevalence and how one can correct these to produce unbiased estimates. Biased sampling here refers to samples that do not reflect population proportions with respect to variables of interest (eg. race, age, gender, SES status etc). The particular motivating example comes from the estimation of population prevalence from COVID-19 testing studies where symptomatic individuals were more likely to get tested than asymptomatic individuals thus leading to an overestimate of prevalence. However, this general framework can be easily adapted to correct for other scenarios of testing disparity in disease surveillance studies. We then move to discuss the role of geocoding as a tool for evaluating contextual risk often in multilevel models. We described some interesting large-scale geocoding work that has been done in the context of public health disparity research and then explore the idea of imputing missing contextual variables in studies linked to (cancer) registry-level data. Finally, we end the chapter with a brief discussion on differential privacy and its impact on health disparities research and describe some ideas on how to do multilevel modeling incorporating differential privacy errors. Technical proofs are available at the end of the chapter.

7.1 Correcting for sampling bias in disease surveillance studies

Disease surveillance studies using population testing are vital to identify and understand important changes in disease dynamics as well as to aid in decision-making for developing mitigation strategies to reduce further spread. However, random sampling protocols can be inefficient and difficult to implement and thus convenience samples are often used instead. For some diseases like COVID-19 which has a large asymptomatic component, this can lead to over-representation of symptomatic individuals [10] which can in turn, lead to over-estimation of disease prevalence since the symptomatic individuals are more likely to test positive.

DOI: 10.1201/9781003119449-7

Much attention has been focused on the issue of correcting for imperfect tests [77, 121]; but less attention has been paid to correcting for biased sampling. One notable exception is [10], where they developed a snowball sampling approach in conjunction with contact tracing in order to set up a better disease surveillance system.

Diaz and Rao (2021)[75] developed a bias-correction method based on the work of [12], a method developed for the correction of publication bias in meta analysis studies. Diaz and Rao (2021)[75] developed the main idea by allowing for several categories of symptoms as a generalization of the two categories (symptomatic and asymptomatic) case.

7.1.1 The model

Diaz and Rao (2021)[75] described a population P of size N with associated partition $\mathcal{P}$ of $2M$ subsets of P each with proportions given by the vector $\mathbf{p}^* := \left(p_1^{(0)}, p_1^{(1)}, p_2^{(0)}, p_2^{(1)}, \ldots, p_M^{(0)}, p_M^{(1)}\right)$, where

$$\sum_{s=1}^{M} \left(p_s^{(0)} + p_s^{(1)}\right) = 1 \text{ and } p_s^{(0)}, p_s^{(1)} \geq 0, \text{ for } s \in \{1, \ldots, M\}.$$

Next define a random variable S^* that takes values in the set $\mathbf{I} := \{1^{(0)}, 1^{(1)}, \ldots, M^{(0)}, M^{(1)}\}$ that, conditioned on $\mathbf{p}^*$, selects an element of the partition $\mathcal{P}$ according to a categorical distribution in the interval $(0,1)$:

$$f_{S^*}\left(s^{(i)} | \mathbf{p}^*\right) = p_s^{(i)},$$

where $s \in \{1, \ldots, M\}$ represents number or degree of symptoms, and $i \in \{0, 1\}$, *prevalence*: $i = 1$ represents infected, while $i = 0$ represents non infected. In the most common scenario there are just the categories —asymptomatic and symptomatic—, so $M = 2$. However, some studies have considered more than two degrees of symptoms (see [346]).

The proportion of people with symptoms $s = s^{(0)} \cup s^{(1)}$ is then given by

$$p_s = p_s^{(0)} + p_s^{(1)}. \tag{7.1}$$

Note that $p_s^{(1)}$ is the probability of being in the category s and being infected, whereas $p_s^{(0)}$ represents the probability of being in the category s and non-infected.

From this notation, the overall probability of being infected can be derived as,

$$p_1^{(1)} + \cdots + p_M^{(1)}.$$

We now can introduce a Bernoulli r.v. T, which is 1 with probability $p(S^*)$.

Further, consider an independent sequence $T_1, \ldots, T_N$, distributed as T. If the individual j belongs to the group s^*, $T_j = 1$, which happens with probability $p(s^*)$, will tell us that the individual j is tested (sampled). The sample size of the testing study is then given by $N_T = \sum_{j=1}^{N} T_j$.

Re-iterating all of the definitions thus far, for $m \in \{1 \ldots, M\}$, we have that:

- $p(m)$ is the probability of being in the category m and being tested.
- $p\left(m^{(1)}\right)$ is the probability of testing for an individual in category m who is infected.
- $\frac{p_m^{(1)}}{p_m}$ is the conditional probability of being infected given m.
- p_m is the real proportion of people with the symptoms.

Without loss of generality, we can assume an ordering by the number of symptoms for the partition of P. This then provides the orderings:

$$p(1) \leq \cdots \leq p(s) \leq \cdots \leq p(M), \tag{7.2}$$

$$p\left(1^{(1)}\right) \leq \cdots \leq p\left(s^{(1)}\right) \leq \cdots \leq p\left(M^{(1)}\right), \tag{7.3}$$

$$\frac{p_1^{(1)}}{p_1} \leq \cdots \leq \frac{p_s^{(1)}}{p_s} \leq \cdots \leq \frac{p_M^{(1)}}{p_M}, \tag{7.4}$$

$$p_1 \geq \cdots \geq p_s \geq \cdots \geq p_M. \tag{7.5}$$

The intuition behind these is that the higher the degree and/or number of symptoms, then the higher the probability of being tested (7.2), the higher the probability of testing infected people (7.3), the higher the probability of being infected inside that group (Eq. 7.4), and the lower the real proportion of people with the symptoms (7.5).

From the conditional distribution of $(S^*|\mathbf{p}^*, T = 1)$, we observe i.i.d. draws of $S|\mathbf{p}$, whose density, because of Bayes theorem, is

$$\begin{aligned} f_{S|\mathbf{p}}(s|\vec{p}) = f_{S^*|\mathbf{p}^*,T}(s|\vec{p}, 1) &= \frac{P[T = 1|S^* = s, \mathbf{p}^* = \vec{p}]}{P[T = 1|\mathbf{p}^* = \vec{p}]} f_{S^*|\mathbf{p}^*}(s|\vec{p}) \\ &= \frac{p(s)}{E[p(S^*)|\mathbf{p}^* = \vec{p}]} p_s. \end{aligned} \tag{7.6}$$

Assume there is no error in testing. Then we know exactly the proportion of infected people in the sample. We also know under which category s each person belongs to. Therefore, for all s, we can derive:

$$\begin{aligned} f_{S|\mathbf{p}}\left(s^{(1)}|\vec{p}\right) = f_{S^*|\mathbf{p}^*,T}\left(s^{(1)}|\vec{p}, 1\right) &= \frac{P\left[T = 1|S^* = s^{(1)}, \mathbf{p}^* = \vec{p}\right]}{P[T = 1|\mathbf{p}^* = \vec{p}]} f_{S^*|\mathbf{p}^*}\left(s^{(1)}|\vec{p}\right) \\ &= \frac{p\left(s^{(1)}\right)}{E[p(S^*)|\mathbf{p}^* = \vec{p}]} p_s^{(1)}. \end{aligned} \tag{7.7}$$

Thus, we obtained in (7.6) the biased estimate of the proportion of people tested —and in (7.7) the biased estimate of the proportion of prevalence) for each s—. The total biased estimator of tested people is

$$\sum_{s=1}^{M} \frac{p(s)}{E[p(S^*)|\mathbf{p}^* = \vec{p}]} p_s, \tag{7.8}$$

and the total biased estimator of prevalence is

$$\sum_{s=1}^{M} \frac{p\left(s^{(1)}\right)}{E[p(S^*)|\mathbf{p}^* = \vec{p}]} p_s^{(1)}. \tag{7.9}$$

7.1.2 Bias correction

The bias correction then amounts to multiplying the quantity on the LHS of (7.6) and (7.7) by the inverse of the quotient on the RHS of each respective equation. Specifically, the bias correction is given by $C(x) f_{S|\mathbf{p}}(x|\vec{p})$, where

$$C(x) := \frac{P\left[T = 1|\mathbf{p}^* = \vec{p}\right]}{p(x)}. \tag{7.10}$$

Replacing x by s and $s^{(1)}$ will give us the bias correction for testing and prevalence, respectively, for each s. Summing over $s^{(1)}$ gives the sampling bias-corrected estimate of disease prevalence. The numerator at the RHS of (7.10) can be estimated as N_T/N, where N_T is the number of people tested, and N is the census population. However, the denominator is unknown, but we can still say some things, depending on the number of symptoms M we are considering.

7.1.2.1 Large values of s

The overall proportion of people tested is N_T/N. We also assume that most of the people tested are symptomatic; therefore, when s approaches M, $\tilde{p}_s := (N_T/N) f_{S|\mathbf{p}}(s|\vec{p})$ is a good estimator of the real proportion of the last value. Finally, since we know that most of the symptomatic people will be infected, and most of them will get tested, then $\tilde{p}_s^{(1)} \approx \tilde{p}_s$ for large values s.

7.1.2.2 Small values of s

When s decreases to 1, the situation is different. According to (7.2), in the absence of symptoms, the probability of being tested is small. Nonetheless, having few tests for small values of s does not mean that the proportion of people infected/uninfected is close to 0. I.e., $p(s)$ might be small, but p_s is large, which according to (7.6) is introducing a heavy bias.

Now, notice that, since $1 \geq C(s) f_{S|\mathbf{p}}(s|\vec{p})$, Diaz and Rao (2021) provide a lower bound for $p(s)$:

$$\frac{N_T}{N} f_{S|\mathbf{p}}(s|\vec{p}) \leq p(s) \tag{7.11}$$

Giving $p(s)$ its lower possible value makes the corrected estimate $C(s) f_{S|\mathbf{p}}(s|\vec{p}) = 1$. However, this implies that for all $s' \neq s$, the estimated probability of being tested is 0, which cannot be true.

In order to solve this, Diaz and Rao (2021)[75] divided $\mathcal{P}$ into three groups: $\mathcal{P}^- \cup \mathcal{P}^m \cup \mathcal{P}^+$, where $\mathcal{P}^-$ and $\mathcal{P}^+$ are the subsets of low and high values of symptoms, respectively; and $\mathcal{P}^m$, the symptoms in between.

According to Section 7.1.2.1, we have already estimated the probability of the elements in $\mathcal{P}^+$. Thus making $p_+ := \sum_{s \in \mathcal{P}^+} \tilde{p}_s$, we propose the following solution for values in $\mathcal{P}^-$:

1. Take the space $\mathcal{P}^- \cup \mathcal{P}^m$, which has probability $1 - p_+$.

2. Letting $\tilde{M}$ be the cardinality of the set $\mathcal{P}^- \cup \mathcal{P}^m$, assign equal probabilities $\tilde{p}_k$ to all $k \in \mathcal{P}^- \cup \mathcal{P}^m$. I.e., $\tilde{p}_s = (1 - p_+) / \tilde{M}$.

The assignation of equal probabilities is justified by our total ignorance of the real proportions. If we are going to consider some other distribution than equiprobability, we must justify the reduction in entropy that is inserting bias.

7.1.2.3 Prevalence

We know that in the asymptomatic population, a non-negligible portion of individuals is infected. Some studies maintain that most of the asymptomatic people are already infected. In such case, $p_s^{(1)} \approx p_s$. Others lean on the side that, for small, s, we have $p_s^{(1)} / p_s$ closer to 0 than to 1, but not necessarily approaching 0. Thus, Diaz and Rao (2021)[75] proposed the following algorithm:

1. If we don't have any information about the asymptomatic category with the disease, generate a random number u according to a uniform distribution in the interval $(0, 1)$.

2. If we have some information about the asymptomatic category with the disease from the biased sample, make u the proportion of prevalence inside the particular category of interest provided by the biased sample (i.e., $u = f_{S|\mathbf{p}}\left(s^{(1)}|\vec{p}\right) / f_{S|\mathbf{p}}(s|\vec{p})$).

3. Make $\tilde{p}_s^{(1)} = u \tilde{p}_s$.

7.1.2.4 Middle values of s

Notice that in the previous algorithm we are not asking to use $\tilde{p}$ for the correction in (7.10) of values in S^m (although it might be done with some care.) This is because for these values we have littel knowledge. Diaz and Rao (2021)[75] recommended collapsing $\mathcal{P}$ to $\mathcal{P}^- \cup \mathcal{P}^+$.

7.1.2.5 $M = 2$

As just suggested, Diaz and Rao (2021)[75] showed that an important simplification occurs when we consider only two groups of symptomatology: asymptomatic ($s = 1$) and symptomatic ($s = 2$). In this case, the analysis is conveniently reduced to:

- $\tilde{p}_2^{(1)} \approx \tilde{p}_2 = (N_T/N) f_{S|\mathbf{p}}(2|\vec{p})$ (from Subsection 7.1.2.1)
- $\tilde{p}_1 = 1 - \tilde{p}_2$ (from Subsection 7.1.2.2).
- $\tilde{p}_1^{(1)} = u\tilde{p}_1$ (from Subsubsection 7.1.2.3).

7.1.3 Estimated variance

Diaz and Rao (2021)[75] also derived the estimation of variation for their bias-corrected prevalance estimate. Again using their notation, let $\mathbf{X}_1, \ldots, \mathbf{X}_n$ be iid multinomial $\mathfrak{M}(1; \mathbf{p}^*)$. Then $\sum_{i=1}^n \mathbf{X}_i \sim \mathfrak{M}(n; \mathbf{p}^*)$. Let $\hat{\mathbf{p}} := n^{-1} \sum_{i=1}^n \mathbf{X}_i$. By the multivariate central limit theorem, we know that

$$\sqrt{n} \cdot \hat{\mathbf{p}} \sim AN(\mathbf{p}^*, \Sigma/n), \tag{7.12}$$

where AN stands for *asymptotically normal*, and $\Sigma = \text{Diag}(\mathbf{p}^*) - \mathbf{p}^* \mathbf{p}^{*T}$.

Now define

$$\mathbf{f}_\mathbf{p} := \left(f_{S|\mathbf{p}}\left(s_1^{(0)} | \vec{p}\right), f_{S|\mathbf{p}}\left(s_1^{(1)} | \vec{p}\right), \ldots, f_{S|\mathbf{p}}\left(s_M^{(0)} | \vec{p}\right), f_{S|\mathbf{p}}\left(s_M^{(1)} | \vec{p}\right) \right),$$

and let $\mathbf{Y}_1, \ldots, \mathbf{Y}_n$ be iid $\mathfrak{M}(1; \mathbf{f}_\mathbf{p})$, so that $\sum_{i=1}^n \mathbf{Y}_i \sim \mathfrak{M}(n; \mathbf{f}_\mathbf{p})$. Applying the Delta method to $\hat{\mathbf{q}} = n^{-1} \sum_{i=1}^n \mathbf{Y}_i$, we obtain that $\sqrt{n} \cdot \hat{\mathbf{q}} \sim AN(\mathbf{f}_\mathbf{p}, \mathbf{V}_n)$, where $\mathbf{V}_n = \frac{1}{n} g'(\mathbf{p}) \mathbf{\Sigma} g'(\mathbf{p})^T$, and $g'(\mathbf{p})$ is

$$g'(\mathbf{p}) = \frac{1}{P[T = 1 | \mathbf{p} = \vec{p}]} \left(p\left(s_1^{(0)}\right), p\left(s_1^{(1)}\right), \ldots, p\left(s_M^{(0)}\right), p\left(s_M^{(1)}\right) \right). \tag{7.13}$$

Notice that the correction in (7.10) applies g^{-1} to $\mathbf{Y}$, which leads back to $\mathbf{X}$. Therefore, asymptotically, we obtain again the distribution in (7.12).

In practice, we start with the biased iid $\tilde{\mathbf{Y}}_1, \ldots, \tilde{\mathbf{Y}}_{N_T}$, which are $\mathfrak{M}(1, \mathbf{f}_\mathbf{p})$, whose sum is $\mathfrak{M}(n, \mathbf{f}_\mathbf{p})$. Letting $\tilde{\mathbf{q}} = N_T^{-1} \sum \tilde{\mathbf{Y}}_i$, we have again by the MCLT that $\sqrt{N_T} \cdot \tilde{\mathbf{q}} \sim AN(\mathbf{f}_\mathbf{p}, \mathbf{V}_{N_T})$. Making $h(\mathbf{f}_\mathbf{p}) = \mathbf{C} \cdot \mathbf{f}_\mathbf{p}$, where $\mathbf{C}$ is a vector with components as in (7.10), we can apply again the Delta method to h, obtaining

$$\sqrt{N_T} \cdot \tilde{\mathbf{q}} \sim AN\left(h(\mathbf{f}_\mathbf{p}), \mathbf{C}\mathbf{V}_{N_T}\mathbf{C}^T\right). \tag{7.14}$$

However, since we are not using $\mathbf{C}$, but $\mathcal{C}$, an M-vector whose last component is $(N_T/N)f_M$ and with the first $M-1$ components being all $\frac{1}{M-1}\left(1-\frac{N_T}{N}f_M\right)$. Then, the variance-covariance matrix becomes

$$\begin{pmatrix} a\sigma_M^2 & a\sigma_M^2 & \cdots & b\sigma_M^2 \\ a\sigma_M^2 & a\sigma_M^2 & \cdots & b\sigma_M^2 \\ \vdots & \vdots & \ddots & \vdots \\ a\sigma_M^2 & a\sigma_M^2 & \cdots & b\sigma_M^2 \\ b\sigma_M^2 & b\sigma_M^2 & \cdots & c\sigma_M^2 \end{pmatrix},$$

where $c=\left(\frac{N_T}{N}\right)^2$, $a=c\left(\frac{1}{M-1}\right)^2$, $b=\frac{c}{M-1}$, and σ_M^2 is the variance of f_M. From this, the estimated variance of the total prevalence estimate can be calculated.

Example 7.1 COVID-19 testing study from Lombardy, Italy

This example comes [75] who analyzed data from [285] where the authors calculated the probability of symptoms and critical disease after SARS-CoV-2 infection in Lombardy, Italy [285] during a time window in 2020. In a sample of 5824 individuals, they identified 932 infections through PCR testing. They also detected 1892 infections using serological assays. Thus, the total of infected individuals was 2824. Among the total of infected, 876 were symptomatic (31%). Focusing only on the PCR group and assuming that 31% of the cases were symptomatic also for the 932 infections detected by PCR. Treating this as the population, the prevalence is then $932/5824 = 0.16$; and among the infected, $0.31(932) = 289$ individuals are symptomatic. The remaining 932-289 = 643 will be infected and are asymptomatic. We will examine four different sampling protocols with varying degrees of sampling bias.

Sampling Protocol 1: The sample consists of 289 infected and symptomatic individuals. In this case, the naïve estimate of prevalence is 1. The bias-corrected estimate will be $\tilde{p}_2 = (N_T/N)1 = 289/5824 \approx 0.05$. And this will also be the correction for $\tilde{p}_2^{(1)}$. Then $\tilde{p}_1 = 1-\tilde{p}_2 = 0.95$, and taking the mean of u we obtain $\tilde{p}_1^{(1)} = 0.5(0.95) = 0.475$. Therefore, the total corrected prevalence is estimated as $\tilde{p}_1^{(1)} + \tilde{p}_2^{(1)} = 0.475 + 0.05 = 0.525$, which still high but corrects heavily the effects of a very bad sample.

Sampling Protocol 2: The sample consists of 384 individuals. Among these, 289 (75%) are infected and symptomatic, and 95 (25%) are asymptomatic. We assume the sample has $95(643/5824) \approx 10$ asymptomatic positive for the virus. So our naïve estimate of prevalence is $(289+10)/384 \approx 0.78$. In this case, $\tilde{p}_2^{(1)} = \tilde{p}_2 = (384/5824)0.75 \approx 0.049$. Now, $\tilde{p}_1 = 1-\tilde{p}_2 = 0.951$; and setting u as $10/95 \approx 0.105$, $p_1^{(1)} = 0.105(0.951) \approx 0.1$. Therefore the total prevalence is corrected to $0.1 + 0.049 = 0.149$, which is very close to the real 0.16.

Sampling Protocol 3: In this scenario, we have 289 symptomatic positive and 289 asymptomatic. We assume the sample has 289(643/5824) $\approx$ 32 asymptomatic and infected individuals. The naïve estimate is $(289+32)/578 \approx 0.55$. However, $\tilde{p}_2^{(1)} = \tilde{p}_2 = (578/5824)0.5 \approx 0.05$; and $\tilde{p}_1 = 0.95$. In this case, $\tilde{p}_1^{(1)} = (32/289)0.95 \approx 0.105$., where $u = 32/289$. Therefore, $0.105 + 0.05 = 0.11$ is the corrected estimate of prevalence.

Sampling Protocol 4: This sample is truly random. Say $N_T = 600$. Among these, 600(289/5824) $\approx$ 30 are symptomatic and positive. Therefore, 570 are asymptomatic. Among the asymptomatic group, we are going to assume 600(643/5824) $\approx$ 66 infected individuals. The naïve sample estimate is thus $(66+30)/600 = 0.16$, which of course is the same as the real prevalence. In this case, the correction will work like this: $p_2^{(1)} = p_2 = (600/5824)0.95 \approx 0.098$. Then $\tilde{p}_1 = 1 - \tilde{p}_2 = 0.902$, and $p_1^{(1)} = (66/570)(0.902) \approx 0.1044$. Therefore, the total prevalence is estimated as $0.1044 + 0.098 = 0.2024$ indicating that the bias correction is small when we want it to be.

7.2 Geocoding

7.2.1 The Public Health Geocoding Project

It is widely acknowledged that there exists a lack of resources at the community level to track the magnitude and trends over time of socioeconomic health inequalities. This is mainly due to this type of data not being routinely collected in U.S. public health surveillance systems outside of birth and death. The main sources come from specialized surveys including the National Health Interview Survey and the Behavioral Risk Factor Surveillance System (BRFSS). As a result, the contribution of economic deprivation to disparities in health remains often hidden. This matters because health statistics that accurately track population disease burden, disability, and death help one understand society better including the existence of health disparities ([204]). Indeed countries like Canada and the UK have developed revised policies to address disparities that emphasize social inequalities in health (e.g., [1]; [2]).

Researchers at Harvard University used the methodology of geocoding residential addresses and extracted area-based socioeconomic measures (ABSMs) whereby both cases and the catchment population are classified by the socioeconomic characteristics of their residential areas. This was given the name the Public Health Disparities Geocoding Project. The purpose of the project was the development of standards and best practices regarding which ABSMs at which level of geography are best suited for monitoring U.S. socioeconomic inequalities in health. The project examined a wide variety of health outcomes ranging from mortality to cancer incidence ([203]) to non-fatal weapons-related injuries ([202]), and focused its attention on the states of Massachusetts and Rhode Island. They also examined socioeconomic gradients in relation to 18 ABSMs choosing those that met stringent inclusion criteria ([204]).

After much research, the PHDGP arrived at the conclusion that the census track poverty level measure (percent of persons below the poverty line) was the most useful for monitoring U.S. socioeconomic inequalities in health.

7.2.2 Geocoding considerations

Geocoding is nothing more than the assignment of a (typically numeric) code to a geographic location. Often this is associated with individual addresses (latitude and longitude) which can then be linked to aggregated areas ranging from census tracts to block groups. Understanding what is termed census geography can be useful in digesting geographical units of analysis. Census tracts and block groups are U.S. Census Bureau defined, standardized, and mostly permanent. Usual ZIP codes are not really able to be linked to anything else since they are U.S. Postal Service administrative units that can change more regularly. In fact, [204] has shown bias due to spatiotemporal mismatches between ZIP codes and U.S. census-defined areas ([203]).

Standalone geocoding software programs are available as well as commercial entities with customized solutions. It is also customary to run quality control analyses to test the accuracy of the geocoding produced. Geocoding requires accurate reference datasets and valid addresses as inputs. Reference datasets are usually classified as network, parcel, or address points data ([373]). In order to protect privacy, addresses are mapped to things like names of buildings, closest intersections, neighborhoods, cities, or counties which represent different scales.

In order to conduct geocoding, matching algorithms are used to determine the location of an input address matched to a range of addresses in a reference dataset. Street geocoding attempts to match the street name of the input address to street names in the reference dataset and then determines the side of the street based on the address number. A final correction is done to output the correct coordinates. For parcel geocoding, the input address is matched to the nearest centroid of a parcel. This technique has been shown to be less accurate as the size of the parcel increases. Finally, address point geocoding tries to mitigate the issues of parcel geocoding where the input address is matched to a point feature rather than a centroid.

The quality of a geocoding procedure is determined by evaluating the match rate which is the percentage of correctly geocoded inputs. Poor match rates may mean that many input addresses will have to be excluded from downstream analyses. However, it should be noted that an increased match rate does not always imply better geocoding. For example, the effect of varying spelling sensitivity is studied in McElroy *et al.* (2003).

Sources of geocoding errors have been studied in some detail and the major sources are input address quality and the quality of the reference dataset ([203], [373]) as well as the quality of the matching algorithms used. Other issues related to positional accuracy and downstream modeling of geocoding errors are discussed in detail in [274].

7.2.3 Pseudo-Bayesian classified mixed model prediction for imputing area-level covariates

When no address information exists, direct geocoding cannot be done. However, we might be able to predict area-level information using a reference dataset consisting of additional observations (from the same areas) that also contain information on individual level covariates. A *linking model* can then be constructed on the reference dataset, and the fitted model can be used to *classify* new observations to areas. Classified mixed model prediction (CMMP) introduced in Chapter 6 could be used. Using these predicted areas, corresponding area level covariates can be attached. For instance, for cancer, the reference dataset may be derived from a statewide registry with the linking covariates being clinical variables in common with the analysis observations (from say a hospital electronic health system), and the registry. After classified predictions are made (to say the area represented at the census tract level), then additional known tract level covariates (e.g., from census or large-scale surveys) can be attached.

In order to conduct the classification, Ma and Jiang (2022)[227] generalized CMMP in what they termed the pseudo-Bayesian classified mixed model prediction (PBCMMP) to allow for uncertainty in the association of the random effects with grouping structure. In doing so, they also discovered that their classification algorithm was provably consistent for classifying test observations to the correct training data groups – a property which the original CMMP did not posses even though CMMP was consistent for the prediction of new mixed effects or future observations.

Suppose that the training data associated with the network satisfy a nested-error regression (NER; [24]) model:

$$y_{ij} \quad = \quad x'_{ij}\beta + \alpha_i + \epsilon_{ij}, \tag{7.15}$$

$i = 1, \ldots, m$, $j = 1, \ldots, k_i$, where i represents the area, k_i is the number of subjects in the training data that belong to area i; y_{ij} is the outcome of interest, x_{ij} is a vector of associated covariates, β is an unknown vector of regression coefficients (the fixed effects), α_i is a area-specific random effect, and ϵ_{ij} is an error. It is assumed that the random effects and errors are independent with $\alpha_i \sim N(0, \sigma^2)$ and $\epsilon_{ij} \sim N(0, \tau^2)$, where $\sigma^2 > 0, \tau^2 > 0$ are unknown variances.

We are interested in the prediction of a mixed effect associated with a new subject. The mixed effect may be a conditional mean, proportion, or other characteristic, given the random effect associated with the subject. Suppose that the new subject belongs to a known group (class) $c_{\rm n}$. Here the subscript n stands for "new". The random effect associated with the new subject, however, is not entirely determined by $c_{\rm n}$—it is subject to some uncertainty. Let $\gamma_{\rm n}$ denote the true class index of the new subject. For the training data, however, the classes match the communities, by assumption, but this is not necessarily true for the new subject. For now, let us assume that $\gamma_{\rm n}$ is an unknown integer between 1 and m. This is called a matched case. Ma and Jiang (2022)[227] assumed that there is a working probability model for $\gamma_{\rm n}$:

$$\pi(\gamma_{\rm n} = i), \quad 1 \leq i \leq m, \tag{7.16}$$

where $\pi(\cdot)$ is a known probability distribution, which is not necessarily the true distribution of $\gamma_{\rm n}$. For example, they proposed consideration of the following working model:

$$\pi(\gamma_{\rm n} = i) \quad = \quad p^{1_{(i=c_{\rm n})}} \left(\frac{1-p}{m-1}\right)^{1_{(i \neq c_{\rm n})}}, \tag{7.17}$$

where p is a given probability; in other words, $\pi(\gamma_{\rm n} = i) = p$ if $i = c_{\rm n}$, and $\pi(\gamma_{\rm n} = i) = (1-p)/(m-1)$ if $i \neq c_{\rm n}$. It is easy to verify that (7.17) is a probability distribution on $\{1, \dots, m\}$. The p in (7.17) may be treated as a tuning parameter, which has an intuitive interpretation: It has to do with one's belief to what extent $c_{\rm n}$ determines $\gamma_{\rm n}$. Ma and Jiang (2022) called $\pi(\cdot)$ a *pseudo-prior.*

Now suppose that the outcomes of interest corresponding to the new subject, $y_{{\rm n}j}, 1 \leq j \leq k_{\rm n}$, satisfy a similar NER model to (7.15), that is,

$$y_{{\rm n}j} \quad = \quad x_{{\rm n}j}'\beta + \alpha_{\gamma_{\rm n}} + \epsilon_{{\rm n}j}, \tag{7.18}$$

$1 \leq j \leq k_{\rm n}$, where $x_{{\rm n}j}$ is the corresponding vector of covariates, and $\epsilon_{{\rm n}j}$s are the new errors that are independent and distributed as $N(0, \tau^2)$, and are independent with $\alpha_{\gamma_{\rm n}}$ and the α_is and ϵ_{ij}s associated with the training data. Note that, given $\gamma_{\rm n} = i$, (7.18) becomes $y_{{\rm n}j} = x_{{\rm n}j}'\beta + \alpha_i + \epsilon_{{\rm n}j}$, $1 \leq j \leq k_{\rm n}$. This means that one can combine the training data and new data into m independent groups:

$$y_1, \dots, y_{i-1}, (y_i, y_{\rm n}), y_{i+1}, \dots, y_m,$$

where $y_i = (y_{ij})_{1 \leq j \leq k_i}$ and $y_{\rm n} = (y_{{\rm n}j})_{1 \leq j \leq k_{\rm n}}$. The pdf of y_u $(u \neq i)$ is given by

$$f(y_u) = \frac{1}{(2\pi)^{k_u/2}|V_u|^{1/2}} \exp\left\{-\frac{1}{2}(y_u - X_u\beta)'V_u^{-1}(y_u - X_u\beta)\right\}, \tag{7.19}$$

where $X_u = (x_{uj}')_{1 \leq j \leq k_u}$ and $V_u = \tau^2 I_{k_u} + \sigma^2 J_{k_u}$ (I_k, J_k denote the $k \times k$ identity matrix and matrix of 1s, respectively). Similarly, given $\gamma_n = i$, the joint pdf of $(y_i, y_{\rm n})$ is given by

$$\begin{aligned} & f(y_i, y_{\rm n}|\gamma_n = i) \\ & = \frac{1}{(2\pi)^{(k_i+k_{\rm n})/2}|V_{i,{\rm n}}|^{1/2}} \exp\left\{-\frac{1}{2}\begin{pmatrix} y_i - X_i\beta \\ y_{\rm n} - X_{\rm n}\beta \end{pmatrix}' V_{i,n}^{-1} \begin{pmatrix} y_i - X_i\beta \\ y_{\rm n} - X_{\rm n}\beta \end{pmatrix}\right\}, \end{aligned} \tag{7.20}$$

where $X_{\rm n} = (x'_{{\rm n}j})_{1\leq j\leq k_{\rm n}}$ and $V_{i,n} = \tau^2 I_{k_i+k_{\rm n}} + \sigma^2 J_{k_i+k_{\rm n}}$. Combining the above results, and with some reorganization of terms, we obtain

$$
\begin{aligned}
f(y|\gamma_{\rm n}=i) &= f(y_i, y_{\rm n}|\gamma_{\rm n}=i)\prod_{u\neq i} f(y_u) \\
&= (2\pi)^{(k.+k_{\rm n})/2}(\tau^2)^{(k.+k_{\rm n}-m)/2}\{\tau^2+(k_i+k_{\rm n})\sigma^2\}^{1/2}\prod_{u\neq i}(\tau^2+k_u\sigma^2)^{1/2} \\
&\quad \times \exp\left\{-\frac{1}{2}\begin{pmatrix} y_i - X_i\beta \\ y_{\rm n} - X_{\rm n}\beta\end{pmatrix}' V_{i,n}^{-1}\begin{pmatrix} y_i - X_i\beta \\ y_{\rm n} - X_{\rm n}\beta\end{pmatrix}\right. \\
&\quad \left. -\frac{1}{2}\sum_{u\neq i}(y_u - X_u\beta)' V_u^{-1}(y_u - X_u\beta)\right\}, \qquad (7.21)
\end{aligned}
$$

where $k. = \sum_{u=1}^m k_u$, and $y = (y'_1, \dots, y'_m, y'_{\rm n})'$.

Ma and Jiang (2022)[227] then derived the pseudo-posterior distribution of γ_n:

$$
{\rm P}_\pi(\gamma_{\rm n} = i|y) = \frac{\pi(\gamma_{\rm n}=i)f(y|\gamma_{\rm n}=i)}{\sum_{j=1}^m \pi(\gamma_{\rm n}=j)f(y|\gamma_{\rm n}=j)}. \qquad (7.22)
$$

The match of γ_n to the training data groups is chosen as the pseudo-posterior mode, that is,

$$
\begin{aligned}
\hat{\gamma}_{\rm n} &= {\rm argmax}_{1\leq i\leq m}{\rm P}_\pi(\gamma_{\rm n}=i|y) \\
&= {\rm argmax}_{1\leq i\leq m}\{\pi(\gamma_{\rm n}=i)f(y|\gamma_n=i)\}. \qquad (7.23)
\end{aligned}
$$

Note. Although the procedure clearly resembles the *maximum posterior*, or Bayesian classification (e.g., [269]), the set-up is not Bayesian. Due to its similarity to the Bayesian classifier, Ma and Jiang termed their procedure matching maximum pseudo-posterior matching (MPPM). Once $\hat{\gamma}_{\rm n}$ is determined, the prediction of the new mixed effect is carried out as in CMMP [178]. Namely, given $\gamma_{\rm n} = i$, the best predictor (BP), in the sense of minimum mean squared prediction error (MSPE), of $\theta_{{\rm n}j} = x'_{{\rm n}j}\beta + \alpha_{\gamma_{\rm n}} = x'_{{\rm n}j}\beta + \alpha_i$ is

$$
{\rm E}(\theta_{{\rm n}j}|y) = x'_{{\rm n}j}\beta + \frac{k_i\sigma^2}{\tau^2 + k_i\sigma^2}(\bar{y}_{i\cdot} - \bar{x}'_{i\cdot}\beta), \qquad (7.24)
$$

where $\bar{y}_{i\cdot} = k_i^{-1}\sum_{j=1}^{k_i} y_{ij}$ and $\bar{x}_{i\cdot} = k_i^{-1}\sum_{j=1}^{k_i} x_{ij}$. The classified mixed effect predictor (CMEP) of $\theta_{{\rm n}j}$, denoted by $\hat{\theta}_{{\rm n}j}$with i replaced by $\hat{\gamma}_{\rm n}$, and β, σ^2, τ^2 replaced by their estimators (e.g., REML estimators; e.g., [173], sec. 1.3.2) based on the training data. The new procedure is called pseudo-Bayesian classified mixed model prediction, or PBCMMP.

7.2.3.1 Consistency and asymptotic optimality of MPPM

Ma and Jiang (2022)[227] established the asymptotic superiority of MPPM mentioned above, as well as consistency of MPPM in terms of the class-index matching. They first consider a simpler, but also realistic situation in some cases (e.g., network data), where m, the number of classes in the training data, is bounded. Later we extend the result to the case that m increases with the sample sizes at an appropriate rate. Throughout this section, we assume a match case, which means that $\gamma_{\rm n}$ matches one of the indexes $1 \le i \le m$.

They assume that a consistent estimator of β, $\hat{\beta}$, is available; however, for the σ^2, τ^2, they only assume that some estimators, $\hat{\sigma}^2, \hat{\tau}^2$, are available, which satisfy

$$0 < a \le \hat{\sigma}^2, \hat{\tau}^2 \le A < \infty, \tag{7.25}$$

where a, A are some known constants.

Note that, for the consistency of $\hat{\beta}$, one does not need $m \to \infty$. In fact, $m \to \infty$ is necessary for the consistency of $\hat{\sigma}^2$ but not for that of $\hat{\beta}$ and $\hat{\tau}^2$. However, it is known that consistent estimator of β is available given any "working" estimators of σ^2 and τ^2, which need not to be consistent. For example, such a result was established earlier in the context of generalized estimating equations (GEE; [221]), and later in the context of generalized linear mixed models (GLMM; e.g., [172], [174]). Ma and Jiang (2022)[227] then defined a quantity $a_i = k_i/(k_i + k_{\rm n}), 1 \le i \le m$. To distinguish MPPM based on different working models, denote the MPPM by $\hat{\gamma}_{{\rm n},\pi}$, where π corresponds to the working model. Let $\gamma_{\rm n}^*$ denote the $\hat{\gamma}_{{\rm n},\pi}$ when π is the true distribution of $\gamma_{\rm n}$ which is purely a theoretical construct. Define

$$\tilde{\gamma}_{\rm n} \quad = \quad \text{argmax}_{1 \le i \le m} f(y|\gamma_{\rm n} = i). \tag{7.26}$$

Note that $\tilde{\gamma}_{\rm n}$ does not depend on π (therefore no index of π is needed).

Theorem 7.1 Theorem 1 (consistency of MPPM). *Suppose that the following hold:*
(i) $m > 1$, $\min_{1 \le i \le m} k_i \to \infty$, $k_{\rm n} \to \infty$, *and*

$$\min_{1 \le i \le m} a_i \ge b \ \text{ for some constant } b > 0; \tag{7.27}$$

(ii) $\bar{x}_{i\cdot} = k_i^{-1} \sum_{j=1}^{k_i} x_{ij}, 1 \le i \le m$ *and* $\bar{x}_{\rm n\cdot} = k_{\rm n}^{-1} \sum_{j=1}^{k_{\rm n}} x_{{\rm n}j}$ *are bounded, so are*

$$b_{ij} \equiv \log\{\pi(\gamma_{\rm n} = j)\} - \log\{\pi(\gamma_{\rm n} = i)\}, \quad 1 \le j \ne i \le m;$$

(iii) $\hat{\beta}$. *Then, Ma and Jiang (2022) stated the following conclusions:*

(I) $\mathrm{P}(\hat{\gamma}_{{\rm n},\pi} = \tilde{\gamma}_{\rm n}) \to 1$ *for any working model* π, *including the true distribution of* $\gamma_{\rm n}$.
(II) MPPM is consistent for any working model π, *that is,* $\mathrm{P}(\hat{\gamma}_{{\rm n},\pi} \ne \gamma_n) \to 0$.

The proof of Theorem 7.1 is given in [227]. If we apply the result to the special case that π is the true distribution of $\gamma_{\rm n}$, we have the following result.

TABLE 7.1: (Taken from Ma and Jiang (2022)[227]): Mean Prob. of Matching and 6-number Summary of MSPE Ratio

	Mean Prob. of Matching		**6-number Summary of MSPE Ratio**					
Case	PBCMMP	CMMP	Min.	Q1	Median	Mean	Q3	Max.
I-1	0.86	0.22	0.52	1.57	2.38	3.95	3.85	19.12
I-2	0.86	0.22	0.43	1.40	2.09	3.96	4.75	19.12
II-1	0.86	0.22	0.60	1.46	2.49	3.95	3.89	19.05
II-2	0.86	0.22	0.57	1.31	2.45	3.96	4.88	19.05
III	0.89	0.19	0.76	1.85	2.58	3.44	3.01	11.22
IV-1	0.84*	0.19*	0.90	1.58	2.60	4.13	5.57	16.24
IV-2	0.84*	0.19*	0.87	1.63	2.61	3.97	4.92	16.24

Corollary 1. Under the conditions of Theorem 1, we have, for any working model π,

$$\mathrm{P}(\hat{\gamma}_{\mathrm{n},\pi} = \gamma_{\mathrm{n}}^{*}) \quad \longrightarrow \quad 1. \tag{7.28}$$

Again the proof is given in [227].

They also conducted comprehensive simulation studies to demonstrate the performance of pseudo-Bayesian CMMP (PBCMMP). Of particular interest is the comparison of PBCMMP to regular CMMP. They studied 7 different scenarios all corresponding to $p = 0.75$ and $p = 0.90$. These scenarios include an example under the setting of [178], the addition of more covariate predictors to this setting, and the addition of noise to the random effect. The following table summarizes the mean probability of correct matching, or probability of approximate matching (results with *), and the six-number summary of the MSPE ratio, that is, the minimum, first quartile, median, mean, third quartile, and maximum of the empirical MSPE of CMMP divided by the empirical MSPE of PBCMMP. Overall, PBCMMP is seen to have a significant advantage over CMMP both in terms of the probability of correct (or approximate) matching and in terms of the MSPE of the prediction.

Example 7.2 Predicting community characteristics for colon cancer patients from the Florida Cancer Data System (FCDS)

Rao and Fan (2017) [303] next analyzed colon cancer cases in a statewide registry breaking up our sample into a training and testing sample. Our goal was to predict community characteristics for a set of test sample individuals as characterized by their census tract community information.

The Florida Cancer Data System (FCDS) is the Florida statewide cancer registry (`fcds.med.miami.edu`). It began data collection in 1981 and in 1994, became part of the National Program of Cancer Registries (NPCR) which is under the administration of the Centers for Disease Control (CDC). Two hundred and thirty hospitals reported approximately 115,000 unduplicated newly diagnosed cases per year. Currently, FCDS contains over 3,000,000 cancer incidence records.

Specifically, at the time of analysis, there were 3,116,030 observations of 144 variables in the original FCDS data set. There were 353,407 observations left after filtering for colon cancer and 314,633 observations left after filtering invalid survival dates. Further filtering to remove curious coding on tumor size, sex, grade, race, smoking status, treatment type, node positivity, radiation treatment, and chemotherapy information, left 45,917 observations for analysis.

There were 2,890 census tracts in the filtered data. We kept the census tracts with the number of observations no smaller than 25, which left us with 18,732 observations among 466 census tracts. We focused our attention on Miami-Dade county which left 210 census tracts for our analysis. We randomly chose 100 census tracts and 25 observations from each tract as our training data for the linking model. The response variable of interest was the square of age.

The coefficients of the variables in the linking model are in Table 7.2. Variables that had small t-values relative to the large sample size of the dataset were removed.[254] The variables that remained in the linking model were race, log survival time, sex, number of positive nodes, smoking history, radiation, and chemotherapy.

For test data, we chose 10 observations (or all the observations in a tract, whichever is smaller), from each of 842 Miami-Dade tracts with no data lost to variable filtering (33 tracts were left out due to variable filtering issues). This left a total test set sample size of 7266 observations. Our predictive geocoding analysis focused on census tracts in the Miami-Dade area. We focused on four community variables: **health insurance coverage status** (estimated percent uninsured based on the total noninstitutionalized population), **employment status** (the estimated unemployment rate for people 16 years of age and older), **median income** in the past twelve months in 2013 inflation-adjusted dollars (based on households), and **educational attainment** (estimated as a percent of the total who did not graduate high school). These were extracted from the 2009-2015 5-Year American Community Survey (ACS) (2014) (`www.census.gove/data/developers/updates/acs-5-yr-sumary-available-2009-2013.html`).

Table 7.3 shows the predictive performance with respect to characterizing community characteristics for test samples using the different predictors: the CMMP using REML estimation, CMMP using the OBP estimate of Jiang et al.,[177] CMMP based on modeling the spatial correlation structure across census tracts, prediction to a randomly chosen census tract and simply using the community variable population mean in each census tract. The table reports the empirical mean squared prediction error (MSPE) averaged across all census tracts as well as its various components (the squared bias, and the variance). The table also reports the variance of the predicted values across census tracts (BT) and the variance of the true community variable values across census tracts (TBT).

Table 7.3 results are illuminating and can be summarized as follows:

1. The CMMP estimators generally significantly outperform the random allocation predictor with respect to MSPE and this is primarily driven by decreased variance in within census tract predictions. This can be attributed

TABLE 7.2: (Taken from Rao and Fan (2017)[303]): Linking model fit

Term	Estimate	t-value	95% CI
Intercept	6539.51	54.59	[6304.71, 6744.33]
Log.surv	-42.22	-6.74	[-54.51, -29.94]
Race	-1003.04	-23.98	[-1085.03, -921.05]
Sex	162.21	7.37	[119.08, 205.34]
Tumor Grade	83.33	4.03	[42.84, 123.84]
Tumor Size	-0.74	-2.21	[-1.41, -0.09]
Number of positive nodes	-23.87	-6.58	[-30.99, -16.76]
Smoking	-297.50	-13.41	[-340.98, -254.03]
Surgery	215.03	2.59	[52.09, 377.97]
Radiation	-436.05	-8.89	[-532.24, -339.87]
Chemo	-953.94	-31.58	[-1013.14, -894.74]

TABLE 7.3: (Taken from Rao and Fan (2017)[303]): Comparison of methods with respect to predictive performance. Reported measures are MSPE, squared bias, average within-tract variance, between-tract (BT) variance, true between-tract (TBT) variance.

Method	MSPE	Bias^2	Variance	BT Variance	TBT Variance
CMMP (REML) – Education	364.22	212.27	154.34	102.47	195.32
CMMP (REML) – Income	1078.92	895.07	186.85	162.76	569.80
CMMP (REML) – Unemployed	51.4	35.11	16.63	10,92	34.50
CMMP (REML) – Uninsured	223.01	163.73	60.18	41.82	131.66
CMMP (OBP) – Education	366.79	209.58	159.66,	87.90	
CMMP (OBP) – Income	1057.50	890.47	169.68	135.60	
CMMP (OBP) – Unemployed	47.99	35.24	12.95	7.22	
CMMP (OBP) – Uninsured	231.67	146.97	86.01	56.45	
CMMP (SP)-Education	360.56	220.81	141.95	105.56	
CMMP (SP)-Income	1089.89	903.20	189.71	154.92	
CMMP (SP)-Unemployed	51.59	35.86	15.98	12.55	
CMMP (SP)-Uninsured	222.50	161.87	61.54	42.02	
Random – Education	434.67	205.71	232.55	232.60	
Random – Income	1048.16	677.63	376.61	370.66	
Random – Unemployed	64.39	35.03	29.81	29.86	
Random – Uninsured	251.30	145.12	107.88	107.07	
Population Mean – Education	202.09	201.09	1.01	0	
Population Mean – Income	680.03	677.89	2.17	0	
Population Mean – Unemployed	35.17	35.11	0.05	0	
Population Mean – Uninsured	143.87	143.62	0.25	0	

to the linking model which borrows strength across tracts amounting to a type of smoothing (and hence variance reduction) for specific tract predictions.

2. The naive population mean predictor actually does very well with respect to MSPE because there is no variance associated with these predictions within tract.

3. Incorporating spatial structure into the CMMP predictor can result in gains in reduced MSPE. But this appears to be only true for the education and uninsured community variables, and the gains are small.

4. Robust estimation using the OBP can produce gains in MSPE but the results are not uniform across all the community variables. Median income and percent unemployed seem to benefit while percent education and percent uninsured do not.

5. Simply focusing on within tract summaries reveals an incomplete picture since by those measures alone, the best predictions would come from the most naive population mean estimator. However, this estimator will assign the same value for all individuals across all census tracts. Clearly, this is overly naive since now between-tract variability will be captured. When examining empirical between tract variance estimates, it is clear that this naive estimator significantly underestimates true tract-to-tract variance. The CMMP estimators fare much better but do still underestimate between-tract variances. This is due to the model fit which captures relatively little of this variance as estimated by the random effect variance component.

Figure 7.1 shows the community variable predictive performance as oriented across census tracts in Miami-Dade. Green coloring indicates highly accurate predictions and as the color shading becomes darker blue, the accuracy of the predictions worsens (as measured by MPSE). Overall, predictions seem to be quite accurate.

The next set of analyses examined the predictive performance of the various estimators while allowing for clustering of census tracts with respect to community variables. The logic here is that even if an individual is incorrectly classified to a given tract, as long as the true tract is similar to the predicted one, then it would still be considered an accurate prediction. In order to allow this robustness to be at play, we clustered census tracts according to the four community variables.

Figure 7.2 shows the gap statistic analysis [294] using the union of the 466 tracts with at least 25 observations after variable filtering and the 875 tracts in the Miami-Dade area. The gap statistic indicated that 3 clusters are a reasonable estimate of the true number of "community clusters". Table 7.4 gives the resulting means of the four community variables by cluster and the number of tracts in each cluster.

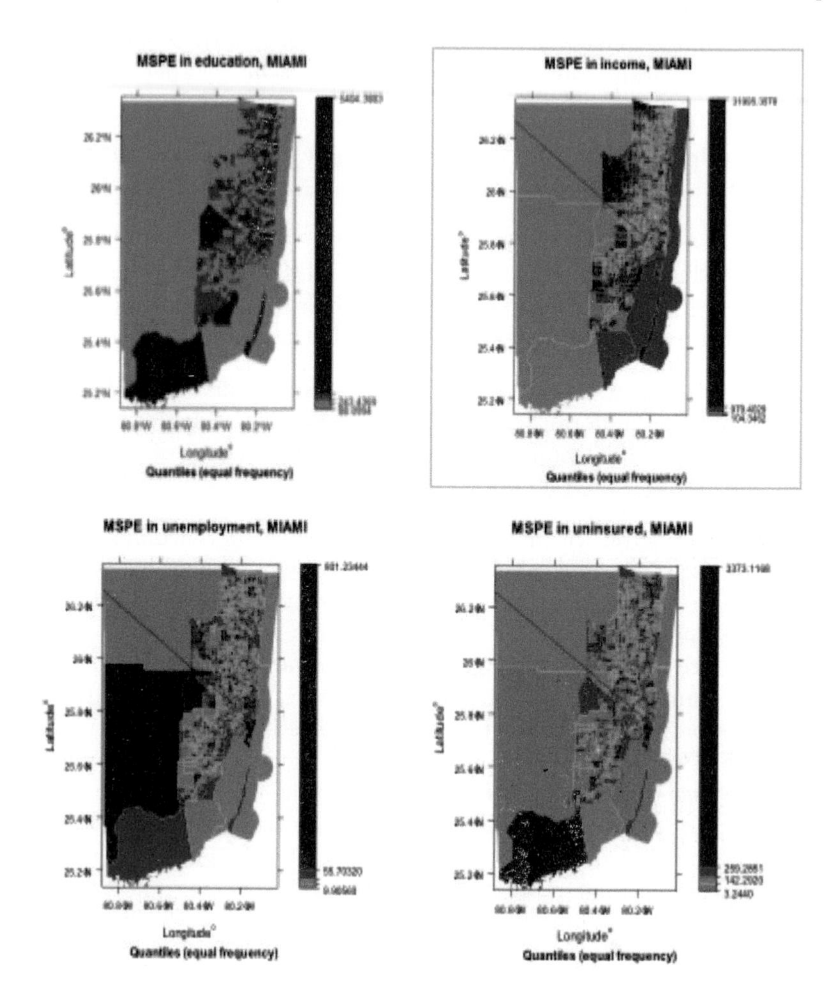

FIGURE 7.1: (Taken from Rao and Fan (2017)[303]): MSPE map for Miami-Dade county – unclustered.

Table 7.5 shows how predictive performance is affected allowing for community clustering. We report only one CMMP estimator (the REML). It's quite clear that clustering improves MSPE performance for all estimators but the relative gains when comparing CMPI to random and population mean estimators increase with clustering. Similar patterns to Table 7.3 are observed when looking at within tract summaries versus between tract summary measures.

Figure 7.3 shows the MSPE spatial plots for Miami-Dade based on community clustering. Now, internal quantiles are fixed from the unclustered analysis

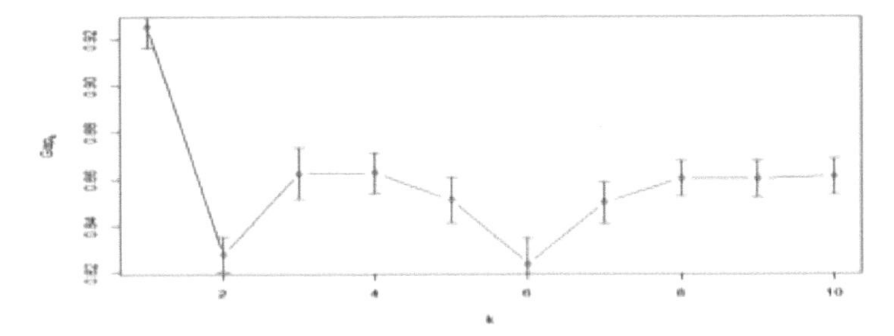

FIGURE 7.2: (Taken from Rao and Fan (2017)[303]): Gap statistic plot showing number of "community clusters" based on four community variables.

so as to be able to compare Figures 7.1 and 7.3 properly. Specifically, the 25th, 50th and 75th percentiles are fixed at the unclustered values. Now, if more green appears, it indicates that clustering is improving MSPE as compared to the unclustered analysis. Figure 7.3 shows that indeed this is the case. Much more green is produced. In conclusion, community clustering adds robustness to the predictive geocoding analysis.

7.3 Differential privacy and the impact on health disparities research

There has been substantial, and increasing, national and global interest in protecting privacy associated with the data. For example, the United States Census Bureau has made new differential privacy (DP) changes in its 2020 decennial enumeration data to protect confidentiality. See, for example, [5, 136].

DP infuses noise into data in a top-down fashion. For instance, it starts by infusing noise into data at the national level and then to the stats and then down to blocks (Santos-Lozada et al. 2020). Specific algorithms have been designed for this purpose (references). For example, the U.S. Census

TABLE 7.4: (Taken from Rao and Fan (2017)[303]): Community variable means by community cluster.

Cluster Number	Education	Median Income	Unemployed	Uninsured	Number of tracts
1	9.87	47.18	11.25	20.98	581
2	11.74	92.20	7.50	11.32	184
3	32.47	34.49	15.11	29.49	366

TABLE 7.5: (Taken from Rao and Fan (2017)[303]): Comparison of methods with respect to predictive performance with clustering. Reported measures are MSPE, squared bias, average within-tract variance, between-tract (BT) variance, true between-tract (TBT) variance.

Method	MSPE	Bias^2	Variance	BT Variance	TBT Variance
CMPI (REML) – Education	297.24	202.81	95.94	59.90	195.32
CMPI (REML) – Income	993.95	696.13	302.25	230.78	569.80
CMPI (REML) – Unemployed	40.75	35.41	5.42	4.36	34.50
CMPI (REML) – Uninsured	171.56	141.95	30.06	24.32	131.66
Random – Education	307.84	203.33	106.15	106.03	
Random – Income	1301.13	688.30	622.33	624.31	
Random – Unemployed	44.98	35.28	9.84	9.87	
Random – Uninsured	204.92	149.47	56.31	56.46	
Population Mean – Education	202.07	200.91	1.17	0	
Population Mean – Income	687.83	684.82	3.05	0	
Population Mean – Unemployed	35.37	35.27	0.10	0	
Population Mean – Uninsured	143.33	143.04	0.28	0	

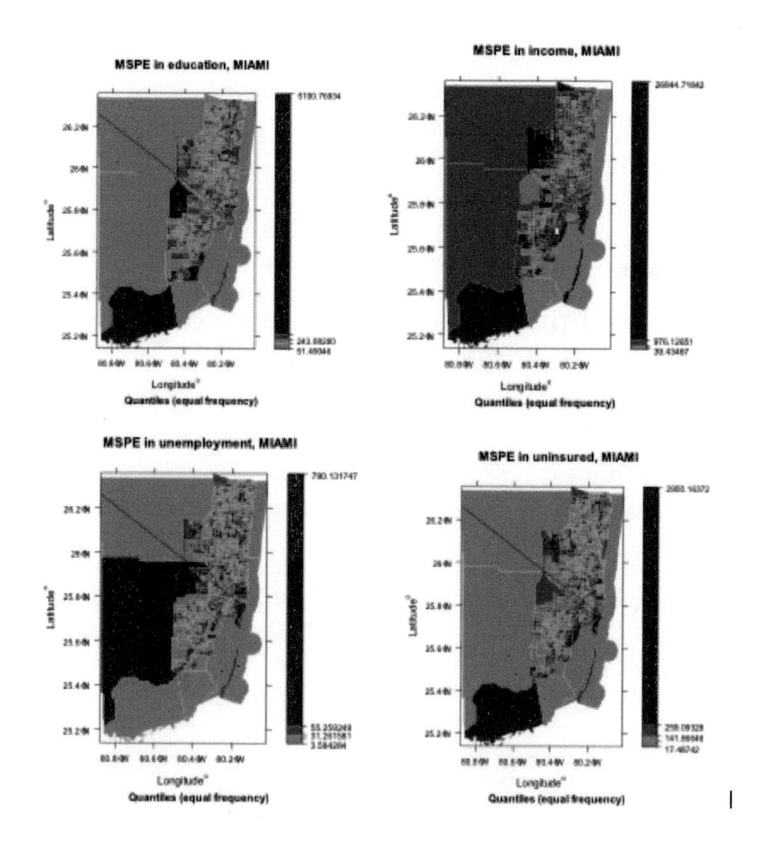

FIGURE 7.3: (Taken from Rao and Fan (2017)[303]): MSPE map for Miami-Dade county – clustered.

Bureau's disclosure avoidance system adopts a particular DP-error infusion algorithm. The Bureau released a 2010 demonstration product to allow the research community to study the utility of the census tabulations under DP errors and to evaluate the trade-offs between accuracy and privacy (reference).

One rationale given for increasing privacy concerns traces back to Title 13 of the United States Code which obliges the U.S. Census Bureau not to release data that could be re-identified (reference). The risk of re-identification has grown with the growth of research into machine learning algorithms, but to date, the success rates are still somewhat low (Santos-Lozada et al. 2020).

The dicennial census has direct implications for tracking health disparities since it's the principal source of information about the U.S. population. Even though its original intent was for political aportionment and legislative redistricting, population counts are used by every level of the federal government, and these influence the distribution of federal funds and grants and other support for local governments. Therefore, problems with census data can have downstream ripple effects in a variety of sectors. Therefore DP errors must be accounted for when estimating quantities that examine health status of populations within the country.

To examine the effect of DP errors on health disparities, Santos-Lozada *et al.* (2020)[323] carried out an empirical study where they estimated county-level population counts, overall and stratified by racial/ethnic groups. They also examined what DP-induced variability in these counts could mean for mortality rate estimates and thus an understanding of racial/ethnic disparities. Mortality rates have a numerator that comes from vital records but the denominator comes from official population counts, and these are also calculated for population subgroups. Thus DP errors could alter mortality rate estimates by altering the accuracy of the denominator quantity.

They compared estimates using the official 2010 population counts to counts under DP error infusion. They asked how county-level mortality rate estimates change for the overall population and three major racial/ethnic groups. Their results indicated high degrees of variation due to the infusion of DP noise and mortality rate estimates were significantly affected in areas with smaller populations and lower levels of urbanization, as well as those non-adjacent to a metropolitan area. Both increases and decreases in counts and mortality rates were observed but the greatest impact was on non-Hispanic Blacks and Hispanics (see Figures 7.4 – 7.5).

7.3.1 Multilevel modeling, mixed model prediction, and incorporating DP errors

DP presents a new challenge to a statistical method, such as multilevel modeling and mixed model prediction (MMP), whose purpose is to borrow strength by utilizing similarities within subpopulations. For example, MMP is widely used in small area estimation (SAE; e.g., [299]). Under a mixed effects model, data are grouped according to area-specific random effects. Here, the areas

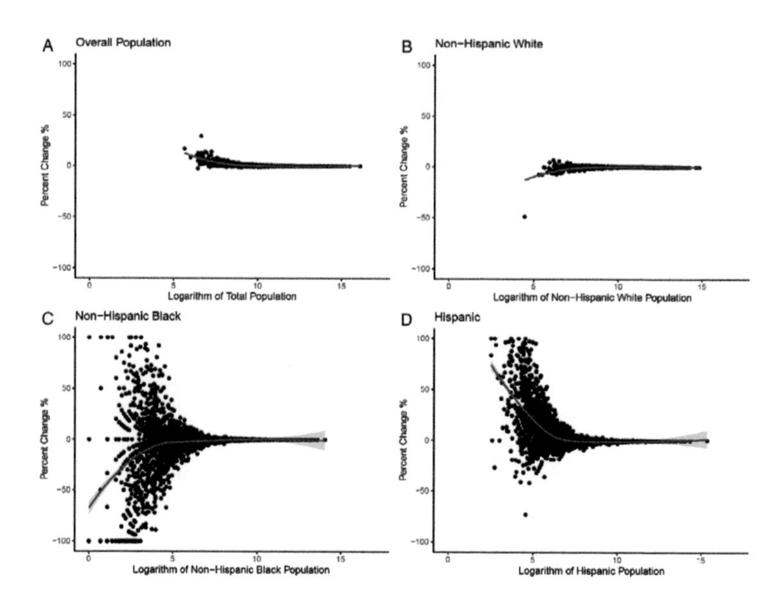

FIGURE 7.4: (Taken from Santos-Lozada et al. (2020)[323]): Differences in 2010 population count estimates with and without DP errors overall and by racial/ethnic subgroups.

may correspond to geographic subpopulations, such as counties, or demographic groups (e.g., race, gender, age-groups) within the geographic subpopulations. Data from the same areas are associated due to sharing the same random effects. This allows one to borrow strength from other areas or sources of information to gain efficiency in inference. However, if the area identities are contaminated via the DP errors, one may encounter difficulties in grouping the data, which is a basis of mixed model analysis, including MMP.

There are different scenarios, in practice, that the group identities are contaminated. Regardless of what scenario, a common feature is that there is uncertainty in an individual's group identity. For example, suppose that the group identity corresponds to a race by gender category within a county. If the group identity is accurate, one knows exactly to which group an individual belongs. However, if the group identity is not accurate [for whatever reason, intentional (e.g., DP) or unintentional (e.g., error in data entry)], the group classification may be in error.

To tackle this problem, we propose a unified approach by relaxing the accurate group identity assumption. Suppose that, in a supposedly grouped data set, each individual has a group label, say, c_n, which is observed. The true group identity, which is unobserved, is denoted by γ_n. Note that c_n is not necessarily equal to c_n. Consider γ_n as a random variable that has a pseudo prior over the possible group indexes, say, $1 \leq i \leq m$, that is, $\mathrm{P}(\gamma_\mathrm{n} =$

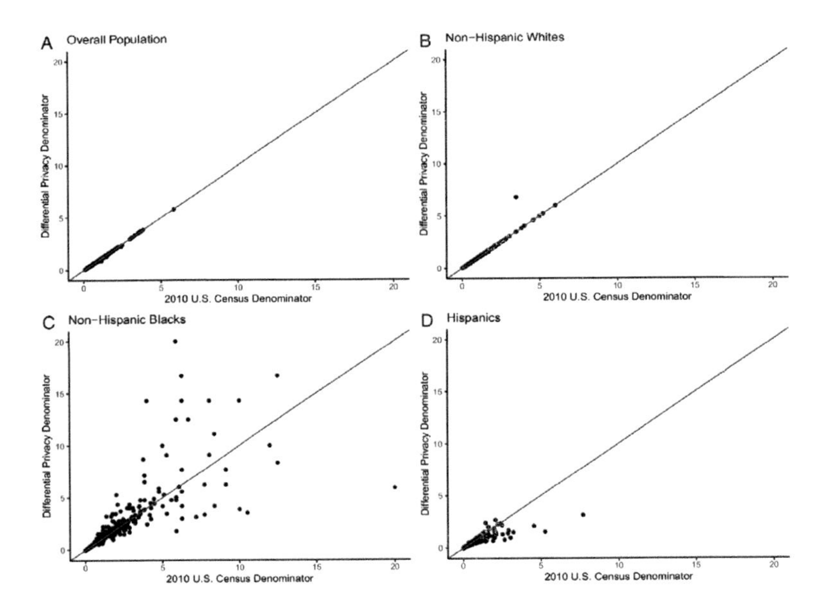

FIGURE 7.5: (Taken from Santos-Lozada et al. (2020)[323]): Differences in 2010 mortality rate estimates with and without DP errors overall and by racial/ethnic subgroups.

$i) = \pi(i), 1 \leq i \leq m$. For example, suppose that, even if the group identity is contaminated, there is still a certain probability, p, that the group label means what it means, that is, one has $\pi(i) = p$ if $i = c_n$. There is also a chance that γ_n equals to one of the indexes other than c_n, and we assume that this is evenly distributed over the other $m-1$ indexes; in other words, we have $\pi(i) = (1-p)/(m-1)$, $i \neq c_n$. In order to carry out the standard mixed model analysis [172], we propose to first find an improved group identity, for each individual, by utilizing information in the data. This is done by computing the pseudo posterior under the pseudo prior, and identifying each individual's group index by maximizing the posterior. This is similar to the Bayesian classifier [269]. Once the group identities are determined, we can carry out the standard mixed model analysis, and MMP built upon the mixed model analysis.

To have some idea about empirical performance, Ma and Jiang (2022) [227] used the pseudo-Bayesian idea to make predictions about the Facebook network. This involves a large social network data regarding Facebook users (available at http://snap.stanford.edu/data/ego-Facebook.html). A node in the network represents a user and an edge a friendship between two users. From Facebook the authors obtained user profile information and network data from 10 ego-networks, consisting of 4039 nodes and 88234 edges. For each node, feature vectors have been provided and their interpretations obscured. For instance, where the original dataset may have contained a feature "political=Democratic Party", the new data would simply contain "political=anonymized feature 1". Therefore, by using the anonymized data it is possible to determine whether two users have the same political affiliations, but not what their individual political affiliations represent. In this dataset, features are '1' if the user has this property in the profile, and '0' otherwise. The authors used a working model with $p = 0.75$, or $p = 0.95$. Because the dimension of feature vectors for each ego-network is different, and the feature value is either 0 or 1, the proportion of features with the value being 1, that is, the number of features equal to 1 divided by the dimension of feature vector, is used as a covariate. The outcome of interest is the log-transformed number of friendships, that is, the number of edges for each node. To assess the predictive performance, and its comparison with CMMP [178] and the standard regression prediction (RP), the authors randomly selected 10% of the data from each community as testing data; the remaining 90% of the data were used as training data. The testing data has size 404 and training data 3635. It is widely believed that there are 10 communities within the network associated with the Facebook data (e.g., [238, 28]). Those 10 communities were used to divide the training data into $m = 10$ groups. For the testing data, however, the community information is known, but is only used as a "prior" according to the pseudo Bayesian model. Table 4 reports the average squared prediction errors, that is, the average of the squared prediction errors over the subset of testing data according to each community for four comparing methods. The first two are the pseudo Bayesian method with $p = 0.95$ and $p = 0.75$, and the last two methods are CMMP and RP, respectively. Note that these are true prediction errors rather than simulated prediction errors.

We expect that, under suitable and, more importantly, practical conditions, methods of the standard mixed model analysis, such as the restricted maximum likelihood (REML; e.g., [172]) remain valid in that the resulting estimators of the fixed effects and variance components maintain good asymptotic properties such as consistency and asymptotic normality. As solid evidence that supports such a claim, we refer to a recent work by Ma and Jiang (2021) [227], in which a pseudo-Bayesian CMMP procedure was developed

TABLE 7.6: Average Squared Prediction Error (Proportion of Correct Matching)

Community	Size	$p = 0.75$	$p = 0.95$	CMMP	RP
1	348	0 (1)	0 (1)	0.788 (0)	0.781
2	225	0.167 (0.957)	0 (1)	1.131 (0)	0.076
3	113	0 (1)	0 (1)	0.562 (0.083)	0.364
4	171	0 (1)	0 (1)	1.036 (0.059)	0.500
5	39	0 (1)	0 (1)	0.062 (0.250)	1.441
6	1016	0.142 (0.980)	0.071 (0.991)	0.510 (0.177)	0.082
7	749	0.229 (0.973)	0.126 (0.987)	0.636 (0.640)	0.479
8	776	0 (1)	0 (1)	0.708 (0.103)	0.021
9	543	0 (1)	0 (1)	0.908 (0.111)	0.392
10	59	0 (1)	0 (1)	0 (1)	1.499

based on such a pseudo prior, It was shown that, asymptotically, the choice of the pseudo prior does not affect consistency of the group matching; neither does it affect consistency of prediction of the group mean, which is a mixed effect under a mixed effects model, under the asymptotic framework that all of the group sizes in the training data as well as in the testing data go to infinity (the number of groups in the training data needs not to go to infinity). In fact, asymptotic efficiency of the PBCMMP, both in terms of the group matching and in terms of prediction of the mixed effect, was established.

There are, however, new challenges with the DP errors. Significant differences are in terms of data size and sparsity. For example, the Census TopDown algorithm, an algorithm developed by the U. S. Census to protect privacy, is designed to handle billions of cells formed by crossing locations (National, State, County, Tract, Block Group, Block; approximately 6 million blocks), ethnicity (2 values), race (63 values), voting age (2 values), and residence type ("household" or group quarters code; 8 values). However. the majority of these cells are empty: Out of approximately 12 billion cells, there are, after all, 309 million people in the United States. A consequence of such sparseness in the data is that, in reality, the prior probability, p, needs to be very low in order to be realistic.

7.4 R software for health disparity research

While the description of statistical methods for health disparity research is important, the implementation of these methods relies on access to well-written, user-friendly, hardened software. In this section, we will focus on R software modules that are available to end users while acknowledging that other software packages can also be used. R (R Core Team 2015) is a free, non-commercial implementation of the original R language developed at AT&T Bell Laboratories based on an object-oriented, function-based approach. It's classified as a development environment and a programming language for statistics and graphics under GNU GPL-2/3 which allows it to be installed on computers without any restrictions. Typically a new release is produced each year with patches further released as necessary during that same year.

The base R system is developed by the R Core Development Team and includes base packages and recommended packages organized in one or more libraries. In addition to these packages are so-called contributed packages which allow members of the broader research community to contribute new packages implementing specialized tasks. These contributed packages are typically grouped into a series of repositories including CRAN (`http://cran.r-project.org/`), Bioconductor (Gentleman *et al.* 2004), Omega (`http://www.omegahat.org/`) and GitHub (`http://github.com`) among others.

7.4.1 Typical R software development and testing/debugging workflow

R software development typically follows the guidelines to R extensions, describing the process of creating R add-on packages, writing R documentation, R's system and foreign language interfaces, and the R API (`http://cran.r-project.org/doc/manuals/R-exts.html`). While R is an excellent tool for statistical research and exploration, it is not always the best choice for optimum run-time performance. A solution is to replace the CPU-bound portions of the program with embedded C++ code. Specialized tools, known as *profilers* can be used to identify *bottlenecks*.

Software testing typically falls into two main categories: *verification* and *validation*. On this basis, one verifies the R software by (i) producing a document that clearly and completely describes the software's expected behaviors and (ii) performing an audit to compare implemented features against those specified in the requirements document. Software validation is done by conducting *white box* testing, a standard testing procedure designed to establish the correctness of explicit logical paths through the program. Finally, integration testing is done to ensure that the package installs correctly to user platforms.

7.4.2 The need for a health disparity R research repository

Below are described individual R packages or libraries or repositories that contain modules for implementing a number of the methods described in earlier chapters. However, not all of these resources are not gathered, organized, and customized for the purposes of health disparity research. Therefore extra work is often required to perform disparity-specific analyses. Similar to the small area estimation and genomics research communities that faced similar issues and developed repositories and packages specific to their purposes, an effort for health disparities researchers should be prioritized.

7.4.3 R packages relevant to Chapter 3

sae: this package ([257]) fits small area estimation models that include the Fay-Herriot model and its extension for spatial and spatiotemporal data. Estimation methods include empirical best linear unbiased predictors (EBLUPs) and empirical best/Bayes (EB) estimates. Additionally, direct and indirect estimators can be fit in this package including the direct Horvitz-Thompson estimator of small area means, the post-stratified synthetic estimator, and the composite estimator. Corresponding estimates of mean squared errors are computed using analytical approximations or via bootstrapping ([256]). Unit level models can also be fit in this package and mean squared error estimates of EBLUPs are given by using parametric bootstrapping.

fence: this package ([192]) performs fence methods variable/model selection for linear and generalized linear mixed models. The simplified adaptive version of the fence procedure ([179]) is also implemented as well as fence methods for non-parametric models ([175]). A specific function can perform fence model selection for small area models and another function can perform invisible fence model selection ([176]) both in the linear mixed model and in more general settings. Simple extractor functions allow for the visualization of fitting results.

7.4.4 R packages relevant to Chapter 4

mediation: this package ([353]) allows investigators to conduct causal mediation analysis using either a model-based approach under a so-called standard design or a design-based approach that is appropriate under different experimental designs. For the model-based approach, the package allows estimation of average causal mediation effects (ACME) as well as other quantities of interest ([156]). It can handle linear models, generalized linear models, censored data, quantile regression, and generalized additive models (GAM). The package also allows for the assessment of treatment and mediator interactions and can handle missing data through the use of multiple imputation algorithms. Moderated mediation analysis can be carried out and even non-binary treatment variables can be analyzed. Finally, sensitivity analyses are made available in order to test sequential ignorability assumptions which are necessary for valid inference. Causal mediation analysis of multilevel data is supported in the package via use of the mixed model functions in R. For designed-based causal mediation analysis, single experiment, parallel, parallel encouragement designs, and crossover encouragement designs are supported. The comprehensive package also allows for the analysis of multiple potential mediators which could be important in identifying the mediation mechanism of primary interest. Other specific causal mediation analyses are also supported in this package.

7.4.5 R packages relevant to Chapter 5

glmnet: this package ([100]) is one of the most widely used packages in machine learning and fits generalized linear models (and related models) via penalized maximum likelihood. Possible solutions include the lasso, elastic net, relaxed lasso, and fused lasso. It can handle linear, logistic, multinomial, Poisson and Cox regression models. It can also be used to fit multi-response linear models. Optimization for regularization is done using cross-validation. The glmnet package uses cyclical coordinate descent ([98]) which iterates through an objective function one predictor at a time while keeping others fixed at their current solution until convergence. The package also efficiently restricts the active set using strong rule theory which can make for highly efficient updates and extremely quick calculation of solution paths.

spikeslab: this package ([169]) implements spike and slab regression shrinkage with high dimensional predictors. It implements the rescaled spike and slab algorithm that involves three steps: i) filtering, ii) Bayesian model averaging and iii) variable selection. The first step filters out all but the top nF variables where n is the sample size and $F > 0$ is a user-specified fraction. Filtering is done based on the absolute values of posterior means. When dealing with very high dimensional data, spikeslab uses an approximate posterior in the filtering step which allows the computational burden to be $O(np)$ operations. The second step involves fitting a rescaled spike and slab model on those variables surviving step 1. This is done using Gibbs sampling making use of a blocking strategy to improve computational times. The posterior means are estimated which are in fact, Bayesian model-averaged estimators. Step 3 performs variable selection in the form of a particular elastic net operation. The ridge regularization parameters are fixed from Step 2 and the solution path with respect to the lasso regularization parameter is determined using the lars R package ([135]). It's important to note that cross-validation is not used in the lasso optimization step because the Step 2 estimator is generally very stable. Instead, simpler AIC model selection methods can be used for optimization. The spikeslab package includes options to specify a high or lower dimensional setting with the former invoking the full three-step algorithm whereas the latter implements only Step 2 and 3 instead. The package also includes wrappers for prediction and sparse principal components spike and slab regression which can be used for multiclass high dimensional data.

keras: this is a model-level library that gives users access to other building blocks for developing deep learning models. It dovetails into an already optimized tensor libraries including TensorFlow, Theano and Microsoft Cognitive Toolkit (CNTK). Using these libraries as backends, keras can run either on CPUs or GPUs. A detailed description of the library and the various ways to set up deep learning models is described in [59].

randomforest: this package ([222]) provides an R interface to the original Fortran programs written by Breiman and Cutler for their random forest algorithm. The algorithm draws n_{tree} bootstrap samples from the original data, then grows classification or regression trees except with a modification at the splitting of each node – that is, randomly try m_{try} of the predictors and choose the best split amongst these. Predictions are then made by averaging (for regression) and majority voting (for classification) over the n_{tree} trees. The package also allows for the estimation of a less biased error rate based on out-of-bag bootstrap observations ([35]). Additional analyses can be conducted post-fitting including extraction of variable importance measures and proximity measures between any two training set observations. Random forests for survival data are implemented in the randomForestSRC package ([170]) which can also handle regression and classification settings. Various visualization tools mapped to an internet browser are also possible.

7.4.6 R packages relevant to Chapter 6

PRISM: this package (`https://github.com/yuhuilin619/prism`) fits PRISM regression models for survival outcomes. It allows for the automatic discovery of non-linear hierarchical interactions between health determinants are multiple levels. The package can conduct inference and prediction for future data. It also provides some tools for data visualization and local variable importance.

Bioconductor: this repository (which is much more comprehensive than a package), was developed for the analysis of high throughput omic data. It's statistical tools are capable of reducing massive datasets to manageable amounts of information, identifying and correcting for technological artifacts, performing rigorous inferential analyses, and analyzing designed experiments. In addition, investigators can focus their work on comprehension of genomic data in terms of reproducibility, visualization, attaching relevant biological annotation, and also in training future genomic scientists. Datasets can range from full sequencing, to microarrays to flow cytometry to proteomics to images. The repository represents a collection of connected packages developed by the Bioconductor Core and other contributors.

7.4.7 R packages relevant to Chapter 7

tidygeocoder: this package ([46]) can make the task of geocoding easier. Typically, geocoding requires an execution of an API query from which one then extracts and formats data. However, API queries can vary quite a lot resulting in wide variation in output formats. The tidygeocoder R package uses a consistent interface for a wide range of geocoding services. A tidy style dataframe format is produced that can easily be incorporated into other projects.

Bibliography

[1] *Health Canada. Toward a Healthy Future – Second Report on Healthy Canadians.* 1999.

[2] *UK Department of Health. Saving Lives: Our Healthier Nation. London: Department of Health.* 1999.

[3] Odd Aalen. Nonparametric inference for a family of counting processes. *The Annals of Statistics*, pages 701–726, 1978.

[4] Alberto Abadie and Guido Imbens. Simple and bias-corrected matching estimators for average treatment effects, 2002.

[5] J.M. Abowd. The U.S. census bureau adopts differential privacy. *Proceedings of the 24th ACM SIGKDD International Conference on Knowledge Discovery and Data Mining*, page 2867, 2018.

[6] K.V. Actkins, S. Stallings, J.S. Rao, M. Aldrich, S. Bland, P. Straub, A. Beeghly-Fadiel, J. Chavez, J. McCauley, S.T. Miller-Hughes, J. Benn-Torres, N.J. Cox, C.H. Wilkins, and L.K. Davis. Racism in the residuals: Disentangling the health effects of race and genetic ancestry in an american hospital population. technical report, Vanderbilt University. 2022.

[7] Nancy E. Adler and David H. Rehkopf. Us disparities in health: descriptions, causes, and mechanisms. *Annual Review of Public Health*, 29:235, 2008.

[8] Murray Aitkin and David Clayton. The fitting of exponential, weibull and extreme value distributions to complex censored survival data using glim. *Journal of the Royal Statistical Society: Series C (Applied Statistics)*, 29(2):156–163, 1980.

[9] William P. Alexander and Scott D. Grimshaw. Treed regression. *Journal of Computational and Graphical Statistics*, 5(2):156–175, 1996.

[10] G. Alleva, G. Arbia, P. D. Falorsi, and A. Zuliani. A sample approach to the estimation of the critical parameters of the SARS-CoV-2 epidemics: an operational design with a focus on the Italian health system. Technical report, University of Sapienza, 2020.

[11] David F. Andrews. Plots of high-dimensional data. *Biometrics*, pages 125–136, 1972.

[12] I. Andrews and M. Kazy. Identification of and correction for publication bias. *American Economic Review*, 109(8):2766–2794, 2019.

[13] S. Assari. The benefits of higher income in protecting against chronic medical conditions are smaller for African Americans than whites. *Healthcare*, 6, 2018.

[14] Zinzi D. Bailey, Nancy Krieger, Madina Agénor, Jasmine Graves, Natalia Linos, and Mary T Bassett. Structural racism and health inequities in the usa: evidence and interventions. *The Lancet*, 389(10077):1453–1463, 2017.

[15] Clare Bambra, Marcia Gibson, Amanda Sowden, Kath Wright, Margaret Whitehead, and Mark Petticrew. Tackling the wider social determinants of health and health inequalities: evidence from systematic reviews. *Journal of Epidemiology & Community Health*, 64(4):284–291, 2010.

[16] E.V. Bandera, V.S. Lee, L. Rodriguez-Rodriguez, et al. Racial/ethnic disparities in ovarian cancer treatment and survival. *Clinical Cancer Research*, 22:5909–5914, 2016.

[17] Rohosen Bandyopadhyay. *Benchmarking the observed best predictor*. University of California, Davis, 2017.

[18] Kirk Bansak and Tobias Nowacki. Effect heterogeneity and causal attribution in regression discontinuity designs. 2022.

[19] Burt S. Barnow and Arthur S. Goldberger. Institute for research on poverty. 1980.

[20] Reuben M. Baron and David A. Kenny. The moderator–mediator variable distinction in social psychological research: Conceptual, strategic, and statistical considerations. *Journal of Personality and Social Psychology*, 51(6):1173, 1986.

[21] Sanjay Basu, James H. Faghmous, and Patrick Doupe. Machine learning methods for precision medicine research designed to reduce health disparities: A structured tutorial. *Ethnicity & Disease*, 30(Suppl 1):217, 2020.

[22] Sanjay Basu, Ankita Meghani, and Arjumand Siddiqi. Evaluating the health impact of large-scale public policy changes: classical and novel approaches. *Annual Review of Public Health*, 38:351, 2017.

[23] Sanjay Basu, Hilary Kessler Seligman, Christopher Gardner, and Jay Bhattacharya. Ending snap subsidies for sugar-sweetened beverages could reduce obesity and type 2 diabetes. *Health Affairs*, 33(6):1032–1039, 2014.

[24] G. E. Battese, R. M. Harter, and W. A. Fuller. An error-components model for prediction of county crop areas using survey and satellite data. *Journal of the American Statistical Association*, 80:28–36, 1988.

[25] Andrew F. Beck, Erika M. Edwards, Jeffrey D. Horbar, Elizabeth A. Howell, Marie C. McCormick, and DeWayne M. Pursley. The color of health: how racism, segregation, and inequality affect the health and well-being of preterm infants and their families. *Pediatric Research*, 87(2):227–234, 2020.

[26] Tarik Benmarhnia, Anjum Hajat, and Jay S. Kaufman. Inferential challenges when assessing racial/ethnic health disparities in environmental research. *Environmental Health*, 20(1):1–10, 2021.

[27] Gérard Biau, Luc Devroye, and Gäbor Lugosi. Consistency of random forests and other averaging classifiers. *Journal of Machine Learning Research*, 9(9), 2008.

[28] P.J. Bickel and P. Sarkar. Hypothesis testing for automated community detection in networks. *Journal of the Royal Statistical Society B*, 78:253–273, 2016.

[29] Arlene S. Bierman, Adalsteinn D. Brown, and Carey M. Levinton. Using decision trees for measuring gender equity in the timing of angiography in patients with acute coronary syndrome: a novel approach to equity analysis. *International Journal for Equity in Health*, 14(1):1–13, 2015.

[30] Linda T. Bilheimer and Richard J. Klein. Data and measurement issues in the analysis of health disparities. *Health Services Research*, 45(5p2):1489–1507, 2010.

[31] Douglas Black. Inequalities in health. *British Medical Journal (Clinical research ed.)*, 282(6274):1468, 1981.

[32] Richard Blundell and Monica Costa Dias. Alternative approaches to evaluation in empirical microeconomics. *Portuguese Economic Journal*, 1(2):91–115, 2002.

[33] Michael Brauer, Jeff T. Zhao, Fiona B. Bennitt, and Jeffrey D. Stanaway. Global access to handwashing: implications for covid-19 control in low-income countries. *Environmental Health Perspectives*, 128(5):057005, 2020.

[34] Paula Braveman and Laura Gottlieb. The social determinants of health: it's time to consider the causes of the causes. *Public Health Reports*, 129(1_suppl2):19–31, 2014.

[35] L. Breiman. Random forests. *Machine Learning*, 45:5–32, 2001.

[36] Leo Breiman. Better subset regression using the nonnegative garrote. *Technometrics*, 37(4):373–384, 1995.

[37] Leo Breiman. Statistical modeling: The two cultures (with comments and a rejoinder by the author). *Statistical science*, 16(3):199–231, 2001.

[38] Leo Breiman, Jerome Friedman, CJ Stone, and RA Olshen. Classification and regression trees. UK ed, 1984.

[39] N.E. Breslow. Discussion of the paper by D.R. Cox. *Journal of the Royal Statistical Society: Series B (Methodological)*, 34:216–217, 1972.

[40] Arleen F. Brown, Grace X Ma, Jeanne Miranda, Eugenia Eng, Dorothy Castille, Teresa Brockie, Patricia Jones, Collins O Airhihenbuwa, Tilda Farhat, Lin Zhu, et al. Structural interventions to reduce and eliminate health disparities. *American Journal of Public Health*, 109(S1):S72–S78, 2019.

[41] John R. Brown and John L. Thornton. Percivall pott (1714–1788) and chimney sweepers' cancer of the scrotum. *British Journal of Industrial Medicine*, 14(1):68, 1957.

[42] Philip J. Brown, Marina Vannucci, and Tom Fearn. Multivariate bayesian variable selection and prediction. *Journal of the Royal Statistical Society: Series B (Statistical Methodology)*, 60(3):627–641, 1998.

[43] Heather H. Burris, Andrea A. Baccarelli, Robert O. Wright, and Rosalind J. Wright. Epigenetics: linking social and environmental exposures to preterm birth. *Pediatric Research*, 79(1):136–140, 2016.

[44] Heather H. Burris and James W. Collins Jr. Commentary: race and preterm birth-the case for epigenetic inquiry. *Ethnicity & Disease*, 20:296–299, 2010.

[45] T. Tony Cai and Jinchi Lv. Discussion: The dantzig selector: Statistical estimation when p is much larger than n. *The Annals of Statistics*, 35(6):2365–2369, 2007.

[46] Cambon, J. and Hernangomez, D. and Belanger, C. and Possenriede, D. tidygeocoder.

[47] Bradley P. Carlin and Thomas A. Louis. *Bayesian methods for data analysis*. CRC Press, 2008.

[48] Iván A. Carrillo, Jiahua Chen, and Changbao Wu. The pseudo-GEE approach to the analysis of longitudinal surveys. *Canadian Journal of Statistics*, 38(4):540–554, 2010.

[49] L. Cavalier. Nonparametric estimation of regression level sets. *Statistics*, 29:131–160, 1997.

[50] David Cesarini, Erik Lindqvist, Robert Östling, and Björn Wallace. Wealth, health, and child development: Evidence from administrative data on swedish lottery players. *The Quarterly Journal of Economics*, 131(2):687–738, 2016.

[51] Edwin Chadwick. *Report on the sanitary condition of the labouring population of Great-Britain: A supplementary report on the results of a special inquiry into the practice of interment in towns...* W. Clowes, 1843.

[52] Amitabh Chandra, Dhruv Khullar, and Thomas H. Lee. Addressing the challenge of gray-zone medicine. *The New England Journal of Medicine*, 372(3):203–205, 2015.

[53] Ranee Chatterjee, Hsin-Chieh Yeh, Tariq Shafi, Cheryl Anderson, James S. Pankow, Edgar R. Miller, David Levine, Elizabeth Selvin, and Frederick L. Brancati. Serum potassium and the racial disparity in diabetes risk: the atherosclerosis risk in communities (aric) study. *The American Journal of Clinical Nutrition*, 93(5):1087–1091, 2011.

[54] Aiyou Chen, Art B. Owen, and Minghui Shi. Data enriched linear regression. *Electronic Journal of Statistics*, 9(1):1078–1112, 2015.

[55] Senke Chen, Jiming Jiang, and Thuan Nguyen. Observed best prediction for small area counts. *Journal of Survey Statistics and Methodology*, 3(2):136–161, 2015.

[56] Nancy F. Cheng, Pamela Z. Han, and Stuart A. Gansky. Methods and software for estimating health disparities: the case of children's oral health. *American Journal of Epidemiology*, 168(8):906–914, 2008.

[57] Marshall H. Chin, Amanda R. Clarke, Robert S. Nocon, Alicia A. Casey, Anna P. Goddu, Nicole M. Keesecker, and Scott C. Cook. A roadmap and best practices for organizations to reduce racial and ethnic disparities in health care. *Journal of General Internal Medicine*, 27(8):992–1000, 2012.

[58] Hugh Chipman. Bayesian variable selection with related predictors. *Canadian Journal of Statistics*, 24(1):17–36, 1996.

[59] F. Chollet and J.J. Allair. Deep learning with R. 2018.

[60] Merlise Clyde, Heather Desimone, and Giovanni Parmigiani. Prediction via orthogonalized model mixing. *Journal of the American Statistical Association*, 91(435):1197–1208, 1996.

[61] W.G. Cochran, W.G. Cochran, and A.S. Bouclier. *Sampling Techniques*. Wiley Series in Probability and Statistics. Wiley, 1977.

[62] William G. Cochran. The effectiveness of adjustment by subclassification in removing bias in observational studies. *Biometrics*, pages 295–313, 1968.

[63] William G. Cochran and Donald B. Rubin. Controlling bias in observational studies: A review. *Sankhyā: The Indian Journal of Statistics, Series A*, pages 417–446, 1973.

[64] Paul B. Cornely. Segregation and discrimination in medical care in the united states. *American Journal of Public Health and the Nations Health*, 46(9):1074–1081, 1956.

[65] National Research Council et al. *Using the American Community Survey: benefits and challenges.* 2007.

[66] David R. Cox. Regression models and life-tables. *Journal of the Royal Statistical Society: Series B (Methodological)*, 34(2):187–202, 1972.

[67] David R. Cox. Partial likelihood. *Biometrika*, 62(2):269–276, 1975.

[68] James Franklin Crow. *An Introduction to Population Genetics Theory.* Scientific Publishers, 2017.

[69] Janet Currie. Healthy, wealthy, and wise: Socioeconomic status, poor health in childhood, and human capital development. *Journal of EconomIc Literature*, 47(1):87–122, 2009.

[70] G. Datta and P. Lahiri. Discussions on a paper by efron and gous, in *model selection (P. Lahiri ed.). IMS Lecture Notes/Monograph*, 38:249–254, 2001.

[71] Gauri Datta, Aurore Delaigle, Peter Hall, and Li Wang. Semi-parametric prediction intervals in small areas when auxiliary data are measured with error. *Statistica Sinica*, 28(4):2309–2335, 2018.

[72] Gauri S. Datta. Model-based approach to small area estimation. *Handbook of Statistics*, 29:251–288, 2009.

[73] Matthew A Davis, Cui Guo, Ketlyne Sol, Kenneth M. Langa, and Brahmajee K. Nallamothu. Trends and disparities in the number of self-reported healthy older adults in the united states, 2000 to 2014. *JAMA Internal Medicine*, 177(11):1683–1684, 2017.

[74] Angus Deaton. Policy implications of the gradient of health and wealth. *Health Affairs*, 21(2):13–30, 2002.

[75] D.A. Díaz-Pachón and J.S. Rao. A simple correction for COVID-19 sampling bias. *Journal of Theoretical Biology*, 512(7):110556, 2021.

[76] Ana V. Diez-Roux. Multilevel analysis in public health research. *Annual Review of Public Health*, 21(1):171–192, 2000.

[77] P.J. Diggle. Estimating prevalence using an imperfect test. *Epidemiology Research International*, page 608719, 2011.

[78] Annette J. Dobson and Adrian G. Barnett. *An introduction to generalized linear models*. Chapman and Hall/CRC, 2018.

[79] Ensheng Dong, Hongru Du, and Lauren Gardner. An interactive web-based dashboard to track COVID-19 in real time. *The Lancet Infectious Diseases*, 2020.

[80] Nianbo Dong, Benjamin Kelcey, and Jessaca Spybrook. Identifying and estimating causal moderation for treated and targeted subgroups. *Multivariate Behavioral Research*, 1–20, 2022, https://doi.org/10/1080/00273171.2022.2046997.

[81] David Donoho. 50 years of data science. *Journal of Computational and Graphical Statistics*, 26(4):745–766, 2017.

[82] Pan Du, Xiao Zhang, Chiang-Ching Huang, Nadereh Jafari, Warren A. Kibbe, Lifang Hou, and Simon M Lin. Comparison of beta-value and m-value methods for quantifying methylation levels by microarray analysis. *BMC Bioinformatics*, 11(1):587, 2010.

[83] Mark R. Duffy, Tai-Ho Chen, W. Thane Hancock, Ann M. Powers, Jacob L. Kool, Robert S. Lanciotti, Moses Pretrick, Maria Marfel, Stacey Holzbauer, Christine Dubray, et al. Zika virus outbreak on yap island, federated states of micronesia. *New England Journal of Medicine*, 360(24):2536–2543, 2009.

[84] David B. Dunson. Commentary: practical advantages of bayesian analysis of epidemiologic data. *American Journal of Epidemiology*, 153(12):1222–1226, 2001.

[85] Laura Dwyer-Lindgren, Parkes Kendrick, Yekaterina O. Kelly, Dillon O. Sylte, Chris Schmidt, Brigette F. Blacker, Farah Daoud, Amal A. Abdi, Mathew Baumann, Farah Mouhanna, et al. Life expectancy by county, race, and ethnicity in the USA, 2000–19: a systematic analysis of health disparities. *The Lancet*, 400(10345):25–38, 2022.

[86] Lynn E. Eberly and George Casella. Estimating bayesian credible intervals. *Journal of Statistical Planning and Inference*, 112(1-2):115–132, 2003.

[87] Lynn E. Eberly, Kristen Cunanan, Olga Gurvich, Kay Savik, Donna Z. Bliss, and Jean F. Wyman. Statistical approaches to assessing health and healthcare disparities. *Research in Nursing & Health*, 38(6):500–508, 2015.

[88] Lynn E. Eberly, James S. Hodges, Kay Savik, Olga Gurvich, Donna Z. Bliss, and Christine Mueller. Extending the Peters–Belson approach for assessing disparities to right censored time-to-event outcomes. *Statistics in Medicine*, 32(23):4006–4020, 2013.

[89] Bradley Efron. The efficiency of cox's likelihood function for censored data. *Journal of the American Statistical Association*, 72(359):557–565, 1977.

[90] Bradley Efron and Robert J. Tibshirani. *An Introduction to the Bootstrap*. CRC press, 1994.

[91] L. El Khoury, T. Gorrie-Stone, M. Smart, et al. Properties of the epigenetic clock. *bioRxiv preprint; doi: http://dx.doi.org/10.1101/363143*, 2018.

[92] Jianqing Fan and Runze Li. Variable selection via nonconcave penalized likelihood and its oracle properties. *Journal of the American Statistical Association*, 96(456):1348–1360, 2001.

[93] Jianqing Fan and Jinchi Lv. Sure independence screening for ultrahigh dimensional feature space. *Journal of the Royal Statistical Society: Series B (Statistical Methodology)*, 70(5):849–911, 2008.

[94] Segun Fatumo, Tinashe Chikowore, Ananyo Choudhury, Muhammad Ayub, Alicia R. Martin, and Karoline Kuchenbaecker. A roadmap to increase diversity in genomic studies. *Nature Medicine*, 28(2):243–250, 2022.

[95] Robert E. Fay III and Roger A. Herriot. Estimates of income for small places: an application of James-Stein procedures to census data. *Journal of the American Statistical Association*, 74(366a):269–277, 1979.

[96] National Center for Health Statistics (US) and National Center for Health Services Research. *Health, United States, 1983*. US Department of Health, Education, and Welfare, Public Health Service, 1994.

[97] Giuliano Franco and Francesca Franco. Bernardino ramazzini: the father of occupational medicine. *American Journal of Public Health*, 91(9):1382–1382, 2001.

[98] J. Friedman, T. Hastie, and R. Tibshirani. Regularization paths for generalized linear models via coordinate descent. *Journal of Statistical Software*, 33:1–22, 2010.

[99] J.H. Friedman, T. Hastie, and R. Tibshirani. *The elements of statistical learning: data mining, inference, and prediction*, volume 2. Springer, 2009.

[100] J. Friedman, T. Hastie, R. Tibshirani, B. Narasimhan, K. Tay, N. Simon, and J. Qian (2021). Package 'glmnet'. CRAN R Repositary.

[101] Emmanuela Gakidou and Gary King. Death by survey: estimating adult mortality without selection bias from sibling survival data. *Demography*, 43(3):569–585, 2006.

[102] N. Ganesh. Simultaneous credible intervals for small area estimation problems. *Journal of Multivariate Analysis*, 100(8):1610–1621, 2009.

[103] Joseph L. Gastwirth. A graphical summary of disparities in health care and related summary measures. *Journal of Statistical Planning and Inference*, 137(3):1059–1065, 2007.

[104] Gilbert C. Gee and Chandra L. Ford. Structural racism and health inequities: Old issues, new directions1. *Du Bois review: social science research on race*, 8(1):115–132, 2011.

[105] Andrew Gelman, John B. Carlin, Hal S. Stern, and Donald B. Rubin. *Bayesian data analysis*. Chapman and Hall/CRC, 1995.

[106] Edward I. George and Robert E. McCulloch. Variable selection via gibbs sampling. *Journal of the American Statistical Association*, 88(423):881–889, 1993.

[107] John Geweke and Richard Meese. Estimating regression models of finite but unknown order. *International Economic Review*, pages 55–70, 1981.

[108] Malay Ghosh and Parthasarathi Lahiri. Robust empirical bayes estimation of means from stratified samples. *Journal of the American Statistical Association*, 82(400):1153–1162, 1987.

[109] Malay Ghosh, Kannan Natarajan, TWF Stroud, and Bradley P. Carlin. Generalized linear models for small-area estimation. *Journal of the American Statistical Association*, 93(441):273–282, 1998.

[110] Malay Ghosh and JNK1278679 Rao. Small area estimation: an appraisal. *Statistical Science*, 9(1):55–76, 1994.

[111] David Buil Gil. *Small area estimation in criminological research: Theory, methods, and applications*. PhD thesis, University of Manchester, 2020.

[112] Corrado Gini. Measurement of inequality of incomes. *The Economic Journal*, 31(121):124–126, 1921.

[113] V.P. Godambe. A unified theory of sampling from finite populations. *Journal of the Royal Statistical Society: Series B (Methodological)*, 17(2):269–278, 1955.

[114] V.P. Godambe. A review of the contributions towards a unified theory of sampling from finite populations. *Revue de l'Institut International de Statistique*, pages 242–258, 1965.

[115] V.P. Godambe. A reply to my critics. *Sankhya Ser. C*, 37:53–76, 1975.

[116] Hüseyin Göksel, David R. Judkins, and William D. Mosher. Nonresponse adjustments for a telephone follow-up to a national in-person survey. *Journal of Official Statistics-Stockholm*, 8:417–417, 1992.

[117] Harvey Goldstein and David J. Spiegelhalter. League tables and their limitations: statistical issues in comparisons of institutional performance. *Journal of the Royal Statistical Society: Series A (Statistics in Society)*, 159(3):385–409, 1996.

[118] A. Gotovos, N. Casati, G. Hitz, and A. Krause. Active learning for level set estimation. *Technical report*, 2013.

[119] B.I. Graubard, R. Sowmya Rao, and Joseph L. Gastwirth. Using the Peters–Belson method to measure health care disparities from complex survey data. *Statistics in Medicine*, 24(17):2659–2668, 2005.

[120] Alastair McIntosh Gray. Inequalities in health. the black report: a summary and comment. *International Journal of Health Services*, 12(3):349–380, 1982.

[121] S. Greenland. Basic methods for sensitivity analysis of biases. *International Journal of Epidemiology*, 25(6):1107–1116, 1996.

[122] Baptiste Gregorutti, Bertrand Michel, and Philippe Saint-Pierre. Correlation and variable importance in random forests. *Statistics and Computing*, 27(3):659–678, 2017.

[123] Samuel M. Gross and Robert Tibshirani. Data shared lasso: A novel tool to discover uplift. *Computational Statistics & Data Analysis*, 101:226–235, 2016.

[124] Kishore Guda, Martina L. Veigl, Vinay Varadan, Arman Nosrati, Lakshmeswari Ravi, James Lutterbaugh, Lydia Beard, James KV Willson, W David Sedwick, Zhenghe John Wang, et al. Novel recurrently mutated genes in African American colon cancers. *Proceedings of the National Academy of Sciences*, 112(4):1149–1154, 2015.

[125] Jinyong Hahn. On the role of the propensity score in efficient semiparametric estimation of average treatment effects. *Econometrica*, 66:315–331, 1998.

[126] Peter Hall and Tapabrata Maiti. On parametric bootstrap methods for small area prediction. *Journal of the Royal Statistical Society: Series B (Statistical Methodology)*, 68(2):221–238, 2006.

[127] Rita Hamad and David H. Rehkopf. Poverty, pregnancy, and birth outcomes: a study of the earned income tax credit. *Paediatric and Perinatal Epidemiology*, 29(5):444–452, 2015.

[128] Noah Hammarlund. Racial treatment disparities after machine learning surgical risk-adjustment. *Health Services and Outcomes Research Methodology*, 21(2):248–286, 2021.

[129] Heidi A. Hanson, Christopher Martin, Brock O'Neil, Claire L. Leiser, Erik N. Mayer, Ken R. Smith, and William T. Lowrance. The relative importance of race compared to health care and social factors in predicting prostate cancer mortality: a random forest approach. *The Journal of Urology*, 202(6):1209–1216, 2019.

[130] Sam Harper and John Lynch. Methods for measuring cancer disparities: using data relevant to healthy people 2010 cancer-related objectives. Technical report, 2005.

[131] Sam Harper and John Lynch. Methods for measuring cancer disparities: using data relevant to healthy people 2010 cancer-related objectives. 2010.

[132] Frank E. Harrell, Robert M. Califf, David B. Pryor, Kerry L. Lee, and Robert A. Rosati. Evaluating the yield of medical tests. *JAMA*, 247(18):2543–2546, 1982.

[133] T. Hastie and R.J. Tibshirani. *Generalized Additive Models*. CRC Press, London, 1990.

[134] Trevor Hastie and Robert Tibshirani. Varying-coefficient models. *Journal of the Royal Statistical Society: Series B (Methodological)*, 55(4):757–779, 1993.

[135] T. Hastie, B. Efron (2007). lars: Least Angle Regression, Lasso and Forward Stagewise. URL http://www-stat.stanford.edu/hastie/Papers/LARS. R package version 0.9-7.

[136] M.B. Hawes. Implementing differential privacy: Seven lessons from the 2020 United States Census. *Harvard Data Science Review*, DOI: 10.1162/99608f92.353c6f99, 2020.

[137] Andrew F. Hayes. Partial, conditional, and moderated mediation: Quantification, inference, and interpretation. *Communication Monographs*, 85(1):4–40, 2018.

[138] James J. Heckman and V. Joseph Hotz. Choosing among alternative nonexperimental methods for estimating the impact of social programs: The case of manpower training. *Journal of the American Statistical Association*, 84(408):862–874, 1989.

[139] James J. Heckman, Hidehiko Ichimura, and Petra Todd. Matching as an econometric evaluation estimator. *The Review of Economic Studies*, 65(2):261–294, 1998.

[140] James J. Heckman, Hidehiko Ichimura, and Petra E. Todd. Matching as an econometric evaluation estimator: Evidence from evaluating a job training programme. *The review of economic studies*, 64(4):605–654, 1997.

[141] James J. Heckman and Edward Vytlacil. Causal parameters, structural equations, treatment effects and randomized evaluations of social programs. *Manuscript, Univeristy of Chicago*, 2000.

[142] Luiz Hespanhol, Caio Sain Vallio, Lucíola Menezes Costa, and Bruno T. Saragiotto. Understanding and interpreting confidence and credible intervals around effect estimates. *Brazilian Journal of Physical Therapy*, 23(4):290–301, 2019.

[143] Robert A. Hiatt and Nancy Breen. The social determinants of cancer: a challenge for transdisciplinary science. *American Journal of Preventive Medicine*, 35(2):S141–S150, 2008.

[144] Sam Hill and Thomas Chalaux. Improving access and quality in the indian education system. 2011.

[145] Keisuke Hirano, Guido W. Imbens, and Geert Ridder. Efficient estimation of average treatment effects using the estimated propensity score. *Econometrica*, 71(4):1161–1189, 2003.

[146] Arthur E. Hoerl and Robert W. Kennard. Ridge regression: applications to nonorthogonal problems. *Technometrics*, 12(1):69–82, 1970.

[147] Arthur E. Hoerl and Robert W. Kennard. Ridge regression: Biased estimation for nonorthogonal problems. *Technometrics*, 12(1):55–67, 1970.

[148] S. Horvath. DNA methylation age of human tissues and cell types. *Genome Biology*, 14::3156, 2013.

[149] Daniel G. Horvitz and Donovan J. Thompson. A generalization of sampling without replacement from a finite universe. *Journal of the American Statistical Association*, 47(260):663–685, 1952.

[150] George Howard, Roger T. Anderson, Gregory Russell, Virginia J. Howard, and Gregory L. Burke. Race, socioeconomic status, and cause-specific mortality. *Annals of Epidemiology*, 10(4):214–223, 2000.

[151] Hilary Hoynes, Doug Miller, and David Simon. Income, the earned income tax credit, and infant health. *American Economic Journal: Economic Policy*, 7(1):172–211, 2015.

[152] Hui Hu, Hong Xiao, Yi Zheng, and Bo Bonnie Yu. A bayesian spatio-temporal analysis on racial disparities in hypertensive disorders of pregnancy in florida, 2005–2014. *Spatial and Spatio-temporal Epidemiology*, 29:43–50, 2019.

[153] E.H. Ibfelt, S.K. Kjaer, C. Høgdall, M. Steding-Jessen, T.K. Kjaer, M. Osler, C. Johansen, K. Frederiksen, and S.O. Dalton. 'socioeconomic position and survival after cervical cancer: influence of cancer stage, comorbidity and smoking among danish women diagnosed between 2005 and 2010. *British Journal of Cancer*, 109(9):2489–2495, 2013.

[154] John Iceland, Daniel H. Weinberg, and Erika Steinmetz. Racial and ethnic residential segregation in the united states. *Census Special Reports: US Census Bureau*, 2002.

[155] John Iceland, Daniel H. Weinberg, and Erika Steinmetz. *Racial and ethnic residential segregation in the United States 1980-2000*, volume 8. Bureau of Census, 2002.

[156] K. Imai, L. Keele, and D. Tingley. A general approach to causal mediation analysis. *Psychological Methods*, 15:309–334, 2010.

[157] Guido W. Imbens. Nonparametric estimation of average treatment effects under exogeneity: A review. *Review of Economics and Statistics*, 86(1):4–29, 2004.

[158] Benjamin Isaac. The invention of racism in classical antiquity. In *The Invention of Racism in Classical Antiquity*. Princeton University Press, 2013.

[159] H. Ishwaran and J. Rao. Decision trees, advanced techniques in constructing. *Encyclopedia of Medical Decision Making. London, UK: SAGE Publishing*, pages 328–332, 2009.

[160] Hemant Ishwaran. Variable importance in binary regression trees and forests. *Electronic Journal of Statistics*, 1:519–537, 2007.

[161] Hemant Ishwaran and Udaya B Kogalur. Consistency of random survival forests. *Statistics & Probability Letters*, 80(13-14):1056–1064, 2010.

[162] Hemant Ishwaran and Min Lu. Standard errors and confidence intervals for variable importance in random forest regression, classification, and survival. *Statistics in Medicine*, 38(4):558–582, 2019.

[163] Hemant Ishwaran and J. Sunil Rao. Detecting differentially expressed genes in microarrays using bayesian model selection. *Journal of the American Statistical Association*, 98(462):438–455, 2003.

[164] Hemant Ishwaran and J. Sunil Rao. Spike and slab gene selection for multigroup microarray data. *Journal of the American Statistical Association*, 100(471):764–780, 2005.

[165] Hemant Ishwaran and J. Sunil Rao. Spike and slab variable selection: frequentist and bayesian strategies. *The Annals of Statistics*, 33(2):730–773, 2005.

[166] Hemant Ishwaran and J. Sunil Rao. Decision tree: introduction – in encyclopedia of medical decision making. 2009.

[167] Hemant Ishwaran and J. Sunil Rao. Generalized ridge regression: Geometry and computational solutions. *Technical report, Division of Biostatistics, University of Miami*, 2010.

[168] Hemant Ishwaran and J. Sunil Rao. Geometry and properties of generalized ridge regression in high dimensions. *Contemporary Mathematics*, 622:81–93, 2014.

[169] Ishwaran, H. Spikeslab.

[170] Ishwaran H. and Kogalur U.B.K. randomforestsrc.

[171] Neal Jeffries, Alan M. Zaslavsky, Ana V. Diez Roux, John W. Creswell, Richard C. Palmer, Steven E. Gregorich, James D. Reschovsky, Barry I. Graubard, Kelvin Choi, Ruth M. Pfeiffer, et al. Methodological approaches to understanding causes of health disparities. *American Journal of Public Health*, 109(S1):S28–S33, 2019.

[172] J. Jiang. Conditional inference about generalized linear mixed models. *Annals of Statistics*, 27:1974–2007, 1999.

[173] J. Jiang. *Linear and Generalized Linear Mixed Models and Their Applications.* Springer-Verlag, New York, 2008.

[174] J. Jiang, H. Jia, and H. Chen. Maximum posterior estimation of random effects in generalized linear mixed models. *Statist. Sinica*, 11:97–120, 2001.

[175] J. Jiang, T. Nguyen, and J.S. Rao. Fence methods for nonparametric small area estimation. *Survey Methodology*, 36:3–11, 2010.

[176] J. Jiang, T. Nguyen, and J.S. Rao. Invisible fence methods and the identification of differentially expressed gene sets. *Statistics and Its Interface*, 4:403–415, 2011.

[177] J. Jiang, T. Nguyen, and J.S. Rao. Observed best prediction via nested-error regression with potentially misspecified mean and variance. *Survey Methodology*, 41:37–45, 2015.

[178] J. Jiang, J. S. Rao, J. Fan, and T. Nguyen. Classified mixed model prediction. *Journal of the American Statistical Association*, 113:269–279, 2018.

[179] J. Jiang, J.S. Rao, Z. Gu, and T. Nguyen. Fence methods for mixed model selection. *Annals of Statistics*, 36:1669–1692, 2008.

[180] Jiming Jiang. Empirical best prediction for small-area inference based on generalized linear mixed models. *Journal of Statistical Planning and Inference*, 111(1-2):117–127, 2003.

[181] Jiming Jiang. *Asymptotic analysis of mixed effects models: theory, applications, and open problems*. Chapman and Hall/CRC, 2017.

[182] Jiming Jiang and P. Lahiri. Empirical best prediction for small area inference with binary data. *Annals of the Institute of Statistical Mathematics*, 53(2):217–243, 2001.

[183] Jiming Jiang, P. Lahiri, and Thuan Nguyen. A unified Monte-Carlo jackknife for small area estimation after model selection. *arXiv preprint arXiv:1602.05238*, 2016.

[184] Jiming Jiang and Partha Lahiri. Mixed model prediction and small area estimation. *Test*, 15(1):1–96, 2006.

[185] Jiming Jiang, Partha Lahiri, and Shu-Mei Wan. A unified jackknife theory for empirical best prediction with M-estimation. *The Annals of Statistics*, 30(6):1782–1810, 2002.

[186] Jiming Jiang and Thuan Nguyen. Comments on: Goodness-of-fit tests in mixed models. *Test*, 18(2):248, 2009.

[187] Jiming Jiang, Thuan Nguyen, and J. Sunil Rao. A simplified adaptive fence procedure. *Statistics & Probability Letters*, 79(5):625–629, 2009.

[188] Jiming Jiang, Thuan Nguyen, and J. Sunil Rao. Best predictive small area estimation. *Journal of the American Statistical Association*, 106(494):732–745, 2011.

[189] Jiming Jiang and J. Sunil Rao. Robust small area estimation: An overview. *Annual Review of Statistics and Its Application*, 7, 2020.

[190] Jiming Jiang and Mahmoud Torabi. Sumca: simple, unified, monte-carlo-assisted approach to second-order unbiased mean-squared prediction error estimation. *Journal of the Royal Statistical Society: Series B (Statistical Methodology)*, 82(2):467–485, 2020.

[191] Jiming Jiang and Weihong Zhang. Robust estimation in generalised linear mixed models. *Biometrika*, 88(3):753–765, 2001.

[192] Jiang, J., Zhao, J., Rao, J. S., Nguyen, T., & Nguyen, M. T. (2017). Package 'fence'. URL: https://cran.r-project.org/web/packages/fence/index.html, version 1.0.

[193] Kevin B. Johnson, Wei-Qi Wei, Dilhan Weeraratne, Mark E. Frisse, Karl Misulis, Kyu Rhee, Juan Zhao, and Jane L. Snowdon. Precision medicine, AI, and the future of personalized health care. *Clinical and Translational Science*, 14(1):86–93, 2021.

[194] Charles M. Judd and David A. Kenny. Process analysis: Estimating mediation in treatment evaluations. *Evaluation Review*, 5(5):602–619, 1981.

[195] John D. Kalbfleisch and Ross L. Prentice. *The statistical analysis of failure time data*. John Wiley & Sons, 2011.

[196] Edward L. Kaplan and Paul Meier. Nonparametric estimation from incomplete observations. *Journal of the American Statistical Association*, 53(282):457–481, 1958.

[197] Robert E. Kass and Duane Steffey. Approximate bayesian inference in conditionally independent hierarchical models (parametric empirical bayes models). *Journal of the American Statistical Association*, 84(407):717–726, 1989.

[198] Jay S. Kaufman. Commentary: Raceritual, regression, and reality. *Epidemiology*, 25(4):485–487, 2014.

[199] Benjamin D. Killeen, Jie Ying Wu, Kinjal Shah, Anna Zapaishchykova, Philipp Nikutta, Aniruddha Tamhane, Shreya Chakraborty, Jinchi Wei, Tiger Gao, Mareike Thies, and Mathias Unberath. A County-level Dataset for Informing the United States' Response to COVID-19. April 2020.

[200] E.M. Kitagawa and P.M. Hauser. *Differential mortality in the United States: A study of socioeconomic epidemiology*. Harvard University Press, 1973.

[201] Phillip S. Kott. Robust small domain estimation using random effects modeling. *Survey Methodology*, 15:3, 1989.

[202] N. Krieger, J.T. Chen, P.D. Waterman, M.J. Soobader, and S.V. Subramanian. Monitoring socioeconomic inequalities in sexually transmitted infections, tuberculosis, and violence: geocoding and choice of area-based socioeconomic measures - the public health disparities geocoding project (us). *Public Health Reports*, 118:240–260, 2003.

[203] N. Krieger, J.T. Chen, P.D. Waterman, M.J. Soobader, S.V. Subramanian, and R. Carson. Geocoding and monitoring of us socioeconomic inequalities in mortality and cancer incidence: does the choice of area-based measure and geographic level matter? *American Journal of Epidemiology*, 156:471–482, 2002.

[204] N. Krieger, P.D. Waterman, J.T. Chen, D.H. Rehkopf, and S.V. Subramanian. *The Public Health Disparities Geocoding Project Monograph*. 2004.

[205] Nancy Krieger. Commentary: On the causal interpretation of race by vanderweele and robinson. *Epidemiology (Cambridge, Mass.)*, 25(6):937, 2014.

[206] Nancy Krieger. Discrimination and health inequities. *International Journal of Health Services*, 44(4):643–710, 2014.

[207] Nancy Krieger, Jarvis T. Chen, Brent A. Coull, Jason Beckfield, Mathew V. Kiang, and Pamela D. Waterman. Jim crow and premature mortality among the us black and white population, 1960–2009: an age–period–cohort analysis. *Epidemiology (Cambridge, Mass.)*, 25(4):494, 2014.

[208] Anton E. Kunst and Johan P. Mackenbach. The size of mortality differences associated with educational level in nine industrialized countries. *American Journal of Public Health*, 84(6):932–937, 1994.

[209] Lynn Kuo and Bani Mallick. Variable selection for regression models. *Sankhyā: The Indian Journal of Statistics, Series B*, 65–81, 1998.

[210] P. Lahiri and J.N.K Rao. Robust estimation of mean squared error of small area estimators. *Journal of the American Statistical Association*, 90(430):758–766, 1995.

[211] Latrice G. Landry, Nadya Ali, David R. Williams, Heidi L. Rehm, and Vence L. Bonham. Lack of diversity in genomic databases is a barrier to translating precision medicine research into practice. *Health Affairs*, 37(5):780–785, 2018.

[212] M. LeBlanc, J. Moon, and C. Kooperberg. Extreme regression. *Biostatistics*, 7:71–84, 2016.

[213] Michael LeBlanc and John Crowley. Survival trees by goodness of split. *Journal of the American Statistical Association*, 88(422):457–467, 1993.

[214] Michael Lechner. Earnings and employment effects of continuous off-the-job training in east germany after unification. *Journal of Business & Economic Statistics*, 17(1):74–90, 1999.

[215] Yann LeCun, D. Touresky, G. Hinton, and T. Sejnowski. A theoretical framework for back-propagation. In *Proceedings of the 1988 Connectionist Models Summer School*, 21–28, 1988.

[216] Fred B. Lempers. Posterior probabilities of alternative linear models. 1971.

[217] Cindy W. Leung, Eric L. Ding, Paul J. Catalano, Eduardo Villamor, Eric B. Rimm, and Walter C. Willett. Dietary intake and dietary quality of low-income adults in the supplemental nutrition assistance program. *The American Journal of Clinical Nutrition*, 96(5):977–988, 2012.

[218] Tama Leventhal and Jeanne Brooks-Gunn. Moving to opportunity: an experimental study of neighborhood effects on mental health. *American Journal of Public Health*, 93(9):1576–1582, 2003.

[219] Y. Li, B.I. Graubard, P. Huang, and J.L. Gastwirth. Extension of the Peters–Belson method to estimate health disparities among multiple groups using logistic regression with survey data. *Statistics in Medicine*, 34(4):595–612, 2015.

[220] Yan Li, Mandi Yu, and Jonathan Zhang. Statistical inference on health disparity indices for complex surveys. *American Journal of Epidemiology*, 187(11):2460–2469, 2018.

[221] K.Y. Liang and S.L. Zeger. Longitudinal data analysis using generalized linear models. *Biometrika*, 73:13–22, 1986.

[222] Liaw, M. A. (2018). Package 'randomforest'. University of California, Berkeley: Berkeley, CA, USA. URL: https://cran.r-project.org/web/packages/randomForest/index.html version 4.7-1.1

[223] Mary J. Lindstrom and Douglas M. Bates. Nonlinear mixed effects models for repeated measures data. *Biometrics*, pages 673–687, 1990.

[224] Markus Loecher. Unbiased variable importance for random forests. *Communications in Statistics-Theory and Methods*, 51(5):1413–1425, 2022.

[225] Wei-Yin Loh. Regression tress with unbiased variable selection and interaction detection. *Statistica Sinica*, pages 361–386, 2002.

[226] Mette Lise Lousdal. An introduction to instrumental variable assumptions, validation and estimation. *Emerging Themes in Epidemiology*, 15(1):1–7, 2018.

[227] H. Ma and J. Jiang. Pseudo-Bayesian classified mixed model prediction. *Journal of the American Statistical Association*, page DOI: 10.1080/01621459.2021.2008944, 2022.

[228] X. Ma, Y. Wang, Zhang M.Q., and Gazdar A.F. DNA methylation data analysis and its application to cancer research. *Epigenomics*, 5:301–316, 2013.

[229] David P. MacKinnon and Linda J. Luecken. How and for whom? mediation and moderation in health psychology. *Health Psychology*, 27(2S):S99, 2008.

[230] David P. MacKinnon, Matthew J. Valente, and Oscar Gonzalez. The correspondence between causal and traditional mediation analysis: The link is the mediator by treatment interaction. *Prevention Science*, 21(2):147–157, 2020.

[231] Adyasha Maharana and Elaine Okanyene Nsoesie. Use of deep learning to examine the association of the built environment with prevalence of neighborhood adult obesity. *JAMA Network Open*, 1(4):e181535–e181535, 2018.

[232] Teri A. Manolio. Using the data we have: improving diversity in genomic research. *The American Journal of Human Genetics*, 105(2):233–236, 2019.

[233] Alejandro Mantero. *Unsupervised Random Forests and Target Outcomes Relationship Exploration*. PhD thesis, University of Miami, 2018.

[234] Yolanda Marhuenda, Isabel Molina, and Domingo Morales. Small area estimation with spatio-temporal Fay–Herriot models. *Computational Statistics & Data Analysis*, 58:308–325, 2013.

[235] Sara Markowitz, Kelli A. Komro, Melvin D. Livingston, Otto Lenhart, and Alexander C. Wagenaar. Effects of state-level earned income tax credit laws in the us on maternal health behaviors and infant health outcomes. *Social Science & Medicine*, 194:67–75, 2017.

[236] Michael Marmot and Richard Wilkinson. *Social determinants of health*. Oup Oxford, 2005.

[237] Edwin P. Martens, Wiebe R. Pestman, Anthonius de Boer, Svetlana V. Belitser, and Olaf H. Klungel. Instrumental variables: application and limitations. *Epidemiology*, pages 260–267, 2006.

[238] J. McAuley and J. Leskovec. Learning to discover social circles in ego networks. *NIPS*, 1:539–547, 2012.

[239] Kelly McConville. *Improved estimation for complex surveys using modern regression techniques*. PhD thesis, Colorado State University, 2011.

[240] Kelly S. McConville, F. Jay Breidt, Thomas Lee, and Gretchen G. Moisen. Model-assisted survey regression estimation with the lasso. *Journal of Survey Statistics and Methodology*, 5(2):131–158, 2017.

[241] Denise Eileen McCoskey. *Race: Antiquity and its legacy*. Bloomsbury Publishing, 2021.

[242] Peter McCullagh and John A. Nelder. *Generalized linear models*. Routledge, 2019.

[243] Warren S. McCulloch and Walter Pitts. A logical calculus of the ideas immanent in nervous activity. *The Bulletin of Mathematical Biophysics*, 5(4):115–133, 1943.

[244] Richard McElreath. *Statistical rethinking: A Bayesian course with examples in R and Stan*. Chapman and Hall/CRC, 2020.

[245] Sara L. McLafferty. Gis and health care. *Annual Review of Public Health*, 24(1):25–42, 2003.

[246] Simon Medcalfe, Catherine P. Slade, and Divesia Lee. Racial segregation as a social determinant of health: Evidence from the state of georgia. *Journal of the Georgia Public Health Association*, 8(1):32–40, 2020.

[247] Nicolai Meinshausen and Greg Ridgeway. Quantile regression forests. *Journal of Machine Learning Research*, 7(6), 2006.

[248] Guillermo Mendez. *Tree-based methods to model dependent data.* Arizona State University, 2008.

[249] Guillermo Mendez and Sharon Lohr. Estimating residual variance in random forest regression. *Computational Statistics & Data Analysis*, 55(11):2937–2950, 2011.

[250] Lucas Mentch and Giles Hooker. Quantifying uncertainty in random forests via confidence intervals and hypothesis tests. *The Journal of Machine Learning Research*, 17(1):841–881, 2016.

[251] Lucas Mentch and Giles Hooker. Formal hypothesis tests for additive structure in random forests. *Journal of Computational and Graphical Statistics*, 26(3):589–597, 2017.

[252] Lynne C. Messer, J. Michael Oakes, and Susan Mason. Effects of socioeconomic and racial residential segregation on preterm birth: a cautionary tale of structural confounding. *American Journal of Epidemiology*, 171(6):664–673, 2010.

[253] J. Meza and P. Lahiri. A note on the Cp statistic under the nested error regression model. *Survey Methodology*, 31(1):105–109, 2005.

[254] A. Miller. *Subset Selection in Regression.* CRC Press, Inc. New York, USA, 2002.

[255] Toby J. Mitchell and John J. Beauchamp. Bayesian variable selection in linear regression. *Journal of the American Statistical Association*, 83(404):1023–1032, 1988.

[256] I. Molina and Y. Marhuenda. sae: An R package for small area estimation. *The R Journal*, 7:1, 2015.

[257] Molina, I., & Marhuenda, Y. (2015). sae: an R package for small area estimation. R J., 7(1), 81.

[258] Stephen J. Mooney and Vikas Pejaver. Big data in public health: terminology, machine learning, and privacy. *Annual Review of Public Health*, 39:95, 2018.

[259] James N. Morgan and John A. Sonquist. Problems in the analysis of survey data, and a proposal. *Journal of the American Statistical Association*, 58(302):415–434, 1963.

[260] Carl Morris and Cindy Christiansen. Fitting weibull duration models with random effects. *Lifetime Data Analysis*, 1(4):347–359, 1995.

[261] Douglass A. Morrison, Gulshan Sethi, Jerome Sacks, William Henderson, Frederick Grover, Steven Sedlis, Rick Esposito, Kodangudi Ramanathan, Darryl Weiman, Jorge Saucedo, et al. Percutaneous coronary intervention versus coronary artery bypass graft surgery for patients with medically refractory myocardial ischemia and risk factors for adverse outcomes with bypass: a multicenter, randomized trial. *Journal of the American College of Cardiology*, 38(1):143–149, 2001.

[262] Ashley I. Naimi and Jay S. Kaufman. Counterfactual theory in social epidemiology: reconciling analysis and action for the social determinants of health. *Current Epidemiology Reports*, 2(1):52–60, 2015.

[263] Ashley I. Naimi, Mireille E. Schnitzer, Erica E.M. Moodie, and Lisa M Bodnar. Mediation analysis for health disparities research. *American Journal of Epidemiology*, 184(4):315–324, 2016.

[264] Claudia Nau, Hugh Ellis, Hongtai Huang, Brian S. Schwartz, Annemarie Hirsch, Lisa Bailey-Davis, Amii M. Kress, Jonathan Pollak, and Thomas A. Glass. Exploring the forest instead of the trees: An innovative method for defining obesogenic and obesoprotective environments. *Health & Place*, 35:136–146, 2015.

[265] Wayne Nelson. Theory and applications of hazard plotting for censored failure data. *Technometrics*, 14(4):945–966, 1972.

[266] Thuan Nguyen, Jiming Jiang, and J. Sunil Rao. Assessing uncertainty for classified mixed model prediction. *Journal of Statistical Computation and Simulation*, 92(2):249–261, 2022.

[267] Trang Quynh Nguyen, Ian Schmid, Elizabeth L. Ogburn, and Elizabeth A. Stuart. Clarifying causal mediation analysis for the applied researcher: effect identification via three assumptions and five potential outcomes. *arXiv preprint arXiv:2011.09537*, 2020.

[268] P. Novak. Checking goodness-of-fit of the accelerated failure time model for survival data. *WDS?10 Proceedings of Contributed Papers, I*, 189–194, 2010.

[269] M.N. Nurty and V.S. Devi. *Pattern Recognition: An Algorithmic Approach*. Springer-Verlag, London, 2011.

[270] All of Us Research Program Investigators. The "all of us" research program. *New England Journal of Medicine*, 381(7):668–676, 2019.

[271] WHO Commission on Social Determinants of Health and World Health Organization. *Closing the gap in a generation: health equity through action on the social determinants of health: Commission on Social Determinants of Health final report.* World Health Organization, 2008.

[272] Jean D. Opsomer, Gerda Claeskens, Maria Giovanna Ranalli, Goeran Kauermann, and F. Jay Breidt. Non-parametric small area estimation using penalized spline regression. *Journal of the Royal Statistical Society: Series B (Statistical Methodology)*, 70(1):265–286, 2008.

[273] Alexander N. Ortega, Stephanie L. Albert, Mienah Z. Sharif, Brent A. Langellier, Rosa Elena Garcia, Deborah C. Glik, Ron Brookmeyer, Alec M. Chan-Golston, Scott Friedlander, and Michael L. Prelip. Proyecto MercadoFRESCO: a multi-level, community-engaged corner store intervention in East Los Angeles and Boyle Heights. *Journal of Community Health*, 40(2):347–356, 2015.

[274] C. Owusu, Y. Lan, M. Zheng, and W. Tang. Geocoding fundamentals and associated challenges. *Geospatial Data Science Techniques and Applications*, 118:41–62, 2017.

[275] Gregory Pappas, Susan Queen, Wilbur Hadden, and Gail Fisher. The increasing disparity in mortality between socioeconomic groups in the united states, 1960 and 1986. *New England Journal of Medicine*, 329(2):103–109, 1993.

[276] Trevor Park and George Casella. The bayesian lasso. *Journal of the American Statistical Association*, 103(482):681–686, 2008.

[277] Jeffrey N. Pearcy and Kenneth G. Keppel. A summary measure of health disparity. *Public Health Reports*, 2016.

[278] Roger Penrose. A generalized inverse for matrices. In *Mathematical Proceedings of the Cambridge Philosophical Society*, volume 51, pages 406–413. Cambridge University Press, 1955.

[279] Roger Penrose. On best approximate solutions of linear matrix equations. In *Mathematical Proceedings of the Cambridge Philosophical Society*, volume 52, pages 17–19. Cambridge University Press, 1956.

[280] R. Peto. Discussion of the paper by D.R. Cox. *Journal of the Royal Statistical Society: Series B (Methodological)*, 34:215–217, 1972.

[281] Danny Pfeffermann. New important developments in small area estimation. *Statistical Science*, 28(1):40–68, 2013.

[282] S. Pignata and J.B. Vermorken. Ovarian cancer in the elderly. *Critical Reviews in Oncology/Hematology*, 49:77–86, 2004.

[283] José C. Pinheiro and Douglas M. Bates. Linear mixed-effects models: basic concepts and examples. *Mixed-effects models in S and S-Plus*, pages 3–56, 2000.

[284] Ganna Pogrebna and Alexander Kharlamov. The impact of cross-cultural differences in handwashing patterns on the covid-19 outbreak magnitude, 2020.

[285] P. Poletti, M. Tirani, D. Cereda, F. Trentini, G. Guzzetta, G. Sabatino, V. Marziano, A. Castrofino, F. Grosso, G. del Castillo, R. Piccarreta, ATS Lombardy COVID-19 Task Force, A. Andreassi, A. Melegaro, M. Gramegna, M. Ajelli, and S. Merler. Probability of symptoms and critical disease after sars-cov-2 infection. 2020.

[286] Dimitris N. Politis, Joseph P. Romano, and Michael Wolf. *Subsampling*. Springer Science & Business Media, 1999.

[287] N.G. Narasimha Prasad and Jon N.K. Rao. The estimation of the mean squared error of small-area estimators. *Journal of the American Statistical Association*, 85(409):163–171, 1990.

[288] N.G.N. Prasad and J.N.K. Rao. On robust small area estimation using a simple random effects model. *Survey Methodology*, 25:67–72, 1999.

[289] Monica Pratesi and Nicola Salvati. Small area estimation: The EBLUP estimator based on spatially correlated random area effects. *Statistical Methods and Applications*, 17(1):113–141, 2008.

[290] Kristopher J. Preacher. Advances in mediation analysis: A survey and synthesis of new developments. *Annual Review of Psychology*, 66:825–852, 2015.

[291] Carla Prins, I. de Villiers Jonker, Francis E. Smit, and Lizelle Botes. Cardiac surgery risk-stratification models. *Cardiovascular Journal of Africa*, 23(3):160–164, 2012.

[292] Maurice H. Quenouille. Approximate tests of correlation in time-series 3. In *Mathematical Proceedings of the Cambridge Philosophical Society*, volume 45, pages 483–484. Cambridge University Press, 1949.

[293] John R. Quinlan et al. Learning with continuous classes. In *5th Australian Joint Conference on Artificial Intelligence*, volume 92, pages 343–348. World Scientific, 1992.

[294] Tibshirani R., Walther G., and Hastie T. Estimating the number of clusters in a data set via the gap statistic. *Journal of the Royal Statistical Society Series B*, 63:411–423, 2001.

[295] J Sunil Rao. Observed best prediction for small area estimation: A review. *Statistics and Applications*, pages 305–314, 2018.

[296] J. Sunil Rao and William J.E. Potts. Visualizing bagged decision trees. In *KDD*, pages 243–246, 1997.

[297] J. Sunil Rao, Hang Zhang, Erin Kobetz, Melinda C. Aldrich, and Douglas Conway. Predicting dna methylation from genetic data lacking racial diversity using shared classified random effects. *Genomics*, 113(1):1018–1028, 2021.

[298] J. Sunil Rao, Hang Zhang, and Alejandro Mantero. Contextualizing COVID-19 spread: a county level analysis, urban versus rural, and implications for preparing for the next wave. *medRxiv*, 2020.

[299] J.N.K. Rao and I. Molina. *Small Area Estimation, 2nd ed.* Wiley, New York, 2015.

[300] John N.K. Rao and Isabel Molina. *Small Area Estimation*. John Wiley & Sons, 2015.

[301] Jon N.K. Rao, Sanjoy K. Sinha, and Laura Dumitrescu. Robust small area estimation under semi-parametric mixed models. *Canadian Journal of Statistics*, 42(1):126–141, 2014.

[302] Jon N.K. Rao and Mingyu Yu. Small-area estimation by combining time-series and cross-sectional data. *Canadian Journal of Statistics*, 22(4):511–528, 1994.

[303] J.S. Rao and J. Fan. Imputation of area-level covariates using registry linking. *Handbook of Statistics*, 37:3–21, 2017.

[304] J.S. Rao, J. Jiang, and T. Nguyen. Distorted variable analysis. A research note. 2022.

[305] J.S. Rao, E. Kobetz, H. Yu, J. Baeker-Bispo, and Z. Bailey. Partially recursively induced structured moderation for modeling racial differences in endometrial cancer survival. *PLoS ONE (to appear)*, 2022.

[306] Stephanie A. Robert and Erin Ruel. Racial segregation and health disparities between black and white older adults. *The Journals of Gerontology Series B: Psychological Sciences and Social Sciences*, 61(4):S203–S211, 2006.

[307] James M. Robins and Ya'acov Ritov. Toward a curse of dimensionality appropriate (CODA) asymptotic theory for semi-parametric models. *Statistics in Medicine*, 16(3):285–319, 1997.

[308] James M. Robins and Andrea Rotnitzky. Semiparametric efficiency in multivariate regression models with missing data. *Journal of the American Statistical Association*, 90(429):122–129, 1995.

[309] Larry L. Rockwood. *Introduction to Population Ecology*. John Wiley & Sons, 2015.

[310] Eugene Rogot. *A mortality study of 1.3 million persons by demographic, social and economic factors: 1979-1985 follow-up: US National Longitudinal Mortality Study*. Number 92. National Institutes of Health, National Heart, Lung, and Blood Institute, 1992.

[311] Paul R. Rosenbaum. Model-based direct adjustment. *Journal of the American Statistical Association*, 82(398):387–394, 1987.

[312] Paul R. Rosenbaum and Donald B. Rubin. The central role of the propensity score in observational studies for causal effects. *Biometrika*, 70(1):41–55, 1983.

[313] Paul R. Rosenbaum and Donald B. Rubin. Reducing bias in observational studies using subclassification on the propensity score. *Journal of the American Statistical Association*, 79(387):516–524, 1984.

[314] Noah A. Rosenberg, Michael D. Edge, Jonathan K. Pritchard, and Marcus W. Feldman. Interpreting polygenic scores, polygenic adaptation, and human phenotypic differences. *Evolution, Medicine, and Public Health*, 2019(1):26–34, 2019.

[315] D.A. Rowbotham, E.A. Marshall, E.A. Vucic, et al. Epigenetic changes in aging and age-related diseases. *Journal of Aging Science*, 3:130:doi:10.4172/2329–8847.1000130, 2014.

[316] R.M. Royall. Linear regression models in finite population sampling theory. in: Foundations of statistical inference, ed. V.P. Godambe and D.A. Sprott, 1971.

[317] R.M. Royall and W.G. Cumberland. An empirical study of prediction theory in finite population sampling: Simple random sampling and the ratio estimator. in: Survey sampling and measurement, ed. namboodiri, n.k. 1977.

[318] D.B. Rubin. *Multiple Imputation for Nonresponse in Surveys*. John Wiley & Sons, New York, 1987.

[319] Donald B. Rubin. Estimating causal effects of treatments in randomized and nonrandomized studies. *Journal of Educational Psychology*, 66(5):688, 1974.

[320] Donald B. Rubin. Bayesian inference for causal effects: The role of randomization. *The Annals of Statistics*, pages 34–58, 1978.

[321] Donald B. Rubin. Causal inference using potential outcomes: Design, modeling, decisions. *Journal of the American Statistical Association*, 100(469):322–331, 2005.

[322] Masahiro Ryo and Matthias C. Rillig. Statistically reinforced machine learning for nonlinear patterns and variable interactions. *Ecosphere*, 8(11):e01976, 2017.

[323] A.R. Santos-Lozada, J.T. Howard, and A.M. Verdery. How differential privacy will affect our understanding of health disparities in the united states. *PNAS*, 117:13405–13412, 2020.

[324] Carl Erik Särndal. Design-consistent versus model-dependent estimation for small domains. *Journal of the American Statistical Association*, 79(387):624–631, 1984.

[325] Barry Schouten and Guido de Nooij. *Nonresponse adjustment using classification trees*. CBS, Statistics Netherlands The Netherlands, 2005.

[326] Saptarshi Sengupta, Sanchita Basak, Pallabi Saikia, Sayak Paul, Vasilios Tsalavoutis, Frederick Atiah, Vadlamani Ravi, and Alan Peters. A review of deep learning with special emphasis on architectures, applications and recent trends. *Knowledge-Based Systems*, 194:105596, 2020.

[327] David M. Seo, Pascal J. Goldschmidt-Clermont, and Mike West. Of mice and men: Sparse statistical modeling in cardiovascular genomics. *The Annals of Applied Statistics*, 1(1):152–178, 2007.

[328] Robert L. Sherbecoe and Gerald A. Studebaker. Supplementary formulas and tables for calculating and interconverting speech recognition scores in transformed arcsine units. *International Journal of Audiology*, 43(8):442–448, 2004.

[329] Mark D. Shriver, Michael W. Smith, Lin Jin, Amy Marcini, Joshua M. Akey, Ranjan Deka, and Robert E. Ferrell. Ethnic-affiliation estimation by use of population-specific DNA markers. *American Journal of Human Genetics*, 60(4):957, 1997.

[330] Corinne N Simonti, Benjamin Vernot, Lisa Bastarache, Erwin Bottinger, David S. Carrell, Rex L. Chisholm, David R. Crosslin, Scott J. Hebbring, Gail P. Jarvik, Iftikhar J. Kullo, et al. The phenotypic legacy of admixture between modern humans and neandertals. *Science*, 351(6274):737–741, 2016.

[331] Chris Skinner and Jon Wakefield. Introduction to the design and analysis of complex survey data. *Statistical Science*, 32(2):165–175, 2017.

[332] Brian D. Smedley, Adrienne Y. Stith, Alan R. Nelson, et al. Racial and ethnic disparities in diagnosis and treatment: a review of the evidence and a consideration of causes. *Unequal Treatment: Confronting Racial and Ethnic Disparities in Health Care*, 2003.

[333] G. Davey Smith, Mel Bartley, and David Blane. The black report on socioeconomic inequalities in health 10 years on. *BMJ: British Medical Journal*, 301(6748):373, 1990.

[334] I.Z. Smith, K.L. Bentley-Edwards, S. El-Amin, and W. Darity. Fighting at birth: Eradicating the Black-White infant mortality gap. *Research report from Duke University's Samuel DuBois Cook Center on Social Equity and Insight Center for Community Economic Development*, 2018.

[335] Paul D. Sorlie, Eric Backlund, and Jacob B. Keller. Us mortality by economic, demographic, and social characteristics: the national longitudinal mortality study. *American Journal of Public Health*, 85(7):949–956, 1995.

[336] Corey Sparks. An examination of disparities in cancer incidence in texas using bayesian random coefficient models. *PeerJ*, 3:e1283, 2015.

[337] D.E. Spratt, T. Chan, L. Waldron et al. Racial/ethnic disparities in genomic sequencing. *JAMA Oncology*, 2:1070–1074, 2016.

[338] Kathleen Sprouffske. *growthcurver: Simple Metrics to Summarize Growth Curves*, 2018. R package version 0.3.0.

[339] Kathleen Sprouffske and Andreas Wagner. Growthcurver: An R package for obtaining interpretable metrics from microbial growth curves. *BMC Bioinformatics*, 17(1):172, 2016.

[340] M.S. Srivastava. On fixed-width confidence bounds for regression parameters and mean vector. *Journal of the Royal Statistical Society: Series B (Methodological)*, 29(1):132–140, 1967.

[341] S.K. Srivastava, A. Ahmad, O. Miree, et al. Racial health disparities in ovarian cancer: not just black and white. *Journal of Ovarian Cancer Research*, 10:58:doi:10.1186/s13048–017–0355–y, 2017.

[342] Jerome F. Strauss III, Roberto Romero, Nardhy Gomez-Lopez, Hannah Haymond-Thornburg, Bhavi P. Modi, Maria E. Teves, Laurel N. Pearson, Timothy P. York, and Harvey A. Schenkein. Spontaneous preterm birth: advances toward the discovery of genetic predisposition. *American Journal of Obstetrics and Gynecology*, 218(3):294–314, 2018.

[343] Winfried Stute. Consistent estimation under random censorship when covariables are present. *Journal of Multivariate Analysis*, 45(1):89–103, 1993.

[344] Winfried Stute and J.L. Wang. The strong law under random censorship. *The Annals of Statistics*, 1591–1607, 1993.

[345] S.V. Subramanian, Jarvis T. Chen, David H. Rehkopf, Pamela D. Waterman, and Nancy Krieger. Racial disparities in context: a multilevel analysis of neighborhood variations in poverty and excess mortality among black populations in massachusetts. *American Journal of Public Health*, 95(2):260–265, 2005.

[346] C.H. Sudre, K. Lee, M. Ni Lochlainn, T. Varsavsky, B. Murray, M.S. Graham, C. Menni, M. Modat, R.C.E. Bowyer, L.H. Nguyen, D.A. Drew, A.D. Joshi, W. Ma, C. Guo, C.H. Lo, S. Ganesh, A. Buwe, J. Capdevila Pujol, J. Lavigne du Cadet, A. Visconti, M. Freydin, J.S. El Sayed Moustafa, M. Falchi, R. Davies, M.F. Gomez, T. Fall, M.J. Cardoso, J. Wolf, P.W. Franks, A.T. Chan, T.D. Spector, C.J. Steves, and S. Ourselin. Symptom clusters in Covid19: A potential clinical prediction tool from the COVID Symptom study app. *medRxiv*, 2020.

[347] Fei Tang and Hemant Ishwaran. Random forest missing data algorithms. *Statistical Analysis and Data Mining: The ASA Data Science Journal*, 10(6):363–377, 2017.

[348] TCGANetwork. Integrated genomic analyses of ovarian carcinoma. *Nature*, 47:609–615, 2011.

[349] David S. TenBrink, Randall McMunn, and Sarah Panken. Project u-turn: increasing active transportation in jackson, michigan. *American Journal of Preventive Medicine*, 37(6):S329–S335, 2009.

[350] H. Theil. *Economics and Information Theory*. Rand McNally and Company, 1967.

[351] Rachel L.J. Thornton, Crystal M. Glover, Crystal W. Cené, Deborah C. Glik, Jeffrey A. Henderson, and David R. Williams. Evaluating strategies for reducing health disparities by addressing the social determinants of health. *Health Affairs*, 35(8):1416–1423, 2016.

[352] Robert Tibshirani. Regression shrinkage and selection via the lasso. *Journal of the Royal Statistical Society: Series B (Methodological)*, 58(1):267–288, 1996.

[353] Tingley, D., Yamamoto, T., Hirose, K., Keele, L., & Imai, K. (2014). Mediation: R package for causal mediation analysis.

[354] D. Toth and J. Eltinge. Simple function representation of regression trees. *Technical report, Bureau of Labor Statistics*, 2011.

[355] Daniell Toth and John L. Eltinge. Building consistent regression trees from complex sample data. *Journal of the American Statistical Association*, 106(496):1626–1636, 2011.

[356] Michael Tsang, Hanpeng Liu, Sanjay Purushotham, Pavankumar Murali, and Yan Liu. Neural interaction transparency (nit): Disentangling learned interactions for improved interpretability. *Advances in Neural Information Processing Systems*, 31, 2018.

[357] Florin Vaida and Suzette Blanchard. Conditional akaike information for mixed effects models. *Corrado Lagazio, Marco Marchi (Eds)*, 101, 2005.

[358] T.J. VanderWeele and I. Shipster. On the definition of a confounder. *Ann. Statist.*, 41:196–220, 2013.

[359] Tyler J. VanderWeele and Miguel A. Hernán. Causal effects and natural laws: towards a conceptualization of causal counterfactuals for nonmanipulable exposures, with application to the effects of race and sex. *Causality: Statistical Perspectives and Applications*, pages 101–113, 2012.

[360] Tyler J. VanderWeele and Whitney R. Robinson. On causal interpretation of race in regressions adjusting for confounding and mediating variables. *Epidemiology (Cambridge, Mass.)*, 25(4):473, 2014.

[361] Ying-Wooi Wan, Genevera I Allen, and Zhandong Liu. Tcga2stat: simple tcga data access for integrated statistical analysis in R. *Bioinformatics*, 32(6):952–954, 2015.

[362] Matt P. Wand. Smoothing and mixed models. *Computational Statistics*, 18(2):223–249, 2003.

[363] Elizabeth Ward, Ahmedin Jemal, Vilma Cokkinides, Gopal K. Singh, Cheryll Cardinez, Asma Ghafoor, and Michael Thun. Cancer disparities by race/ethnicity and socioeconomic status. *CA: A Cancer Journal for Clinicians*, 54(2):78–93, 2004.

[364] David P. Weikart et al. Preschool intervention–a preliminary report of the perry preschool project. 1967.

[365] T. Wiecki. Mcmc sampling for dummies. *URL http://twiecki.github.io/blog/2015/11/10/mcmc-sampling*, 2015.

[366] R.M. Willet and R.D. Nowak. Minimax optimal level set estimation. *Technical report*, 2016.

[367] David R. Williams, Manuela V. Costa, Adebola O. Odunlami, and Selina A. Mohammed. Moving upstream: how interventions that address the social determinants of health can improve health and reduce disparities. *Journal of Public Health Management and Practice*, 14(6):S8–S17, 2008.

[368] Stacey J. Winham, Colin L. Colby, Robert R. Freimuth, Xin Wang, Mariza de Andrade, Marianne Huebner, and Joanna M Biernacka. Snp interaction detection with random forests in high-dimensional genetic data. *BMC Bioinformatics*, 13(1):1–13, 2012.

[369] Taylor Winter, Benjamin Riordan, Anthony Surace, Damian Scarf, and Paul Jose. A tutorial on the use of informative bayesian priors for minority research. 2020.

[370] Mitchell D. Wong, Martin F. Shapiro, W. John Boscardin, and Susan L. Ettner. Contribution of major diseases to disparities in mortality. *New England Journal of Medicine*, 347(20):1585–1592, 2002.

[371] Sewall Wright. The method of path coefficients. *The Annals of Mathematical Statistics*, 5(3):161–215, 1934.

[372] Yu Ye, Jason C. Bond, Laura A. Schmidt, Nina Mulia, and Tammy W. Tam. Toward a better understanding of when to apply propensity scoring: a comparison with conventional regression in ethnic disparities research. *Annals of Epidemiology*, 22(10):691–697, 2012.

[373] P.A. Zandbergen. A comparison of address point, parcel and street geocoding techniques. *Computers, Environment and Urban Systems*, 32:214–232, 2008.

[374] Xinzhi Zhang, Eliseo J. Pérez-Stable, Philip E. Bourne, Emmanuel Peprah, O. Kenrik Duru, Nancy Breen, David Berrigan, Fred Wood, James S. Jackson, David WS Wong, et al. Big data science: opportunities and challenges to address minority health and health disparities in the 21st century. *Ethnicity & Eisease*, 27(2):95, 2017.

[375] Zhong Zhao. Using matching to estimate treatment effects: Data requirements, matching metrics, and monte carlo evidence. *Review of Economics and Statistics*, 86(1):91–107, 2004.

[376] Hui Zou and Trevor Hastie. Regularization and variable selection via the elastic net. *Journal of the Royal Statistical Society: Series B (Statistical Methodology)*, 67(2):301–320, 2005.

Index

Note: **Bold** page numbers refer to tables and *italic* page numbers refer to figures.

B

C

L

M

U

V

W

For Product Safety Concerns and Information please contact our
EU representative GPSR@taylorandfrancis.com Taylor & Francis
Verlag GmbH, Kaufingerstraße 24, 80331 München, Germany